PLASMAPHERESIS: THERAPEUTIC APPLICATIONS AND NEW TECHNIQUES

Plasmapheresis: Therapeutic Applications and New Techniques

Editors

Yukihiko Nosé, M.D., Ph.D.
Department of Artificial Organs
Cleveland Clinic Foundation
Cleveland, Ohio

Paul S. Malchesky, M.S.
Department of Artificial Organs
Cleveland Clinic Foundation
Cleveland, Ohio

James W. Smith, M.D., Ph.D.
Department of Artificial Organs
Cleveland Clinic Foundation
Cleveland, Ohio

Randall S. Krakauer, M.D.
Department of Rheumatic and
Immunologic Disease
Cleveland Clinic Foundation
Cleveland, Ohio

Raven Press ■ New York

Raven Press, 1140 Avenue of the Americas, New York, New York 10036

Made in the United States of America

Library of Congress Cataloging in Publication Data

Main entry under title:

Plasmapheresis, therapeutic applications and new
  techniques.

  Includes bibliographical references and index.
  1. Plasmapheresis. 2. Plasma exchange (Therapeutics)
I. Nose, Yukihiko. [DNLM: 1. Plasmapheresis. 2. Plasma-
pheresis—Methods. WH 460 P7155]
RM173.P56   1983   615'.39   82-42896
ISBN 0-89004-980-7

Great care has been taken to maintain the accuracy of the information contained in the volume. However, Raven Press cannot be held responsible for errors or for any consequences arising from the use of the information contained herein.

Materials appearing in this book prepared by individuals as part of their official duties as U.S. Government employees are not covered by the above-mentioned copyright.

Preface

Plasma exchange or plasma processing techniques for autoimmune, hematologic, and metabolic diseases are becoming increasingly more acceptable methods of therapy. The availability of centrifugal cell separators and membrane plasma filters have made this possible. Hematologists, blood bankers, nephrologists, neurologists, hepatologists, and others have applied this type of therapeutic technology. The literature in each of these specialties reports the use of plasmapheresis. However, depending upon the area of specialty, the preferred method and technology of plasma treatment is different. For instance, the hematologists and blood bankers prefer to use a centrifugal apparatus, while nephrologists prefer to use membrane devices. There has also been a geographical difference in emphasis and scope of plasma treatment technology. In the United States, where early development of the centrifugal devices occurred, most of the clinical studies have been performed by centrifugal techniques. Membrane plasma separators were developed first in Japan and Europe. Subsequently, the Japanese and European experiences in plasma therapy with membrane systems dominate the literature. Only recently have membrane filters been approved for clinical use in the United States.

Realizing this imbalance, the International Society for Artificial Organs has tried to present the therapeutic applications and techniques of plasmapheresis on a global scale. Fifty-five chapters on these subjects are presented in this volume. Emphasis is placed on providing an overview of therapeutic apheresis, current technology, and clinical applications for rheumatic and immunologic diseases, transplantation, renal, hematologic and hepatic diseases.

The Editors

Acknowledgments

The editors acknowledge their debt to Prof. Dr. Horst Klinkmann, President of the International Society for Artificial Organs, and to the members of the International Organizing Committee who have helped to make this publication an overall representation of the current art of technology:

Jean-Louis Funck-Brentano	Paris, France
Hans J. Gurland	Munich, Federal Republic of Germany
Noboru Inoue	Tokyo, Japan
John Verrier Jones	Halifax, Nova Scotia, Canada
Edward F. Leonard	New York, New York, U.S.A.
C. Martin Lockwood	London, England
Kenji Maeda	Nagoya, Japan
Kazuo Ota	Tokyo, Japan
Alvaro A. Pineda	Rochester, Minnesota, U.S.A.
Heinz Gunter Sieberth	Koln, Federal Republic of Germany
Mitsuru Suzuki	Chiba, Japan
Zenya Yamazaki	Tokyo, Japan

Special appreciation is given to Mary Ann Edsall, Executive Director of the ISAO, who not only coordinated the first International Symposium on Plasmapheresis, but also assisted in the publication of this volume.

Contents

Current Technology: On-Line Plasma Treatment

Rheumatic and Immunologic Diseases

Contributors

M. Abe
Kawasumi Laboratories, Inc.
4–7–1, Shiba, Minato-ku
Tokyo, Japan

T. Abe
Teikyo University
11–1, Kaga 2-chome
Itabashi-ku
Tokyo 173, Japan

Y. Abe
Department of Artificial Organs
Cleveland Clinic Foundation
9500 Euclid Avenue
Cleveland, Ohio 44106

T. Agishi
Kidney Center
Tokyo Women's Medical College
10 Kawada-cho, Shinjuku-ku
Tokyo, Japan

Peter Ahrenholtz
University of Rostock
Klinik für Innere Medizin
DDR-25, Rostock 1
German Democratic Republic

D. Alcalay
Service de Réanimation Médicale
et de Nephrologie
C.H.U. Poitiers
86021 Poitiers Cedex, France

G. Alcalay
Service de Réanimation Médicale
et de Nephrologie
C.H.U. Poitiers
86021 Poitiers Cedex, France

M. Alijani
Georgetown University
School of Medicine
Washington, D.C. 20007

H. Amemiya
Kidney Center
Tokyo Women's Medical College
10 Kawada-cho, Shijuku-ku
Tokyo, Japan

B. Amir-Ansari
Institute of Urology
London University
Shaftesbury Avenue
London W.C.2, England

M. Anderson
Fenwal Laboratories
Division of Travenol
Laboratories, Inc.
Route 120 and Wilson Road
Round Lake, Illinois 60073

Chantal Andre
Department of Immuno-Hematology
Hôpital Henri Mondon
94 010 Creteil, France

G. Delbert Antwiler
Cobe Laboratories, Inc.
1201 Oak Street
Lakewood, Colorado 80215

Mattias Aurell
Medical Department V
Sahlgren's Hospital
S-413 45 Goteborg, Sweden

Nakanobu Azuma
Tokyo Tokatsu Clinic
822 Kinokuchi Matudoshi
Chiba, Japan

R. Bambauer
Department of Nephrology
Universität des Saarlandes
D-6650 Homburg/Saar
Federal Republic of Germany

G. Bazzato
Nephrology and Dialysis Department
Umberto I Hospital
50–30174 Mestre, Italy

E. Behm
Department of Medicine
W. Pieck University, Rostock
E.-Heydemann Strasse
GDR-2500, Rostock
German Democratic Republic

Rosemarie Beress
II Medizinische Universitätsklinik
Metzstrasse 53
D 2300 Kiel
Federal Republic of Germany

D. Bernard
Laboratoire d'Immunologie
Hôpital Nord
Marseille, France

V. A. Blanchette
Canadian Red Cross
Blood Tranfusion Service
Ottawa Centre
85 Plymouth Street
Ottawa, Ontario K1S 3E2 Canada

Matthias Blumenstein
Medizinische Klinik I
Klinikum Grosshadern
University of Munich
D-8000 Munich 70
Federal Republic of Germany

D. H. Buchholz
Fenwal Laboratories
Division of Travenol
Laboratories Inc.
Route 120 and Wilson Road
Round Lake, Illinois 60073

George W. Buffaloe
Cobe Laboratories, Inc.
Research and Development
1201 Oak Street
Lakewood, Colorado 80215

Hans-Christian Burck
Abteilung für Intensivmedizine
und Dialyse
Stadtisches Krankenhaus Kiel
D 2300 Kiel
Federal Republic of Germany

Leonard Calabrese
Department of Rheumatic and
Immunologic Disease
9500 Euclid Avenue
Cleveland, Ohio 44106

J. P. Cassuto
Service de Médecine Interne A
Departement d'Hematologie
Hôpital de Cimiez
avenue Victoria
06031 Nice Cedex, France

E. Cassuto-Viguier
Clinique Nephrologique
Hôpital Pasteur
avenue de la Voie Romaine
06031 Nice Cedex, France

L. Chan
Department of Medicine
University of Ottawa
Ottawa, Canada

John Clough
Department of Rheumatic and
Immunologic Disease
Cleveland Clinic Foundation
9500 Euclid Avenue
Cleveland, Ohio 44106

U. Coli
Nephrology and Dialysis Department
Umberto I Hospital
50–30174 Mestre (VE), Italy

J. J. Conte
Service de Nephrologie et d'Hemodialyse
C.H.U. Toulouse-Purpan
Place du Docteur Baylac
31059 Toulouse Cedex, France

Frank Corbin
Cobe Laboratories, Inc.
1201 Oak Street
Lakewood, Colorado 80215

F. W. Darr
American Red Cross Blood Services
2025 E Street, N.W.
Washington, D.C. 20006

R. Ben Dawson
Apheresis Center
Blood Transfusion Labs
University of Maryland Hospital
Baltimore, Maryland 21201

Marc De Clippele
Department of Internal Medicine
Renal Division
University Hospital
De Pintelaan 185
B-9000 Gent, Belgium

Ch. Dittrich
Department of Chemotherapy
University of Vienna
Lazarettgasse 14
A-1090 Vienna, Austria

P. Doenecke
Department of Cardiology
Universität des Saarlandes
D-665-Homburg/Saar
Federal Republic of Germany

Ronald E. Domen
Department of Pathology
The Ohio State University
410 West 10th Avenue
Columbus, Ohio 43210

J. M. Dueymes
Service de Nephrologie et d'Hemodialyse
C.H.U. Toulouse-Purpan
Place du Docteur Baylac
31059 Toulouse Cedex, France

P. DuJardin
Service de Medecine Interne A
Departement d'Hematologie
Hôpital de Cimiez
Avenue Victoria
06031 Nice Cedex, France

H. Duplay
Clinique Nephrologique
Hôpital Pasteur
Avenue de la Voie Romaine
06031 Nice Cedex, France

Bennett B. Edelman
Apheresis Center
Blood Transfusion Labs
University of Maryland Hospital
Baltimore, Maryland 21201

Conny Edenö
Medical Department V
Sahlgren's Hospital
S-413 45 Göteborg, Sweden

R. Elsen
Cordis Dow B.U.
Blvd. du Souverain 191
1160 Brussels, Belgium

Hans-Hartwig Euler
II Medizinische Universitätsklinik
Metzstrasse 53
D 2300 Kiel
Federal Republic of Germany

Ross R. Erickson
Cobe Laboratories, Inc.
1201 Oak Street
Lakewood, Colorado 80215

Dieter Falkenhagen
University of Rostock
Klinik für Innere Medizin
DDR-25 Rostock 1
German Democratic Republic

A. Fracasso
Nephrology and Dialysis Department
Umberto I Hospital
50–30174 Mestre (VE), Italy

Yoshizo Fujimori
2nd Department of Surgery
University of Tokyo
7–3–1 Hongo Bunkyo-ku
Tokyo 113, Japan

T. Furuta
New Product Development Laboratory
Asahi Chemical Industry Co., Ltd.
1–2, Yurakucho 1-chome
Chiyoda-ku
Tokyo, Japan

M. Gelfand
Georgetown University
  School of Medicine
Washington, D.C. 20007

W. M. Glöckner
Abteilung Innere Medizine II
an der Rhein. -Westf. Technische.
Hochschule Aachen
Goethestrasse 27/29
5100 Aachen
Federal Republic of Germany

W. Graninger
Department of Chemotherapy
University of Vienna
Lazarettgasse 14
A-1090 Vienna, Austria

Richard Greenstreet
Cleveland Clinic Foundation
9500 Euclid Avenue
Cleveland, Ohio 44106

Patricia Griffith
Clinical Center Blood Bank
National Institutes of Health
Bethesda, Maryland 20205

Klaus Gülzow
II Medizinische Universitätsklinik
Metzstrasse 53
D 2300 Kiel
Federal Republic of Germany

Hans J. Gurland
Nephrology Division
Klinikum Grosshadern
Medizinische Klinik I
University of Munich
D-8000 Munich 70
Federal Republic of Germany

Rupert Habersetzer
Nephrology Division
Klinikum Grosshadern
Medizinische Klinik I
University of Munich
D-8000 Munich 70
Federal Republic of Germany

Michael H. Hall
Department of Surgery
Division of Cardiovascular Surgery
North Shore University Hospital
Manhasset, New York 11030

H. G. Hartmann
Department of Nephrology
Universität des Saarlandes
D-6650 Homburg/Saar
Federal Republic of Germany

Y. Hasuo
Kidney Center
Tokyo Women's Medical College
10 Kawada-cho, Shinjuku-ku
Tokyo, Japan

Andreas Hauff
Free University
Klinikum Steglitz
Hindenburgdamm 30
D-1000 Berlin 45
Federal Republic of Germany

G. B. Helfrich
Georgetown University
  School of Medicine
Washington, D.C. 20007

C. Helphingstine
Fenwal Laboratories
Division of Travenol
Laboratories Inc.
Route 120 and Wilson Road
Round Lake, Illinois 60073

Hans Herlitz
Medical Department V
Sahlgren's Hospital
S-413 Goteborg, Sweden

Stephen P. Heyse
Office of Program Planning
and Evaluation
National Institute of Arthritis, Diabetes,
Digestive and Kidney Diseases
National Institutes of Health
Bethesda, Maryland 20205

V. Hogan
Blood Transfusion Service
Canadian Red Cross
Blood Transfusion Service
Ottawa Centre
85 Plymouth Street
Ottawa, Ontario K1S 3ES Canada

T. Horiuchi
Department of Artificial Organs
Cleveland Clinic Foundation
9500 Euclid Avenue
Cleveland, Ohio 44106

Ichiro Iizuka
2nd Department of Surgery
University of Tokyo
7-3-1 Hongo Bunkyo-ku
Tokyo 113, Japan

K. Inagaki
New Product Development Laboratory
Asahi Chemical Industry Co., Ltd.
1-2, Yurakucho 1-chome
Chiyoda-ku
Tokyo, Japan

Noboru Inoue
Director, Internal Medicine
National Oji Hospital
Akabadai 4-17-56
Kita-ku, Tokyo, Japan

Rouben M. Jiji
Apheresis Center
Blood Transfusion Labs
University of Maryland Hospital
Baltimore, Maryland 21201

A. M. Joekes
Institute of Urology
London University
Shaftesbury Avenue
London W.C. 2, England

John Verrier Jones
Department of Medicine
Division of Rheumatology
Dalhousie University
Victoria General Hospital
Halifax, Nova Scotia B34 2Y9 Canada

Størker Jørstad
Department of Nephrology
University of Trondheim
7034 Trondheim -NTH, Norway

G. A. Jutzler
Department of Nephrology
Universität des Saarlandes
D-6650 Homburg/Saar
Federal Republic of Germany

Fukuei Kanai
2nd Department of Surgery
University of Tokyo
7-3-1 Hongo Bunkyo-ku
Tokyo, Japan

I. Kaneko
Kidney Center
Tokyo Women's Medical College
10 Kawada-cho, Shinjuku-ku
Tokyo, Japan

R. Kardish
Canadian Red Cross
Blood Transfusion Service
Ottawa Centre
85 Plymouth Street
Ottawa, Ontario K1S 3E2, Canada

C. Katsume
Department of Artificial Organs
Cleveland Clinic Foundation
9500 Euclid Avenue
Cleveland, Ohio 44106

S. Kawaguchi
Department of Internal Medicine
Nagoya University Branch Hospital
1–4, Daiko-cho 1-chome
Higashi-ku, Nagoya 461 Japan

A. Kawanishi
Department of Internal Medicine
Nagoya University Branch
1–4, Daiko-cho 1-chome
Higashi-ku, Nagoya 461 Japan

K. Kayashima
Department of Artificial Organs
Cleveland Clinic Foundation
9500 Euclid Avenue
Cleveland, Ohio 44106

M. Kazama
Teikyo University
11–1, Kaga 2-chome
Itabashi-ku
Tokyo 173, Japan

Frieder Keller
Free University
Klinikum Steglitz
Hindenburgdamm 30
D-1000 Berlin 45
Federal Republic of Germany

Melanie S. Kennedy
Department of Pathology
The Ohio State University
410 West 10th Avenue
Columbus, Ohio 43210

H. Kierdorf
Abteilung Innere Medizin II
an der Rhein. -Westf. Technische
* Hochschule Aachen*
Goethestrasse 27/29
5100 Aachen
Federal Republic of Germany

Mutsumi Kimura
Toray Industries, Inc.
2, Nihonbashi-Muromachi, 2-chome
Chuo-ku, Tokyo 103, Japan

Harvey G. Klein
Clinical Center Blood Bank
Building 104, Room 1E 33
National Institutes of Health
Bethesda, Maryland 20205

Lutz Kleine
II Medizinische Universitätsklinik
Metzstrasse 53
D 2300 Kiel
Federal Republic of Germany

Horst Klinkmann
University of Rostock
Klinik für Innere Medizin
DDR-25 Rostock 1
German Democratic Republic

M. Koehler
Departments of Haemostaseology
Universität des Saarlandes
D-6650 Homburg/Saar
Federal Republic of Germany

Peter J. Kragel
Apheresis Center
Blood Transfusion Labs
University of Maryland Hospital
Baltimore, Maryland 21201

Randall J. Krakauer
Cleveland Clinic Foundation
9500 Euclid Avenue
Cleveland, Ohio 44106

Gottfried Kreutz
Free University
Klinikum Steglitz
Hindenburgdamm 30
D-1000 Berlin 45
Federal Republic of Germany

Claus Laessing
Abteilung für Intensivmedizine
und Dialyse
Stadtisches Krankenhause Kiel
D 2300 Kiel
Federal Republic of Germany

I. Lafreniere
Department of Medicine
University of Ottawa
Ottawa, Canada

S. Landini
Nephrology and Dialysis Department
Umberto I Hospital
50–30174 Mestre (VE), Italy

Claudine le Berre
Regional Blood Bank
Allee P. J. Gineste
35000 Rennes, France

G. LeBlond
Hôpital St.-Marguerite
Blvd. de St.-Marguerite 270
13274 Marseille, Cedex 2, France

Catherine le Pogamp
Department Obstetrics A
2 rue Hôtel Dieu CHU
35043 Rennes, France

Patrick le Pogamp
Department of Nephrology
rue Henri Le Guilloux CHU
35043 Rennes, France

R. Lenzhofer
Departments of Chemotherapy
University of Vienna
Lazarettgasse 14
A-1090 Vienna, Austria

Edward F. Leonard
Artificial Organs Research Laboratory
355 Engineering Terrace
Columbia University
New York, New York 10027

A. Lin
Department of Laboratory Medicine
School of Medicine
University of Minnesota
Minneapolis, Minnesota 55455

Olgierd Lindan
International Center for Artificial Organs
and Transplantation
8937 Euclid Avenue
Cleveland, Ohio 44106

Donn D. Lobdell
Cobe Laboratories, Inc.
1201 Oak Street
Lakewood, Colorado 80215

C. M. Lockwood
Department of Medicine
Royal Postgraduate Medical School
Hammersmith Hospital
London W12 OHS, England

Helmut Loffler
II Medizinische Universitätsklinik
Metzstrasse 53
D 2300 Kiel
Federal Republic of Germany

Michael J. Lysaght
Nephrology Division
Medizinische Klinik I
Klinikum Grosshadern
University of Munich
D-8000 Munich, 70
Federal Republic of Germany

K. Maeda
Department of Internal Medicine
Nagoya University Branch Hospital
1–4, Daiko-cho 1-chome
Higashi-ku, Nagoya 461 Japan

P. S. Malchesky
Department of Artificial Organs
Cleveland Clinic Foundation
9500 Euclid Avenue
Cleveland, Ohio 44106

B. Mamoli
Department of Neurology
University of Vienna
Lazarettgasse 14
A-1090 Vienna, Austria

D. Mandel
Department of Rheumatic and
* Immunologic Disease*
Cleveland Clinic Foundation
9500 Euclid Avenue
Cleveland, Ohio 44106

S. Matsubara
Department of Artificial Organs
Cleveland Clinic Foundation
9500 Euclid Avenue
Cleveland, Ohio 44106

Takao Matsugane
Tokyo Tokatsu Clinic
822 Hinokuchi Matudoshi
Chiba, Japan

Valerie A. McCahon
Apheresis Center
Blood Transfusion Labs
University of Maryland Hospital
Baltimore, Maryland 21201

N. McCombie
Department of Medicine
University of Ottawa
Ottawa, Canada

J. McCullough
Department of Laboratory Medicine
School of Medicine
University of Minnesota
Minneapolis, Minnesota 55455

Paul R. McCurdy
American Red Cross Blood Services
2025 E Street, N.W.
Washington, D.C. 20006

R. J. McKendry
Department of Medicine
Ottawa General Hospital
Ottawa, Ontario, Canada

Bruce McLeod
Rush-Presbyterian-St. Luke's Medical
* Center*
Chicago, Illinois 60612

Hans Georg Mertens
Department of Neurology
University of Wurzburg
Josef-Schneider-Strassell
D-8700 Würzburg
Federal Republic of Germany

Florence E. Metrinko
Apheresis Center
Blood Transfusion Labs
University of Maryland Hospital
Baltimore, Maryland 21201

Carmine G. Moccio
Department of Surgery
* Division of Cardiovascular Surgery*
North Shore University Hospital
Manhasset, New York 11030

Martin Molzahn
Free University
Klinikum Steglitz
Hindenburgdamm 30
D-1000 Berlin 45
Federal Republic of Germany

E. Montas
Hôpital St.-Marguerite
Blvd. de St.-Marguerite 270
13274 Marseille, Cedex 2, France

P. Morachiello
Nephrology and Dialysis Department
Umberto I Hospital
50–30174 Mestre (VE), Italy

M. Morioka
Teiko University
11–1, Kaga 2-chome
Itabashi-ku
Tokyo 173, Japan

Henric Mulec
Medical Department V
Sahlgren's Hospital
S-413 45 Göteborg, Sweden

A. Murisasco
Hôpital St.-Marguerite
Blvd. De St.-Marguerite 270
13274 Marseille, Cedex 2, France

Roy L. Nelson
Department of Surgery
Division of Cardiovascular Surgery
North Shore University Hospital
300 Community Drive
Manhasset, New York 11030

Arthur W. Nienhuis
Clinical Center Blood Bank
Building 104, Room 1E33
National Institutes of Health
Bethesda, Maryland 20205

T. Niwa
Department of Internal Medicine
Nagoya University Branch Hospital
1-4, Daiko-cho 1-chome
Higashi-ku, Nagoya 461 Japan

Takuo Nobuto
Tokyo Tokatsu Clinic
822 Hinokuchi Matudoshi
Chiba, Japan

Tachio Nogi
Toray Industries, Inc.
2, Nihonbashi-Muromachi, 2-chome
Chuo-ku, Tokyo 103, Japan

Y. Nosé
Department of Artificial Organs
Cleveland Clinic Foundation
9500 Euclid Avenue
Cleveland, Ohio 44106

Toshitsugu Oda
Tokyo University Hospital
7-3-1 Hongo, Bunkyo-ku
Tokyo 113, Japan

Gerd Offermann
Free University
Klinikum Steglitz
Hindenburgdamm 30
D-1000 Berlin 45
Federal Republic of Germany

Yoshihiro Okada
Tokyo University Hospital
7-3-1, Hongo, Bunkyo-ku
Tokyo 113, Japan

J. P. Ortonne
Service de Dermatologie
Hôpital Pasteur
Avenue de la Voie Romaine
06031 Nice Cedex, France

Bernd Osten
University of Rostock
Klinik für Innere Medizin
DDR-25 Rostock 1
German Democratic Republic

K. Ota
Kidney Center
Tokyo Women's Medical College
10 Kawada-cho-Shinjuku-ku
Tokyo, Japan

Z. K. Papadopolou
Georgetown University
School of Medicine
Washington, D.C. 20007

M. Path
Department of Laboratory Medicine
School of Medicine
University of Minnesota
Minneapolis, Minnesota 55455

D. Patte
Service de Réanimation Médicale
et de Nephrologie
C.H.U. Poitiers
86021 Poitiers Cedex, France

B. W. Pechan
Georgetown University
School of Medicine
Washington, D.C. 20007

D. K. Peters
Department of Medicine
Royal Postgraduate Medical School
Hammersmith Hospital
London W12 OHS, England

T. Philips
Georgetown University
School of Medicine
Washington, D.C. 20007

Alvaro A. Pineda
Mayo Clinic Blood Bank
200 First Street, S.W.
Rochester, Minnesota 55901

J. Porten
Fenwal Laboratories
Division of Travenol
Laboratories, Inc.
Route 120 and Wilson Road
Round Lake, Illinois 60073

J. P. Pourrat
Service de Nephrologie et d'Hemodialyse
C.H.U. Toulouse-Purpan
Place du Docteur Baylac
31059 Toulouse Cedex, France

O. Pourrat
Service de Réanimation Médicale
et de Nephrologie
C.H.U. Poitiers
86021 Poitiers Cedex, France

C. D. Pusey
Department of Medicine
Royal Postgraduate Medical School
Hammersmith Hospital
London W12 OHS, England

J. F. Quaranta
Service de Médecine Interne A
Departement d'Hematologie
Hôpital de Cimiez
Avenue Victoria
06031 Nice Cedex, France

David H. Randerson
Nephrology Division
Klinikum Grosshadern
University of Munich
D-8000 Munich 70
Federal Republic of Germany

Sabine Reeck
Free University
Klinikum Steglitz
Hindenburgdamm 30
D-1000 Berlin 45
Federal Republic of Germany

Paul A. Reuther
Department of Neurology
University of Wurzburg
Josef-Schneider-Strasse 11
D-8700 Wurzburg
Federal Republic of Germany

Jean Revuz
Department of Dermatology
Hôpital Henri Mondor
94 010 Creteil, France

F. Righetto
Nephrology and Dialysis Department
Umberto I Hospital
50–30174 Mestre (VE), Italy

Severin Ringoir
Department of Internal Medicine
Renal Division
University Hospital
De Pintelaan 185
B-9000 Gent, Belgium

William H. Roberts
Department of Pathology
The Ohio State University
410 West 10th Street
Columbus, Ohio 43210

G. A. Rock
Canadian Red Cross
Blood Transfusion Service
Ottawa Centre
85 Plymouth Street
Ottawa, Ontario K1S 3E2 Canada

Reinhard Rohkamm
Department of Neurology
University of Wurzburg
Josef-Schneider-Strasse 11
D-8700 Wurzburg
Federal Republic of Germany

Jean Claude Roujeau
Department of Dermatology
Hôpital Henri Mondor
94 010 Creteil, France

Walter Samtleben
Nephrology Division
Klinikum Grosshadern
Medizinische Klinik I
University of Munich
D-8000 Munich 70
Federal Republic of Germany

Takemasa Sanjo
Tokyo University Hospital
7–3–1, Hongo, Bunkyo-ku
Tokyo 113, Japan

F. Scanferla
Nephrology and Dialysis Department
Umberto I Hospital
50–30174 Mestre (VE), Italy

K. Schmengler
Department of Cardiology
Universität des Saarlandes
D-6650 Homburg/Saar
Federal Republic of Germany

Baerbel Schmidt
Medizinische Klinik I
Klinikum Grosshadern
University of Munich
D-8000 Munich 70
Federal Republic of Germany

Matthias Schmidt
Fachbereich Humanmedizin der
*   Johann Wolfgang Goethe Universität*
Theodor-Stern-Kai 1
D-6006 Frankfurt 70
Federal Republic of Germany

Reinhard Schmidt
University of Rostock
Klinik für Innere Medizin
DDR-25 Rostock 1
German Democratic Republic

Eberhard Schmitt
University of Rostock
Klinik für Innere Medizin
DDR-25 Rostock 1
German Democratic Republic

P. Schneider
Department of Medicine
W. Pieck University, Rostock
E.-Heydemann Strasse
GDR-2500, Rostock
German Democratic Republic

Georg Schultze
Free University
Klinikum Steglitz
Hindenburgdamm 30
D-1000 Berlin 45
Federal Republic of Germany

Eva H. Schwartz
Apheresis Center
Blood Transfusion Labs
University of Maryland Hospital
Baltimore, Maryland 21201

Alberto C. Seiguer
Apheresis Center
Blood Transfusion Labs
University of Maryland Hospital
Baltimore, Maryland 21201

R. Sezaki
Department of Internal Medicine
Nagoya University Branch Hospital
1–4, Daiko-cho 1-chome
Higashi-ku, Nagoya 461 Japan

M. Shibata
Department of Internal Medicine
Nagoya University Branch Hospital
1–4, Daiko-cho 1-chome
Higashi-ku, Nagoya 461 Japan

T. Shinzato
Department of Internal Medicine
Nagoya University Branch Hospital
1–4, Daiko-cho 1-chome
Higashi-ku, Kanoya 461 Japan

H.-G. Sieberth
Abteilung Innere Medizine II
an der Rhein. -Wesf. Technische
Hochschule Aachen
Goethestrasse 27/29
5100 Aachen
Federal Republic of Germany

Leif C. Smeby
Institute of Biophysics
University of Trondheim
7034 Trondheim-NTH, Norway

J. Smith
Department of Laboratory Medicine
School of Medicine
University of Minnesota
Minneapolis, Minnesota 55455

James W. Smith
Cleveland Clinic Foundation
9500 Euclid Avenue
Cleveland, Ohio 44106

E. Snyder
Department of Laboratory Medicine
Yale University School of Medicine
New Haven, Connecticut 06510

Takeshi Sonoda
Toray Industries, Inc.
2, Nihonbashi-Muromachi, 2-chome
Chu-ku, Tokyo 103, Japan

J. Starre
Department of Artificial Organs
Cleveland Clinic Foundation
9500 Euclid Avenue
Cleveland, Ohio 44106

D. Stolz
Department of Nephrology
Universität des Saarlandes
D-6650 Homburg/Saar
Federal Republic of Germany

Akinori Sueoka
Department of Artificial Organs
Cleveland Clinic Foundation
9500 Euclid Avenue
Cleveland, Ohio 44106

N. Sugino
Kidney Center
Tokyo Women's Medical College
10 Kawada-cho, Shijuku-ku
Tokyo, Japan

Mitsuru Suzuki
Tokyo Tokatsu Clinic
822 Hinokuchi Matudoshi
Chiba, Japan

Tatsuo Suzuta
Tokyo Medical College
6–7–1, Nishishinjuku, Shinjuku-ku
Tokyo 160, Japan

Thor M. Svartaas
Institute of Biophysics
University of Trondheim
7034 Trondheim-NTH, Norway

Tatsuhiko Takahama
2nd Department of Surgery
University of Tokyo
7–3–1 Hongo Bunkyo-ku
Tokyo 113, Japan

Masatoshi Takahashi
Tokyo Medical College
6–7–1, Nishishinjuku, Shinjuku-ku
Tokyo 160, Japan

Yehuda Tamari
Department of Surgery
Division of Cardiovascular Surgery
North Shore University Hospital
300 Community Drive
Manhasset, New York 11030

Dieter Tessenow
University of Rostock
Klinik für Innere Medizin
DDR-25 Rostock 1
German Democratic Republic

W. Tessenow
Department of Medicine
W. Pieck University, Rostock
E.-Heydemann Strasse
GDR-2500, Rostock
German Democratic Republic

Anthony J. Tortolani
Department of Surgery
Division of Cardiovascular Surgery
North Shore University Hospital
300 Community Drive
Manhasset, New York 11030

G. Touchard
Service de Réanimation Médicale et de
*   Nephrologie*
C.H.U. Poitiers
86021 Poitiers Cedex, France

René Touraine
Department of Dermatology
Hôpital Henri Mondor
94 010 Creteil, France

M. Ueno
Department of Artificial Organs
Cleveland Clinic Foundation
9500 Euclid Avenue
Cleveland, Ohio 44106

M. Usuda
Department of Internal Medicine
Nagoya University Branch Hospital
1–4, Daiko-cho 1-chome
Higashi-ku, Nagoya 461 Japan

Raymond VanHolder
Department of Internal Medicine
Renal Division
University Hospital
DePintelaan 185
B-9000 Gent, Belgium

Tatsuo Wada
2nd Department of Surgery
University of Tokyo
7–3–1 Hongo Bunkyo-ku
Tokyo 113, Japan

M. Wahlen
Department of Paediatrics
Universität des Saarlandes
D-6650 Homburg/Saar
Federal Republic of Germany

Gregory P. Wanger
Department of Pathology
The Ohio State University
410 West 10th Avenue
Columbus, Ohio 43210

Gunnar Westberg
Medical Department V
Sahlgren's Hospital
S-413 45 Goteborg Sweden

Dieter Wiebecke
Transfusion Center
University of Wurzburg
Josef-Schneider-Strasse 11
D-8700 Wurzburg
Federal Republic of Germany

J. Wojcicki
Department of Artificial Organs
Cleveland Clinic Foundation
9500 Euclid Avenue
Cleveland, Ohio 44106

Arjeh J. Wysenbeek
Cleveland Clinic Foundation
9500 Euclid Avenue
Cleveland, Ohio 44106

K. Yabe
Tokyo University Hospital
7–3–1, Hongo, Bunkyo-ku
Tokyo 113, Japan

N. Yamawaki
Asahi Chemical Industry Co., Ltd.
1–2, Yurakucho 1-chome, Chiyoda-ku
Tokyo, Japan

Z. Yamazaki
2nd Department of Surgery
Tokyo University Hospital
7–3–1, Hongo, Bunkyo-ku
Tokyo 113, Japan

Makoto Yoshiba
Tokyo University Hospital
7–3–1, Hongo, Bunkyo-ku
Tokyo 113, Japan

Neal S. Young
Clinical Center Blood Bank
Building 104, Room 1E33
National Institutes of Health
Bethesda, Maryland 20205

J. Zeitelhofer
Department of Neurology
University of Vienna
Lazarettgasse 14
A-1090 Vienna, Austria

Plasmapheresis, edited by Y. Nosé, P. S.
Malchesky, J. W. Smith, and R. S. Krakauer.
Raven Press, New York © 1983.

Introduction to Therapeutic Apheresis

Y. Nosé, H. E. Kambic, and S. Matsubara

Department of Artificial Organs, The Cleveland Clinic, Cleveland, Ohio 44106

The biotechnology for on-line plasma separation and on-line plasma treatment has opened a new era, expanding the application of extracorporeal technology to modern therapeutic medicine. Plasmapheresis is finding its way into the treatment of an increasing number of autoimmune, hematologic, and metabolic diseases that are considered difficult to treat by conventional medicine. Today, plasmapheresis technology offers a new treatment modality, and is emerging as a tool for the elucidation of disease processes. With the increasing need for alternative processing of plasma components, the use of plasmapheresis techniques is expanding.

In this chapter, currently available centrifugal cell separators and membrane plasma filters, in addition to the variety of on-line plasma treatment schemes, are introduced. The state-of-the-art technologies for therapeutic plasma exchange and plasma treatment are reviewed. The status of the emerging clinical plasma therapies is reported, with an outlook to the future utilization of plasmapheresis as an alternative treatment for end-stage diseases. Research problems remain. These include system modeling, on-line monitoring of the system, efficient optimization procedures, and the identification and quantification of removed plasma factors. With the rapidly growing number of research groups in industry and academia that are studying different aspects of the problem in this emerging field of medicine, it appears that the answers may be close at hand.

PLASMA EXCHANGE

Plasma exchange involves the nonspecific removal of plasma factors, reduction of their circulating concentrations, and improvement of the clinical state of the patient. The major limitations of the method include (a) the requirement of plasma products, (b) loss of essential plasma solutes, (c) potential contamination by plasma substitutes, and (d) loss of blood cellular elements, particularly platelets. Factors in the application of plasma exchange are (a) exchange volumes that may vary from minimal to extensive, (b) variations in the type of replacement fluid (albumin, fresh frozen plasma, or purified protein solutions), (c) intensity of exchange procedures, the rate and volume of exchange, and the frequency of exchange, and (d) differences in therapeutic applications and procedures. Despite many unknown factors and limitations, plasma exchange is gaining in popularity. The following sections of this volume will attempt to clarify some of the above-mentioned areas.

In 1980, it was estimated that about 40,000 therapeutic plasma exchange procedures were carried out in the United States and that this number will increase yearly (Fig. 1). Growth is related to the cost-effectiveness of the procedure, compared to conventional treatments. Plasma exchange has been employed in a wide variety of disease states, which may be generally categorized as metabolic or immunologic. The literature cites over 50 diseases treated by plasmapheresis (1) (Table 1). While many studies have been anecdotal in nature, plasma exchange is highly recommended in certain diseases (2) (Table 2). Through further investigation, the role of plasma exchange in therapy will be more clearly understood scientifically; however, several deterrents to the use of plasma exchange exist.

Procedurally, plasma exchange is an invasive treatment and one that is generally considered as a last resort. As in most invasive treatments, there are risks. Blood access is required, and contamination of, or reaction to, the infusion solution (plasma or its products, such as albumin) are ever-present potential problems. The potential magnitude of these problems is related to the clinical area in question. In the renal and hematological areas, these problems may generally be considered less important, since comparable procedures are part of the routine treatment of patients.

The potential number of patients for plasmapheresis is shown in Table 3, but this number may be too low if the procedures prove effective and application is expanded to include nonhospitalized patients. For example, the potential number

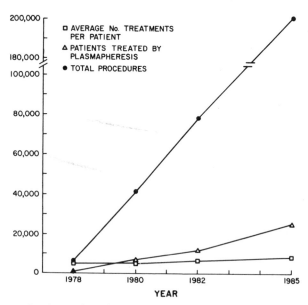

FIG. 1. Therapeutic plasmapheresis procedures performed in the United States from 1978, and projections through the year 1985.

TABLE 1. *Diseases treated with therapeutic apheresis—plasmapheresis (plasma exchange)*

Medical discipline	Protein-related	Antibody-related	Immune complex-related
Hematology	Waldenstrom's macroglobulinemia	Idiopathic thrombocytopenic purpura Factor VIII auto-antibody Rh disease Autoimmune hemolytic anemia	Thrombotic thrombocytopenic purpura
Rheumatology	Raynaud's disease	Systemic lupus erythematosus	Rheumatoid arthritis Systemic lupus erythematosus Scleroderma Other
Neurology		Myasthenia gravis Multiple sclerosis Polymyositis Polyneuropathy	Guillain-Barré syndrome
Oncology	Multiple myeloma	Other cancers	
Nephrology		Progressive nephritis Glomerulonephritis Goodpasture's syndrome	Transplant rejection (?) Polyarteritis nodosa
Other	Toxins Poisons Hypercholesterolemia Thyrotoxicosis Primary biliary Cirrhosis Hypertriglyceridemia Hepatic insufficiency	Chronic active hepatitis Diabetes mellitus Pemphigus vulgaris Asthma	

of rheumatoid arthritic patients alone is well over one-half million. In 1981, over 6 million liters of plasma were collected in the United States to supply the international marketplace (Table 4). If plasma exchange is successful in the wide variety of diseases being investigated, various disease states will be competing for the supply. Diseases associated with deficiencies in clotting factors, which require plasma components, would also be competing with those diseases associated with plasma excess. Thus, plasma exchange may have a high probability for effective therapeutic treatment of metabolic and immunologic disorders, but this method must be practical and cost-effective.

The recent introduction of membrane plasmapheresis has provided an alternative solution to these problems. Membrane systems of the hollow-fiber geometry that are presently being investigated generate a plasma product that has minimal or no platelets. Thus, blood cell losses are minimal. For the same devices, large solutes

TABLE 2. *Classification of diseases treated by plasmapheresis*

Proven
Exogenous intoxications
Thyroid storm
Myasthenic crisis
Goodpasture's syndrome
Justified
Hemophilia with antibodies to factor VIII
Thrombotic thrombocytopenic purpura
Paraproteinemia
Pemphigus vulgaris
Immune complex GN
Promising
Systemic lupus erythematosus
Rheumatoid arthritis
Guillain-Barré syndrome
Rhesus disease
Possible
Familial hypercholesterolemia
Renal allograft rejection

Adapted from Gurland, H. J., *Trans. Am. Soc. Artif. Intern. Organs,* 28:356, 1981.

(immunoglobulins, rheumatoid factor, albumin, and total protein fraction) have been shown clinically to have over 95% passage into the plasma.

While membrane systems provide certain advantages, the selection of the membrane, its design into a module, and the determination of operating parameters have not yet been optimized. The development stage of membrane systems for plasmapheresis is similar to that of hemodialysis in the late 1950s.

The major deterrent to plasma exchange, whether carried out by centrifuges or membranes, is the requirement for plasma products. To remove those solutes of interest, techniques must be devised that will not place a major demand on the plasma products' supply (Table 5).

CENTRIFUGAL APHERESIS

Following the development of the various types of cell centrifuge apparatuses, the introduction of the NCI/IBM Blood Cell Separator made possible the processing of plasma and white cells by uninterrupted whole blood flow through the centrifugal apparatus. The on-line production of plasma and white cell components allows for therapeutic plasma exchange or therapeutic leukopheresis. G. T. Judson (Fig. 2) and E. J. Freireich were co-inventors of the NCI/IBM Blood Cell Separator (Fig. 3). The instrument was first shown publicly in October 1965. Judson, a research engineer with the International Business Machines Corporation (IBM), and Freireich, at the National Cancer Institute (NCI), designed and fabricated this mechanical device that can therapeutically remove white blood cells (WBCs). The initial em-

TABLE 3. Hospitalized patient populations[a] and procedures used in the United States, 1981

Medical discipline	Plasma exchange	Plasma exchange and/or cytapheresis	Cytapheresis
Hematology	Waldenstrom's—2,000 Thrombocytopenic purpuras—16,000		Sickle cell—48,000 Polycythemia—5,000
Rheumatology	Lupus—23,000 Other—11,000	Rheumatoid arthritis—136,000	
Neurology	Guillain-Barré—9,000 Myasthenia gravis—9,000 Polymyositis—7,000	Multiple sclerosis—41,000	
Nephrology	Nephritis—20,000 Glomerulonephritis—18,000 Goodpasture's—5,000 Transplant rejection—(?)		
Oncology	Multiple myeloma—52,000		Some leukemias—17,000
Other	Miscellaneous—8,000		
Total patient population—180,000		177,000	70,000

[a]Total apheresis patient population, 427,000; plasma exchange patient population, 180,000–357,000.

TABLE 4. Sources and use of plasma in the United States (in millions of liters)

	1975	1977	1979	1981	1983[a]	1985[a]	1987[a]	Average annual growth (%)	
								1975–1979	1979–1987
Sources of plasma									
Totals from whole blood for transfusion as whole plasma; for fractionation	1.1	1.5	1.8	2.1	2.4	2.7	3.0	12	6
From plasmapheresis	2.0	2.6	3.4	4.3	5.5	7.0	9.0	15	13
Imported from third world countries	0.3	0.2	—	—	—	—	—	—	—
Total plasma collected	3.4	4.3	5.2	6.4	7.9	9.7	11.9	11	11
Uses of plasma									
Total of plasma for fractionation from whole blood from plasmapheresis imports	3.0	3.6	4.3	5.4	6.7	8.3	10.2	10	11
For transfusion	0.4	0.5	0.5	0.5	0.5	0.5	0.5	—	—
Exported to Europe and Japan	—	0.2	0.4	0.5	0.7	0.9	1.2	—	15
Total usage	3.4	4.3	5.2	6.4	7.9	9.7	11.9	11	11

[a]Estimated values.

TABLE 5. *Comparison of plasma replacement fluids*

Source	Advantages	Disadvantages
Albumin	Depletion of inflammatory mediators	Cost
Plasma protein fraction (PPF)	Ease and convenience of use	Hypotensive reactions (with PPF)
		Reduction in coagulation factors
Fresh frozen plasma (FFP)	Maintains normal plasma factors	Hepatitis
		Allergic reactions
		Citrate toxicity
		ABO incompatibility
		Sensitization to protein, RBC by HLA antigens
Crystaloids	Cost	Protein depletion

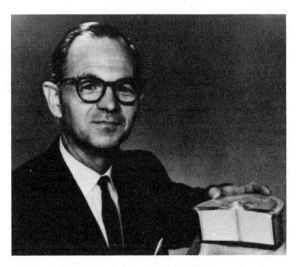

FIG. 2. G. T. Judson, co-inventor of NCI/IBM Blood Cell Separator.

phasis on WBC removal later shifted to plasma removal. This procedure became popular after the introduction of the disposable separation chamber. Currently, there are three companies producing centrifugal apparatuses in the United States that are routinely utilized for therapeutic plasma exchange purposes (3) (Table 6).

Extracorporeal circulation was used for plasmapheresis and/or cytopheresis. Several varieties of centrifugal apparatuses are available, including the intermittent-flow and the continuous-flow instruments (Table 6). Intermittent-flow devices require repetitive shutdown for cell or plasma retrieval. Continuous-flow devices are operated continuously, withdrawing blood, separating and retaining specific blood components, and reinfusing the remaining blood components to the patient.

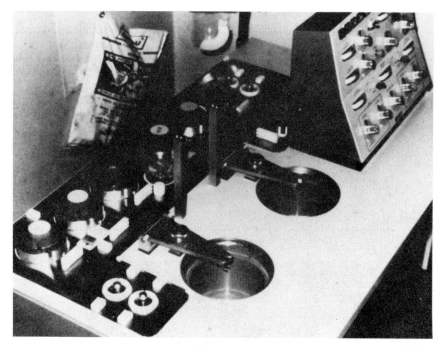

FIG. 3. NCI/IBM Two-Bowl Experimental Blood Cell Separator. The first bowl separated plate-let-rich plasma and packed red blood cells. The second bowl concentrated platelets. The most difficult problem in the development of the blood cell separator was the unique engineering feature of the two rotating seals, through which whole blood and the separated components pass with minimal trauma. The final seal design incorporated saline lubrication to prevent intrusion of cells between contacting surfaces.

In consequence of the developmental collaboration between IBM and NCI, the 2990–6 Experimental Blood Cell Separator evolved (supported in part by federal funds). IBM made these machines to order under a special program, but elected not to market them. The American Instrument Company (Aminco) acquired the technical file of the separator shortly before the company was purchased by Travenol Laboratories in 1969. Travenol then stripped down the blood cell separator and, in 1970, under the leadership of Robert Eisel, marketed the Continuous-Flow Cell-trifuge Blood Cell Separator.

In the centrifuge bowl (Fig. 4), which is not disposable, the whole blood input travels down a central core, peripherally along the bottom, and ascends the sides (where the separation occurs). Ports cut into the faceplate permit collection from the bottom of the packed red cell layer, from the top of the plasma layer, and from the plasma red cell interface where buffy coat concentration occurs.

In 1978, IBM introduced the model 2997 Blood Cell Separator. It incorporates the basic ideas of continuous flow centrifugation, selective separation by means of collection ports and concentric channels, and a rotating seal (Fig. 5). IBM also made this model available with a buffer system similar to that in Freireich's original

TABLE 6. *Automated blood cell separation systems*

Type	Manufacturer	Models	Introduced	Components separated	Membrane type
Continuous-flow centrifuge	Fenwal	CS-3000	1979	Cells, plasma	None
	(Traverol)	Celltrifuge 11	1981	Cells, plasma	None
	IBM Biomedical	2997	1977	Cells, plasma	None
Intermittent-flow centrifuge	Haemonetics	30	1973	Cells, plasma	None
		V-50	1980	Cells, plasma	None
		PEX	1980	Cells, plasma	None
Continuous-flow membrane	Cobe Laboratories		1981	Plasma only	Sheet
	Parker-Hannifin	Cryomax	1979	Plasma only	Hollow fiber
	Fenwal (Traverol)		1981	Plasma only	Hollow fiber

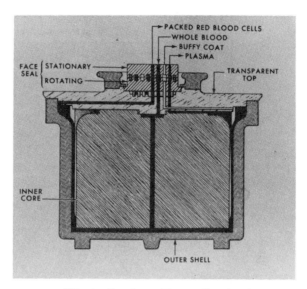

FIG. 4. Nondisposable centrifuge bowl.

design. In this system, the centrifuge bowl is replaced with a separation channel, consisting of a semirigid rectangular plastic tube attached at both ends to the input–collection chamber, forming a closed loop. The breakthrough in design is the division of this chamber by a restrictive barrier. As whole blood enters the input end of the channel and travels around to the input–collection chamber, it is separated by the centrifugation into components.

The specificity of the model 2997 was enhanced in 1980 by the addition of a variation of the separation channel. The dual-stage separation channel was introduced as a means of obtaining platelet concentrate with minimum lymphocyte contamination.

The apex of hemapheresis technology was reached in 1979 when Fenwall Laboratories marketed their CS-3000 Blood Cell Separator. This third generation of blood cell separators was developed by combining more automation, in the form of a microprocessor to control machine operation, with a sealless system. Whole blood separation and consequent component collection is performed within the centrifuge by means of specifically designed chambers interconnected by a single five-lumen umbilical (Fig. 6). This articulation permits blood flow from the donor vein into the separation bag of the centrifuge, transfer of component-rich plasma within the centrifuge to the collection bag, and subsequent return of recombined fractions to the recipient vein.

The separation chambers for the CS-3000 are unique for the component desired. The blood processing pathway, including the bowl, is completely disposable. No rotating seals are utilized, thus reducing the threat of leaks and contamination during the procedure (Fig. 7).

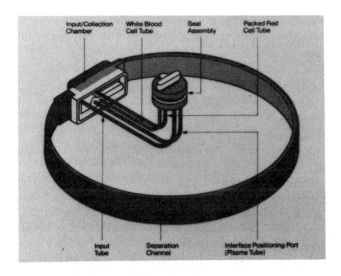

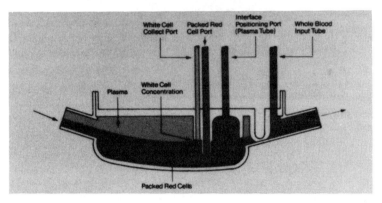

FIG. 5. Collection ports, concentric channels, and rotating seal of the IBM 2997 Blood Cell Separator.

The Haemonetics disposable bowl, developed by the Haemonetics Corporation (Braintree, MA), permits the safe and effective processing of the blood of both donors and patients, with rapid separation of that blood into its component parts. This device is an intermittent-flow centrifuge, and, because of its simple design, it remains one of the most popular tools for centrifugal plasma therapy. The bowl is a sterile, disposable chamber, available in a variety of sizes, that processes the blood of donor or patients. The bowl has two parts, one rotating and one stationary. Blood from the donor or patient enters at the top of the bowl, flows to the bottom, and is distributed to the periphery by centrifugal force. Separation of blood components occurs depending on the density of each component. The red cells, being heaviest, are found at the outside of the bowl. Plasma, the lightest component, is drawn to the center of the bowl, where it overflows and can be collected through

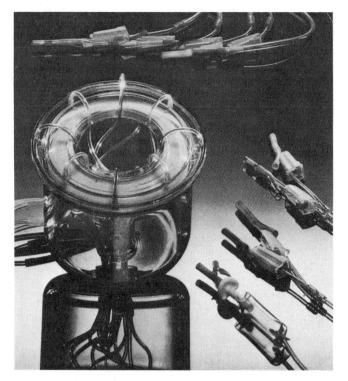

FIG. 6. Completely disposable separation chamber of the Fenwal CS-3000 Blood Cell Separator.

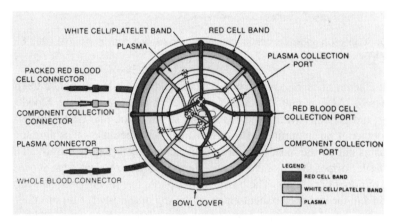

FIG. 7. Blood processing pathway within the bowl. Whole blood is removed from the donor/patient via the inlet line and mixed with the desired anticoagulant. Whole blood enters the disposable bowl and separates into its components. The desired component is harvested. The remaining components are combined and returned to the donor/patient via the return line.

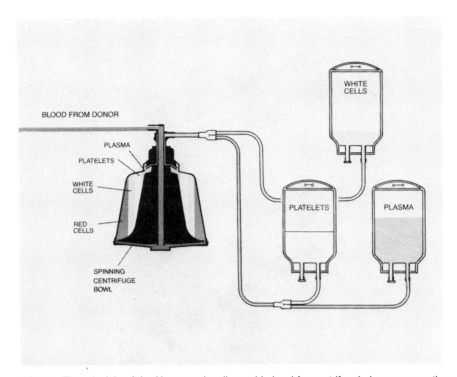

FIG. 8. The principle of the Haemonetics disposable bowl for centrifugal plasma separation.

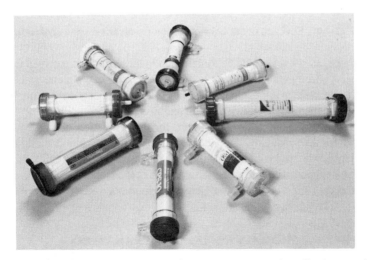

FIG. 9. Eight of the hollow-fiber membrane plasma separators produced by the manufacturers listed in Table 7.

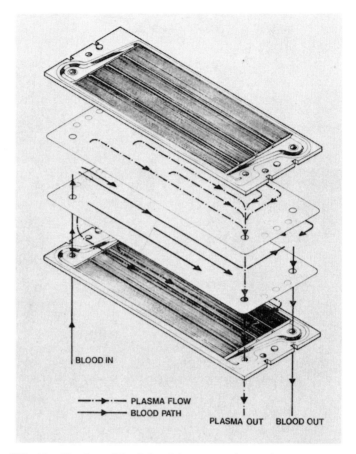

BLOOD IN

— · —▶— · — PLASMA FLOW
————▶———— BLOOD PATH

PLASMA OUT   BLOOD OUT

FIG. 10. Structure of the Cobe plate-type membrane plasma separator.

the outlet port, as shown in Fig. 8. Platelets and white cells fall between the plasma and red cells. Through the use of the sterile bowl, needed components can be rapidly collected while the remainder can be returned to the donor or patient. This flexibility in the Haemonetics bowl allows the collection of blood components from donors for transfusion to patients who need them, for the reinfusion of surgical patients' blood, and for treatment by the therapeutic exchange of blood components. In several therapeutic applications, such as plasmapheresis, the mobility of the Haemonetics system and ability to place the machine at the patient's bedside are definite benefits for the direct treatment of patients having a variety of immunological diseases.

MEMBRANE PLASMA SEPARATORS

As of April 1982, 10 companies have developed membrane plasma separator modules (Figs. 9–11). Based on our evaluation of seven of the modules and in-

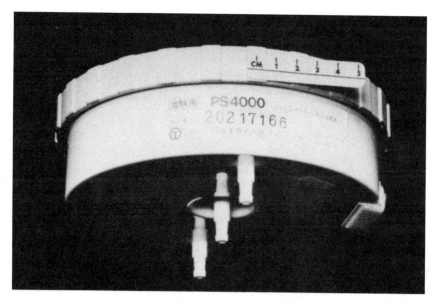

FIG. 11. Terumo pile-type membrane plasma separator.

formation provided by the manufacturers, all appear to satisfy the clinical criteria for safe and effective plasma separators (Fig. 12). Ten basic requirements for a plasma separator have been established (4). The available membrane plasma separators can separate cell-free plasma at a level of over 30 ml/min at a blood flow of 100 ml/min when the hematocrit ranges from 30 to 40% without hemolysis. The sieving coefficients are over 95% of total plasma protein, over 80% for immuno-complexes, and 90% for immunoglobulins. A stable and reproducible plasma separation rate is maintained for the duration of operation (3–5 hr). All separators are applicable for a wide range of blood flows (50–200 ml/min), show better blood compatibility than do cellulose base hemodialysis membranes, and are available as disposable sterile products. Most are of the hollow-fiber design (Fig. 13), but some are of the plate type, resembling a disposable hemodialyzer.

A membrane plasma filter does not require bulky, expensive hardware to be operable. Although most manufacturers of membrane plasma separators have introduced a designated system for use with their filters, a special system or specific apparatus is not required if the hollow-fiber plasma filter is to be used. A standard blood pump, as is generally used for hemodialysis, is adequate. Because of its simplicity and ease of operation, membrane plasma separation therapy is gaining in popularity.

As early as 1960, membrane plasma separation was attempted using "Japanese filter paper" (5). The availability of microporous polymeric hollow fibers in 1972 (6), and microporous polymeric sheet membranes by 1974 (7,8) spurred the development of membrane plasma filters by our group. A membrane with 0.2–0.6

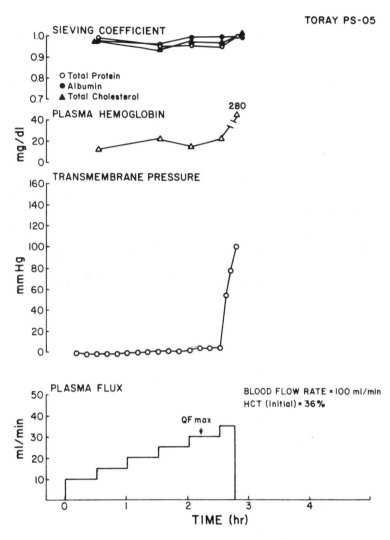

FIG. 12. *In vitro* performance test data for Toray Plasmax plasma separator.

μm nominal porosity satisfies the requirements of a plasma filter membrane (Fig. 14). Since 1977, the Asahi hollow-fiber devices with cellulose acetate membrane of 0.1–0.2 nominal porosity, applied in ascites treatment, have been further evaluated for their applicability in membrane plasmapheresis. Our experimental results showed that the Asahi ascites device could be used for plasmapheresis (9). The first clinical applications were made by Yamazaki and his group in Japan (10). Further, extensive experimental and clinical studies have been conducted to improve this system for on-line separation of plasma from whole blood by our group (11–20) and others. Studies show that it is extremely important, in order to achieve

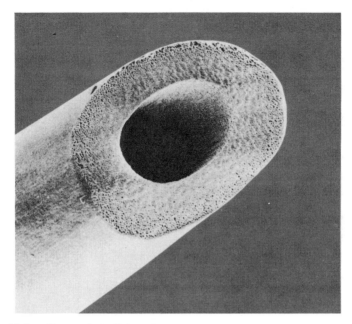

FIG. 13. Hollow fiber made by Enka AG and used by Fresenius, Takeda, and Travenol for their plasma separators.

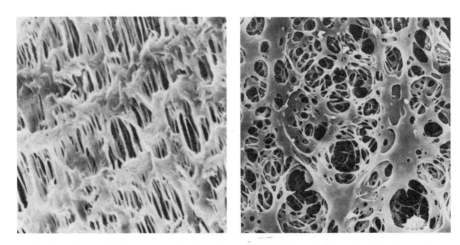

FIG. 14. **Left:** Membrane structure of Mitsubishi polyethylene hollow-fiber membrane, which is distinctly different from the pore structure of the other hollow-fiber membranes (×10,000). **Right:** Scanning electron microscopic image of Toray PS-05 hollow-fiber membrane (inner surface, ×10,000).

TABLE 7. *Available plasma filters, membrane and module*

Membrane

Filter	Type	Max. pore size (μm)	Material	ID (μm)	Wall thickness (μm)	Effective length (mm)	Effective surface area (m²)
Asahi Hi-05	HF	0.2	Cellulose diacetate	330	75	157	0.5
Kuraray PVA SA	HF	0.4	Polyvinyl alcohol	330	125	275	0.6
Toray Plasmax PS-05	HF	0.4	PMMA	370	85	175	0.5
Mitsubishi MPS	HF	0.2	Polyethylene	270	60	175	0.65
Fresenius Plasmaflux	HF	0.55	Polypropylene	330	140	200	0.5
Takeda separator	HF	0.55	Polypropylene	330	140	155	0.2
Travenol CPS-10TM	HF	0.55	Polypropylene	320	150	214	0.17
Teijin TP-50	HF	0.2	Cellulose diacetate base	330	75	150 (?)	0.5
Cobe Centry TPE	Plate	0.6	Polyvinyl chloride derivative	NA	—	NA	0.13
Terumo pile type	Plate	0.45	Cellulose acetate	NA	170	NA	0.4

Module

Filter	Container Material	Container Dimensions LXφ (mm)	Sealant	Priming volume (ml)	Sterilization method	Wet or dry
Asahi Hi-05	Polycarbonate	255 × 43	Polyurethane	65	Ethylene oxide	Glycerin, dry
Kuraray PVA	Polycarbonate Polypropylene	380 × 67	Polyurethane	80	Steam autoclave	Water, wet
Toray Plasmax PS-05	Polystyrene	240 × 73	Polyurethane	59	γ-Ray	Water, wet
Mitsubishi MPS	Polycarbonate	225 × 53	Polyurethane	60	Formaldehyde	Formaldehyde, wet
Fresenius Plasmaflux	Macrolon	250 × 50	Polyurethane	54	Ethylene oxide	Surfactant, dry
Takeda separator	Polycarbonate	245 × 56	Polyurethane	21	Ethylene oxide	Surfactant, dry
Travenol CPS-10TM	—	—	—	22	—	—
Cobe Centry TPE	—	—	—	—	Ethylene oxide gas	Dry
Terumo pile type	Polycarbonate	25 × 150	Silicone rubber adhesive	80	Ethylene oxide gas	Dry

HF, hollow-fiber; NA, not available; PMMA, polymethylmethacrylate.

TABLE 8. *Plasma sorption systems*

System	Application/diseases	Plasma factors removed
Activated charcoal and anionic resins	Poisoning Primary biliary cirrhosis Hepatic coma (liver failure)	Poison Bile acid Toxins, including mercaptans, and bilirubin
Heparin-agarose columns	Hypercholesterolemia	Cholesterol
A & B antigen	Bone-marrow transplant	Anti A & Anti B isoagglutinins
DNA collodian charcoal columns	Systemic lupus erythematosus	DNA antibody and immune complexes
Protein A columns and filters	Cancer (colon, carcinoma, breast cancer) Multiple myeloma Hemolytic anemia Probable effectiveness in myasthenia gravis and hemophilia (factor VIII)	IgG antibodies and immune complexes

effective plasma separation, that the filter be operated under the proper conditions. Transmembrane pressure, shear rate, rate of plasma removal, and hematological conditions are extremely crucial. It is also particularly important to stress that these devices should be operated with the lowest transmembrane pressures possible. Table 7 lists the features of acceptable plasma filters as of April 1982. The relevant features and specifications of each filter type are included.

PLASMA TREATMENT

Plasma exchange requires discarding the separated plasma and replacing it by an infusion of a plasma substitute. It is possible, however, to eliminate the infusion of a plasma substitute if the plasma is treated to remove selective pathological molecules. On-line plasmapheresis is defined as a treatment modality consisting of (a) the removal of whole blood from the patient, (b) separation of plasma from the cellular blood components, (c) subjecting the separated plasma to specific procedures, like cooling and perfusion through columns with adsorbents or specific membranes, and (d) the subsequent reunion of the treated plasma with the cellular blood components and its return to the patient.

Sorbent Treatment

Since 1974, our group has been utilizing membrane plasma separators with biological and nonbiological sorbents for hepatic assist purposes (6–21). At first, freshly sliced liver tissues were used; later, these were replaced with activated charcoal and anion resins. For treatment of various diseases, not only have activated charcoal (22) and anion resins been used, but also heparin-agarose (23), insolubilized

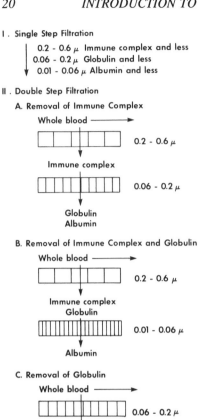

I . Single Step Filtration

0.2 - 0.6 μ Immune complex and less
0.06 - 0.2 μ Globulin and less
0.01 - 0.06 μ Albumin and less

II . Double Step Filtration

A. Removal of Immune Complex

Whole blood ⟶

0.2 - 0.6 μ

Immune complex

0.06 - 0.2 μ

Globulin
Albumin

B. Removal of Immune Complex and Globulin

Whole blood ⟶

0.2 - 0.6 μ

Immune complex
Globulin

0.01 - 0.06 μ

Albumin

C. Removal of Globulin

Whole blood ⟶

0.06 - 0.2 μ

Globulin

0.01 - 0.06 μ

Albumin

FIG. 15. Cascade membrane technology for selective removal of macromolecules. General objectives for success of this technology are filter membranes of various porosities suitable for the selective removal of macromolecules from blood (6).

A & B antigens (24), DNA collodian charcoal (25), and protein A with filters (26). Table 8 and Fig. 15 describe the various plasma sorption systems.

Cascade Membrane Filtration

Once plasma is separated from the cellular components, it is easy to remove certain toxic substances or measure the blood levels of essential substances, as well as to add to this system. If we know certain macromolecules should be removed, we can use cascade membrane technology (6) to selectively remove molecules of a few million daltons molecular weight (e.g., immune complexes), a few hundred thousand daltons molecular weight (e.g., gammaglobulin fractions), or below 100,000 daltons molecular weight (e.g., albumin fractions). Aiming for separation of these various types of macromolecules, several industrial firms have developed macromolecular filters of various porosities over the last 6 years. At this time, various membranes with the selectivity to do these tasks are available or becoming available (Fig. 15).

Cryofiltration

Selective separation of globulin fraction or larger molecules from albumin or smaller molecules is theoretically possible, but the molecular size of albumin and globulin are quite similar in dimension and it is rather difficult to effectively separate them by simple membrane filtration systems. Realizing that cryoprotein is very often present in the autoimmune disease state treated by plasmapheresis, an attempt was made to utilize the phenomenon of cold separation to accelerate the effective separation of albumin and globulin. Cryofiltration was developed by Malchesky and Nosé in 1980 (6,27,28), and since then they have continued to expand its clinical applications. A detailed description of the current art of technology and its clinical application are cited elsewhere in this volume. Cryogel removed from the plasma by this process is quite different from cryoprotein. About 10 g of cryogel can be removed even from a healthy individual by a single, standard cryofiltration process.

CONCLUSION

Recent progress in plasma separation and plasma treatment technologies has provided us with a powerful tool in therapeutic medicine for diseases that were once considered difficult to treat by conventional methods. Following chapters of this volume report the current status of clinical applications of this new technology, as described by practitioners of diverse medical specialties.

REFERENCES

1. Horiuchi, T., Kambic, H., Takatani, S., and Nosé, Y., eds: *Topics in Plasmapheresis: A Bibliography of Therapeutic Applications and New Techniques.* International Center for Artificial Organs and Transplantation, Cleveland, 1982.
2. Gurland, H. J., Samtleben, W., Blumenstein, M., Randerson, D. H., and Schmidt, B.: Clinical applications of macromolecular separations. *Trans. Am. Soc. Artif. Intern. Organs*, 27:356, 1981.
3. Kambic, H., and Nosé, Y.: *Plasmapheresis: Historical Perspective, Therapeutic Applications and New Frontiers.* International Center for Artificial Organs and Transplantation, Cleveland, 1982.
4. Nosé, Y., and Malchesky, P. S.: Technical aspects of membrane plasma treatment. *Artif. Organs*, 5 (Suppl):86, 1981.
5. Nosé, Y.: An experimental artificial liver utilizing extracorporeal metabolism with sliced or granulated canine liver [Discussion]. *Trans. Am. Soc. Artif. Intern. Organs*, 9:362, 1963.
6. Nosé, Y., Malchesky, P. S., and Smith, J. W.: Hybrid artificial organs: Are they really necessary? *Artif. Organs*, 4:285, 1980.
7. Nosé, Y., Koshino, I., Castino, F., Yoshida, K., Carse, C., Kambic, H., Scheucher, K., Kretz, A. P., and Malchesky, P. S.: Further assessment of liver tissue materials for extracorporeal hepatic assist. In: *Artificial Liver Support*, edited by Williams, R., and Murray-Lyons, I. M. Pitman Medical Press, Turnbridge Wells, U.K., 1975, p. 202.
8. Castino, F., Scheucher, K., Malchesky, P. S., Koshino, I., and Nosé, Y.: Microemboli-free blood detoxification utilizing plasma filtration. *Trans. Am. Soc. Artif. Intern. Organs*, 22:637, 1976.
9. Ouchi, K., Piatkiewicz, W., Malchesky, P. S., Hermann, R., and Nosé, Y.: An efficient specific and blood compatible sorbent system for hepatic assist. *Trans. Am. Soc. Artif. Intern. Organs*, 24:246, 1978.
10. Yamazaki, Z., Fujimori, Y., Sanjo, K., Kojima, Y., Sugiura, M., Wada, T., Inoue, N., Sakai, T., Oda, T., Kominami, N., Fujisaki, U., and Kataoka, K.: New artificial liver support systems (plasma perfusion detoxification) for hepatic coma. *Artif. Organs*, 2(Suppl):273, 1978.

11. Malchesky, P. S., Ouchi, K., Piatkiewicz, W., and Nosé, Y.: Membrane plasma filtration systems with multiple reactors for hepatic assist. *Artif. Organs*, 2 (Suppl):265, 1978.
12. Asanuma, Y., Smith, J. S., Malchesky, P. S., Hermann, R. E., Carey, W. D., Ferguson, D. R., and Nosé, Y.: Preclinical evaluation of membrane plasmapheresis with on-line bilirubin removal. *Artif. Organs*, 3:279, 1979.
13. Nosé, Y., and Malchesky, P. S.: Therapeutic application of plasmapheresis. In: *Plasma Forum*, edited by Warner, W. L. American Blood Resources Association, 1979, p. 47., Berkeley, CA.
14. Zawicki, I., Smith, J. W., Harasaki, H., Asanuma, Y., Malchesky, P. S., and Nosé, Y. (1981): Axial distribution of particle deposition in capillary membrane filter. *Artif. Organs*, 5:241.
15. Asanuma, Y., Smith, J. W., Suwa, S., Zawicki, I., Harasaki, H., Dixon, A. C., Malchesky, P. S., and Nosé, Y.: Membrane plasmapheresis: Platelet and protein effects on filtration. *Proc. ESAO*, 6:308, 1979.
16. Nosé, Y., Malchesky, P. S., Asanuma, Y., Smith, J. W., Carey, W. D., Ferguson, D. R., and Hermann, R. E. (1980): Procedures and methodology of hemoperfusion as hepatic assist. In: *Hemoperfusion, Kidney, Liver Support and Detoxification*, Part I, edited by Sideman, S., and Chang, T. M. S., p. 265. Hemisphere Publishing, Washington, D.C.
17. Asanuma, Y., Malchesky, P. S., Smith, J. W., Zawicki, I., Carey, W. D., Ferguson, D. R., Hermann, R. E., and Nosé, Y.: Removal of protein bound toxins from critical care patients. *Clin. Toxicol.*, 17:571, 1980.
18. Nosé, Y., Malchesky, P. S., Asanuma, Y., and Zawicki, I.: Plasma filtration perfusion on hepatic patients: Its optimal operating conditions. In: *Therapeutic Plasma Exchange*, edited by Gurland, H. J., Heinze, V., and Lee, H. A. Springer-Verlag, Berlin, 1980, p. 125.
19. Asanuma, Y., Malchesky, P. S., Zawicki, I., Smith, J. W., Carey, W. D., Ferguson, D. R., Hermann, R. E., and Nosé, Y.: Clinical hepatic support by on-line plasma treatment with multiple sorbents. Evaluation of system performance. *Trans. Am. Soc. Artif. Intern. Organs*, 26:400, 1980.
20. Malchesky, P. S., Asanuma, Y., Hammerschmidt, D. E., and Nosé, Y.: Complement removal by sorbents in membrane plasmapheresis with on-line plasma treatment. *Trans. Am. Soc. Artif. Intern. Organs*, 26:541, 1980.
21. Nosé, Y., Malchesky, P. S., Koshino, I., Castino, F., and Scheucher, K.: Hepatic Assist II: Devices for use with sorbent and biological reactors. In: *Artificial Organs*, edited by Kenedi, R. M., Courtney, J. M., Gaylor, J. D. S., and Gilchrist, T. Macmillan Press, New York, 1976, p. 378.
22. Chang, T. M. S.: Blood compatible coating of synthetic immunoadsorbents. *Trans. Am. Soc. Artif. Intern. Organs*, 26:546, 1980.
23. Lupien, P. J., Moorjani, S., and Awad, J.: A new approach to the management of familial hypercholesterolemia: Removal of plasma cholesterol based on the principle of affinity chromatography. *Lancet*, I:1261, 1976.
24. Bensinger, W. I., Baker, D. A., Buckner, C. D., Clift, R. A., and Thomas, E. D.: Immunoadsorption for removal of A and B blood-group antibodies. *N. Engl. J. Med.*, 304:160, 1981.
25. Terman, D. S., Petty, D., and Harbeck, R.: Specific removal of DNA antibodies in vivo by extracorporeal circulation over DNA immobilized in collodion charcoal. *Clin. Immunol. Immunopathol.*, 8:90, 1977.
26. Bansal, S. C., Bansal, B. R., Thomas, H. L., Siegel, P. D., Rhoads, J. E., Cooper, D. R., Terman, D. S., and Mark, R.: Ex vivo removal of serum IgG in a patient with colon carcinoma: Some biochemical, immunological and histological observations. *Cancer*, 42:1, 1978.
27. Malchesky, P. S., Asanuma, Y., Zawicki, I., Blumenstein, M., Calabrese, L., Kyo, A., Krakauer, R., and Nosé, Y.: On-line separation of macromolecules by membrane filtration with cryogelation. In: *Plasma Exchange*, edited by H. G. Sieberth, p. 133. F. K. Shattauer-Verlag, Stuttgart, 1980.
28. Nosé, Y., Malchesky, P. S., and Asanuma, Y.: Augment solute reduction in diseases treated by extracorporeal detoxification system: X-effect hypothesis. In: *Artificial Liver Support*, edited by Burnner, G., and Schmidt, F. W. Springer-Verlag, Berlin, 1980, p. 181.

Plasmapheresis, edited by Y. Nosé, P. S.
Malchesky, J. W. Smith, and R. S. Krakauer.
Raven Press, New York © 1983.

Current Status in Europe

Hans J. Gurland

*Med. Klinik I, Nephrology Division, Klinikum Grosshadern, University of Munich,
D-8000 Munich 70, Federal Republic of Germany*

Although apheresis has increasingly been applied worldwide, and especially in Europe, reliable figures on modes of treatment, patient numbers, and outcome are lacking. Consequently, an overview of the current status in Europe must be based primarily on estimates, even though this type of analysis will inevitably result in a journalistic rather than a scientific report. Following is a review of data obtained from three main sources: (a) published articles on therapeutic plasma exchange, analyzed with emphasis on those containing case reports; (b) four firms, two that serve the market for apheresis by centrifugal techniques and two that distribute products for apheresis by membrane filtration, provided their market estimates for Europe, and in particular for the Federal Republic of Germany; and (c) Dr. Wing, chairman of the Registration Committee of the European Dialysis and Transplant Association, supplied preliminary 1981 data on the use of plasmapheresis for reversible renal failure in Europe.

Since this chapter is concerned with apheresis in Europe, Europe is contrasted with "other continents". The 800 publications that appeared between 1977 and 1981 are grouped according to the region of their origin, and are further divided into nonspecific publications (Fig. 1). Until 1979 Europe and the other continents remained on an almost equal level, then in 1980 and 1981 Europe gained considerably, probably as a consequence of the introduction of membrane plasma separation. The following figures and tables deal only with publications containing case reports; figures were obtained by analyzing and tallying case reports.

Regarding the areas of application, nephrology leads with 26% of the cases, followed by neurology with 21%, rheumatic and vascular diseases with 19%, and hematology with 13% (Fig. 2).

The first report on therapeutic plasma exchange was published in 1952, and the number of cases reported at the end of 1981 was 1,924 (Table 1). Worldwide, the majority of patients has been reported by the United States followed by the United Kingdom, France, and the Federal Republic of Germany.

Since membrane plasmapheresis was not employed until mid-1979, the 1,281 patients described worldwide in 1980 and 1981 are divided into those treated by centrifugal techniques and those treated by membrane plasma exchange (Table 2). At the time of this writing, this new method already represented 15% of the total

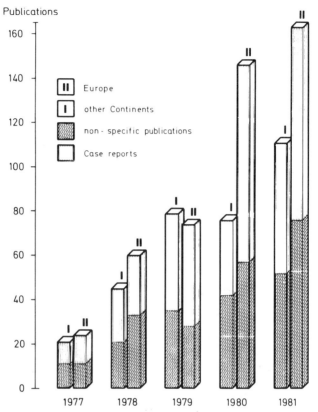

FIG. 1. Growth of literature dealing with therapeutic plasma exchange. Total publications 1977–1981, $N = 800$.

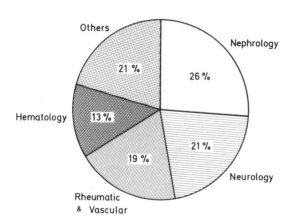

FIG. 2. Areas of application. Total cases reported in the literature, $N = 1,924$.

TABLE 1. *Case reports on therapeutic plasma exchange in the literature from 1952 to 1981 (1,924 cases)*

	Europe (N = 1,185)		Other continents (N = 739)		
	N	%		N	%
UK	403	34	USA	573	77
France	322	27	Japan	59	8
FRG	210	18	Australia	58	8
Italy	100	8	Canada	39	5
Other countries	150	13	Other countries	10	2

TABLE 2. *Case reports on therapeutic plasma exchange in the literature from 1980 to 1981 (1,281 cases)*

Treatment	N	%
Centrifugal techniques	1,093	85
Membrane plasma exchange	188	15

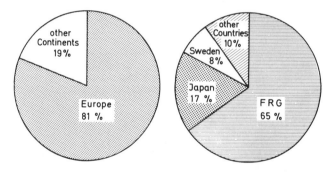

FIG. 3. Cases treated by membrane plasma exchange. Publications 1980/81; 188 cases.

treatments, which is even more impressive, considering that the case reports on patients treated in 1981 will not be published for a year or more.

As can be seen from Fig. 3, Europe accounts for 81% of the 188 cases of membrane plasma exchange. Looking at individual countries in which the membrane technique has become established, the Federal Republic of Germany leads with 65% of the cases, followed by Japan with 17%, and Sweden with 8%. All other countries make up only a small 10%.

After discussing data extracted from the literature, figures obtained from commercial sources will be examined. According to estimates, approximately 400 centrifugal separators are in use for therapeutic plasma exchange in Europe. The largest number is to be found in the Federal Republic of Germany, but Italy and France are well represented also. Calculation of the available centrifuges per million of the population reveals a relatively uniform distribution with about 1 centrifuge for 1–1.5 million people in most European countries (Table 3).

Table 4 only refers to the Federal Republic of Germany. It is of special interest because the largest number of membrane plasma exchanges are being performed in this country. According to the estimate of the firms, there were 95 centers practicing therapeutic plasma exchange in 1981, 79% of which are primarily performing membrane plasma exchange, while 21% employ the centrifugal technique. Out of the approximately 3,500 treatments performed in 1981, 70% were allotted to the membrane plasma exchange and 30% to the centrifuge.

Table 5 shows the preliminary results of a survey still in progress as of this writing. The question directed exclusively to renal units reads: "Did you use plasmapheresis in your center in 1981 for acute (reversible) renal failure due to the following conditions?" The findings for Europe agree closely with those for the Federal Republic alone. Rapidly progressive glomerulonephritis is being treated by 17% of the responding units, rejection of renal transplant by 5%, and other causes of renal failure by 14% in Europe and 19% in the Federal Republic of Germany.

TABLE 3. *Estimated number of centrifuges used for therapeutic plasma exchange in Europe (obtained from commercial sources) (N = 400)*

Country	%	Centrifuges (per mil. pop.)
FRG	28	1.8
Italy	22	1.5
France	19	1.4
UK	14	1.0
Benelux	6	0.9
Scandinavia	5	1.0
Others	6	0.1

TABLE 4. *Therapeutic plasma exchange in the FRG in 1981[a]*

Centers performing:	Centrifugal technique N = 20	Membrane plasma exchange N = 75
<10 Treatments/yr	7	27
≤50 Treatments/yr	4	29
>50 Treatments/yr	9	19
Total treatments	~1,000	~2,500

[a]Estimated number of centers and treatments performed (obtained from commercial sources).

TABLE 5. E.D.T.A. Dialysis and transplant registry[a]

Condition	Europe (N = 878 centers) response		FRG (N = 168 centers) response	
	N	%	N	%
Rapidly progressive glomerulonephritis	148	17	28	17
Rejection of renal transplant	47	5	8	5
Other causes of acute renal failure	127	14	32	19

[a] Question: Did you use plasmapheresis in your center in 1981 for acute (reversible) renal failure due to the folllowing conditions?

The various data discussed essentially confirm what we already knew: that therapeutic plasma exchange is performed more and more every year, and that membrane plasma exchange, especially in Europe, accounts for an important share. One has to admit, however, that many of the current indications are still controversial. Controlled studies are lacking and will be difficult to undertake for rare diseases.

The problem of insufficient information about treatment protocols and treatment results could be mitigated by a registry. Thus, I believe the time has come to set up a worldwide registry on apheresis, and there is not a more suitable and appropriate location for such a registry than the International Center for Artificial Organs and Transplantation in Cleveland.

ACKNOWLEDGMENTS

The author would like to acknowledge the cooperation of Bellco Medizintechnik GmbH, Freiburg i.Br., Diamed GmbH, Cologne, Fresenius MTS, St. Wendel, and Haemonetics GmbH, Munich, in supporting this paper with market estimates on the use of apheresis in Europe.

Plasmapheresis, edited by Y. Nosé, P. S. Malchesky, J. W. Smith, and R. S. Krakauer. Raven Press, New York © 1983.

Current Status in Japan

N. Inoue

Department of Internal Medicine, National Oji Hospital, Kita-ku, Tokyo, Japan

Plasma exchange is currently coming into use as a new therapeutic tool to treat or to modify various intractable diseases. Since the late 1970s, techniques to obtain large amounts of plasma by making use of the principle of ultrafiltration through macroporous membranes and continuous or intermittent flow centrifugation during extracorporeal circulation have been developed and widely used in Japan. It is estimated that about 20,000 therapeutic plasma exchange procedures were performed in Japan in 1981. In June of 1981, the Japanese Society for Therapeutic Plasmapheresis was formed and held its first symposium in Tokyo, the goal of which was to promote the effective spread and growth of therapeutic plasma exchange. The meeting was attended by 450 professionals from various disciplines, and views and experiences in this fast developing field were exchanged. The current status of therapeutic plasma exchange in Japan, with primary regard to the information obtained from this meeting, is described in this chapter.

HISTORICAL ASPECTS

Plasmapheresis was first introduced to Japan in 1962 by Murakami (1), who reviewed the introductory application of plasmapheresis in the United States. Since then, plasmapheresis has been carried out for the following purposes: (a) to obtain large quantities of plasma; (b) to obtain platelet-rich plasma or platelet concentrate; (c) to obtain leukocyte-rich plasma or leukocyte concentrates; and (d) to treat patients' disorders (therapeutic plasmapheresis).

Recent development of technology for efficient plasma separation has made plasma exchange procedures much easier for its application to patients' disorders. The historical highlights of plasmapheresis in Japan are shown in Table 1.

TECHNICAL ASPECTS

The technical aspects of on-line plasma exchange therapy can be divided into four main divisions: (a) plasma separation by means of centrifuge or membrane; (b) substitution of replacement fluid; (c) selective removal of unnecessary substances in plasma; and (d) blood access for extracorporeal circulation.

TABLE 1. *History of plasmapheresis in Japan*

1962	Introduction of plasmapheresis in USA by Dr. Murakami
1963	The need for research on plasmapheresis was recognized by the Japanese Ministry and Welfare
1970	Japanese Ministry and Welfare approved the practice of plasmapheresis to isolate a concentrated protein, antihemophilic factor from plasma of a single donor for whom the risk of hepatitis is minimum
1976	Therapeutic plasmapheresis utilizing the on-line blood cell processor (Celltrifuge or Haemonetics Model 30S)
1977	Development of a plasma separator with macroporous membrane
1980	International Symposium on plasma exchange in Cologne
1981	First meeting on therapeutic plasmapheresis in Tokyo

TABLE 2. *The current methods for plasmapheresis available in Japan*

Plasma separation	Apparatus	Manufacturer
Membrane (plasma separator)	Plasmaflo Hi-05	Asahi Medical
	Plasmax	Toray
	Plasma separator	Kuraray
	Plasmaflux	Fresenius
Centrifugal	Knigtmage	Green Cross
	Haemonetics Model 30, 50, and PEX	Haemonetics
	Celltrifuge	Fenwall
	CS 3000 Blood Cell Separator	Fenwall
	IBM 2997 Blood Cell Separator	IBM
Selective removal of macromolecules in plasma	Cryomax	Parker Hannifin
	Double filtration plasmapheresis	Kawasumi

Plasma Separation

The available methods for plasmapheresis in Japan are listed in Table 2. There are two methods for on-line plasmapheresis—centrifugal separation and ultrafiltration through macroporous membrane. The advantages and disadvantages of these methods are discussed below, and outlined in Table 3 (2).

On-line plasmapheresis by means of centrifugal separation of plasma from whole blood is performed with blood processors such as Haemonetics (Model 30s, 50 and PEX), Celltrifuge, CS 3000 blood cell separator, and IBM 2997. It is estimated that about 150 of these automated blood cell separation systems were distributed throughout Japan by late 1981. Since all of these apparatuses are expensive and large, this method of plasmapheresis is only available in university hospitals or in other large hospitals. It was initially used by groups of hematologists engaged in cytopheresis and blood component transfusion. The major difficulties with this method for clinical application are loss of platelets as well as the excessive time required for the procedures.

TABLE 3. *Advantages and disadvantages of centrifugal and membrane separation*

Factors	Centrifugal	Membrane
Separation characteristics	Large and small molecular proteins are equally removed	Small molecular proteins are more effectively removed
Platelet	Considerable loss	Minimal loss
Hemolysis	Rare	Observed depending on condition
Apparatus	Expensive, available to component transfusion	Applicable to dialysis machine, not available to component transfusion
Disposables	Relatively inexpensive	Expensive
Blood access	Not necessary	Necessary depending on patient condition

From Ota, ref. 2, with permission.

TABLE 4. *Specifications of plasma separators available for clinical application*

	Plasmaflo Hi-05	Plasmax	Plasmacure	Plasmaflux PS-500
Membrane	CA	PMMA	PVA	PP
Surface area (m²)	0.5	0.5	0.6	0.5
Max. pore size (μm)	0.2	0.5	0.4	0.5
Wall thickness (μm)	60	85	200	140
Inner diameter (μm)	330	370	400	330
Sterilizing method	EOG	γ-Ray	Autoclave	EOG
Manufacturer	Asahi Medical	Toray	Kuraray	Fresenius

CA, cellulose diacetate; PMMA, polymethylmethacrylate; PVA, polyvinyl alcohol; PP, polypropylene.

Membrane plasma separation is performed with ultrafiltration through a plasma filter having the capacity to generate high flow rates of platelet-free plasma. In Japan, for patients with intractable ascites, a cellulose acetate hollow fiber filter has been utilized as a filter of ascites in the ascites reinfusion system (3). However, this device could not be utilized for plasmapheresis due to its low sieving coefficients for protein fractions.

The collaboration of researchers at the University of Tokyo and the Asahi Medical Company has been instrumental in developing a high performance membrane plasma filter (4). Various plasma separators with high performance have been developed by other Japanese industries such as Toray (Plasmax), Kuraray (Plasmacure), Mitsubishi Rayon (MPS), Teijin (TP50), Terumo (disc type), and others. The specifications of available plasma separators for clinical application are listed in Table 4.

These devices have been used mainly by doctors in dialysis centers who are skilled in extracorporeal circulation. Since each plasma separator differs in material and in pore size of the membrane, the optimal operating conditions for the efficient plasma separation differ accordingly. Transmembrane pressure, shear rate, rate of plasma removal, and hematological conditions are particularly important. In comparison to conventional hemodialysis, the lowest operable transmembrane pressures are preferable for the passage of large molecular weight plasma solutes (5).

Substitution of Replacement Fluid

Four kinds of replacement fluid have been used in Japan: fresh frozen plasma (FFP), plasma protein fraction (PPF), electrolyte solution, and plasma expanders such as low molecular dextran and hydroxyethyl starch (HES). Although FFP and PPF are most frequently used, the high cost and shortage of these fluids present major obstacles in plasma exchange therapy. It is estimated that about 1–2% of plasma preparations have been used for plasma exchange therapy during 1979–1980. However, the recent increase of plasma exchange procedures will disturb the supply balance of plasma preparations in the near future. The risk of infection with hepatitis virus is also a serious problem. According to the recent reports in Tokyo, the incidences of hepatitis following administration of FFP were 5–16%.

Supplementation of essential or missing factors is of prime importance in the management of patients treated with repeated plasma exchange. The development of low cost replacement fluids should be considered.

Selective Removal of Unwanted Macromolecules

In order to avoid the side effects as well as the economical problems associated with the replacement fluid, there is a great need for techniques of the selective removal of unwanted macromolecules in plasma. A double filtration plasmapheresis utilizing a second filter for unwanted macromolecules, which is capable of separating albumin from gamma globulins efficiently, has been developed (6), and work is now in progress on the development of the second filter with high performance for this purpose. Suzuki and colleagues are treating patients with rheumatoid arthritis by the continuous cryofiltration method, which was developed by Malchesky and Nosé in Cleveland, Ohio, and their successful results are presented elsewhere in this volume.

Blood Access for Extracorporeal Circulation

Blood access for extracorporeal circulation must be secured in order to perform the efficient plasma exchange procedure with either the membrane or centrifugal method. A blood flow rate of 40–60 ml/min is necessary for efficient plasmapheresis. Percutaneous venous access, either femoral or subclavian, is commonly used for temporary access. Arteriovenous shunts, arteriovenous fistula, and exteriorization of blood vessels are used for long-term access.

CLINICAL ASPECTS

In Japan, plasma exchange has been used as a new therapeutic tool to deal with diseases and morbidities where humoral factors play an important role in the life-threatening or acute fulminating stage.

Since the beneficial effects of plasma exchange on several immunologically mediated diseases were proven, more than 20 diseases treated by plasma exchange have been reported in Japan in 1981, and this number is increasing.

At present, we are analyzing the accumulated data in order to establish proper therapeutic protocols. The need for more rigid standards applicable to this procedure is obvious.

The indications for plasma exchange therapy are listed in Table 5. The cases indicated for plasma exchange are divided into four groups as follows: (a) intoxi-

TABLE 5. *Indications for plasma exchange*

Intoxication
    Drugs (digitoxin, L-thyroxin)
    Poisons (paraquat, methylparathion,
     mushroom)
    Aluminum and dialysis dementia
Metabolic and hormonal disorders
    Thyrotoxic crisis
    Malignant exophthalmus
    Familial hypercholestrolemia
    Primary biliary cirrhosis
    Hyperbilirubinemia
    Acute hepatic failure
Immunologically mediated disease
    Antibody mediated disease
      Goodpasture's syndrome
      Myasthenia gravis
      Idiopathic thrombocytopenic purpura
      Autoimmune hemolytic anemia
      Anti-factor VIII antibody
      Guillain–Barré's syndrome
      Transplant rejection
      Pemphigus vulgaris
    Immune complex mediated disease
      Systemic lupus erythematosus
      Polyarteritis nodosa
      Cutaneous vasculitis
      Rheumatoid arthritis
      Rapidly progressive glomerulonephritis
      Dermatomyositis
Miscellaneous
    Psoriasis
    Paraproteinemia
    Malignant tumor
    Multiple sclerosis
    Wegener's granulomatosis
    Raynaud's phenomenon

cation with poisons and drugs refractory to the conventional methods of blood purification; (b) metabolic and hormonal disorders; (c) immunologically mediated diseases; and (d) miscellaneous patients including hyperviscosity syndrome.

Intoxication

Plasma exchange therapy is considered to be effective for the removal of poisons and drugs that are protein bound. Successful treatments of patients with overdoses of digitoxin and L-thyroxin were reported.

It is postulated that the delayed development of progressive pulmonary fibrosis, which is the usual cause of death, following intoxication of parathion, might be prevented with plasma exchange when compared with charcoal hemoperfusion. This appears to be one of the beneficial effects of plasma exchange on immunological reactions that occur in the lung.

Metabolic and Hormonal Disorders

The efficient correction of various metabolic disturbances that do not respond to the conventional therapy can be carried out by plasma exchange.

Liver Disease

Plasma exchange with membrane plasmapheresis was first applied by our group in Tokyo to patients with fulminant hepatic failure. Plasma exchange is advantageous in that it cannot only remove protein bound toxins but can also supplement substances that are deficient due to hepatic failure. In comparison to the results obtained by charcoal hemoperfusion, the occurrences of bleeding were obviously decreased and the survival time prolonged, although the survival rate showed no remarkable improvement. The plasma level of substances with large pool sizes in the body such as bilirubin or amino acids could not be normalized in the nonsurviving cases by the application of daily 5-liter plasma exchanges, although most of clinical parameters for hepatic synthetic function could be maintained at a certain level.

These results indicate that the correction of metabolic disturbances was insufficient for nonsurviving cases. However, at present, plasma exchange is considered to be the most promising method for short-time substitution of hepatic function for patients with acute hepatic failure.

Cirrhotic patients with acute decompensation, who did not respond to conventional therapy, were also treated with plasma exchange, and satisfactory results were obtained.

Yoshiba and co-workers have reported the effective use of plasma exchange for acute hepatic failure. Details of this work are presented elsewhere in this volume.

Hyperlipidemia

Successful treatment with plasma exchange in patients with homozygous familiar hypercholesterolemia has been reported (7). According to their results, with 2-liter plasma exchanges at 2- or 3-week intervals, serum cholesterol and high-density lipoprotein cholesterol were controlled at certain levels, xanthoma disappeared, and anginal attacks were reduced.

Hyperlipidemia in primary biliary cirrhosis was treated by plasma exchange with satisfactory results.

Other Metabolic Disturbances

Thyrotoxic crisis, malignant exophthalmus, and intractable pruritis in cholestasis are considered to be indicated for plasma exchange therapy.

Immunologically Mediated Disease

Plasma exchange is regarded as an immunotherapy to control an acute phase of various immunologically mediated diseases by removal of circulating pathologically related macromolecules such as antigen, antibody, immune complex, and other serum factors causing tissue damage. Many clinicians and researchers in various fields employed this new therapeutic tool in the treatment of patients with immunologically mediated diseases and morbidities uncontrolled by conventional therapy.

Among immunologically mediated disease are rheumatoid arthritis, myasthenia gravis, systemic lupus erythematosus, idiopathic thrombocytopenic purpura, antifactor VIII antibody diseases, rhesus disease, renal allograft rejection, multiple sclerosis, and pemphigus vulgaris. In comparison with high incidences of Goodpasture's syndrome and rapidly progressive glomerulonephritis in Europe, there were very few reports of the treatment of these diseases in Japan.

Plasma exchange in immunologically mediated diseases has been performed according to the following criteria: (a) active and progressive stage; (b) high serum level of immunological parameters such as antibody, immune complex, cryoglobulin, and others; and (c) no definitive improvement following various conventional therapy including steroid and immunosuppressants.

On the basis of their results on plasma exchange in 61 patients with rheumatic disorders and other immunologically mediated diseases, Shiozawa et al. (8) postulated that plasma exchange therapy is effective for the normalization not only of humoral immunity but also of cellular immunity.

Since the beneficial effects of plasma exchange are only temporary in the majority of patients with immunologic disorders, intermittent plasma exchange in combination with drug therapy is required for the management of patients. Long-term treatment by intermittent plasma exchange for rheumatoid arthritis, systemic lupus erythematosus, and myasthenia gravis has been reported with successful results. However, the development of a technology for the selective removal of pathologically related macromolecules appears to be a prerequisite for the chronic application of plasma exchange. In order to achieve this purpose, continuous cryofiltration, double filtration plasmapheresis, and plasma perfusion over newly developed immunoadsorbents are being studied in clinical trials.

The optimal frequency and volume of plasma processed in plasma exchange in different diseases is still being debated. Randomized clinical trials with control of the appropriate parameters will offer a more precise evaluation of the effectiveness of this therapy.

Miscellaneous Diseases

The remarkable effects of plasma exchange on hyperviscosity syndrome in various diseases such as paraproteinemia, rheumatoid arthritis, and systemic lupus erythematosus have been reported.

There are several groups who have been actively engaged in plasma exchange therapy for patients with advanced cancer. They observed a partial reduction in tumor mass as well as improvements in immunological parameters for cellular immunity, although the exact nature of the humoral factors in these patients remains uncertain.

Side Effects

Side effects of plasma exchange can be divided into four groups: (a) infection (hepatitis); (b) circulatory disturbances during extracorporeal circulation; (c) bleeding (depletion of coagulation factors, anticoagulant); and (d) allergic reactions (rash, urticaria, fever, chills, shivering). Although no fatal side effects have been reported, it should be emphasized that the main cause of adverse effects is closely related to the replacement fluids used.

CONCLUSION

Plasma exchange is a new therapeutic tool to control patients with immunologic and metabolic disorders at an acute or life-threatening stage, when conventional therapies prove unsuccessful. It is of importance for chronic application to develop technologies for the selective removal of unwanted macromolecules. Since results of the therapy have been promising, plasma exchange therapy can be of great assistance if properly understood and utilized.

REFERENCES

1. Murakami, S., and Tokunaga, E. (1967): *Practice of Blood Transfusion*. Chugai Igaku, Tokyo, p. 31.
2. Ota, K. (1981): Present status and future prospect of plasmapheresis. In: *Therapeutic Plasmapheresis (I)*, edited by T. Oda, p. 15. Schattauer Verlag, Stuttgart, New York.
3. Inoue, N., Yamazaki, Z., Oda, T., Sugiura, M., Wada, T., Fujisaki, Y., and Hayano, F. (1979): Treatment of intractable ascites by continuous reinfusion of the sterilized, cell-free and concentrated ascitic fluid. *Trans. Am. Soc. Artif. Intern. Organs*, 23:698.
4. Yamazaki, Z., Fujimori, Y., Sanjo, K., Sugiura, M., Wada, T., Inoue, N., Kominami, T., Fujisaki, Y., and Hayano, F. (1977): New artificial liver support for hepatic coma. *Trans. Am. Soc. Artif. Intern. Organs*, 6:99.
5. Nosé, Y., and Malchesky, P. S. (1981): Therapeutic membrane plasmapheresis. In: *Therapeutic Plasmapheresis (I)*, edited by T. Oda, p. 3. Schattauer Verlag, Stuttgart, New York.
6. Agishi, T., Kaneko, I., Hasuo, Y., Hayasaka, Y., Sanaka, T., Ota, K., Amemiya, H., Sugino,

N., Abe, M., Ono, T., Kawai, S., and Yamane, T. (1980): Double filtration plasmapheresis. *Trans. Am. Soc. Artif. Intern. Organs*, 26:406.

7. Kikkawa, T., Kishino, B., Fushimi, H., Nishikawa, M., and Yamamoto, A. (1981): Plasma exchange therapy for homozygous familial hypercholestrolemia. In: *Therapeutic Plasmapheresis (I)*, edited by T. Oda, p. 127. Schattauer Verlag, Stuttgart, New York.

8. Shiozawa, K., Yamagata, J., Shiokawa, Y., Yuasa, S., and Hashimoto, H. (1981): Plasma exchange for rheumatoid arthritis. In: *Therapeutic Plasmapheresis (I)*, edited by T. Oda, p. 165. Schattauer Verlag, Stuttgart, New York.

Plasmapheresis, edited by Y. Nosé, P. S.
Malchesky, J. W. Smith, and R. S. Krakauer.
Raven Press, New York © 1983.

Current Status in North America

Alvaro A. Pineda

Mayo Clinic Blood Bank, Rochester, Minnesota 55905

The utilization of plasma exchange and cytapheresis as techniques to treat or modify disease has increased tremendously since the advent of continuous and intermittent blood flow centrifugation technology. These centrifugation systems, generically known as blood cell separators, or simply cell separators, were originally developed to collect large quantities of platelets or granulocytes from single donors. The separators have been utilized to remove selectively from patients' blood component excesses that characterize a number of disease states, thus finding a direct therapeutic application (1). The removal of cellular fractions (cytapheresis) is highly selective compared with the removal of plasma components which requires sacrificing plasma as a whole with all its components. Unlike cytapheresis, in the North American continent, plasma exchange has rapidly evolved as an accepted or experimental method of treatment for a wide variety of disorders. A perusal of the English literature reveals reports of the use of plasma exchange to treat 52 different diseases or syndromes, encompassing dermatologic, endocrine, neurologic, rheumatologic, gastroenterologic, cardiovascular, nephrologic, hematologic, and other, unclassified disorders.

Historically, the introduction of new and expensive technology into clinical research and practice, particularly if the disease is dangerous and the technique appealing, has created advocates and adversaries. It has not been any different with plasma exchange, a technique that permits large volumes of plasma to be quickly removed with minimal morbidity and almost no mortality. In 1978, it was estimated that approximately 20,000 therapeutic apheresis (TA) procedures were performed in the United States (2). There is every indication that the number of TA procedures has registered a marked annual increase since 1978. For instance, since 1978, the Mayo Clinic Apheresis Laboratory has experienced an increase in TA procedures of 146, 52, and 23% for the years 1979, 1980, and 1981, respectively. Because TA is an expensive treatment and carries with it a number of inherent risks, efforts to control its use and to evaluate its benefits have surfaced.

Efforts to regulate the use of TA are particularly directed at plasma exchange, which is the most expensive of the apheresis modalities and represents the bulk of apheresis activity. Controlling efforts largely inspired by financial concerns emanate mostly from nonmedical quarters (external pressures). In addition, controlling pressures are also being exercised by the medical community at large (internal pressures).

The latter are mainly motivated by a desire to establish the therapeutic role of apheresis on a sound scientific basis. Unquestionably, there is a need, because of scientific and financial concerns, to develop guidelines for the rational use of TA. Not to be forgotten, however, is the role played by the largely anecdotal reports of TA. Criticized by many, they may in fact be the germinal seed that grows under scientific guidance, as has occurred with other therapeutic modes in the past.

EXTERNAL PRESSURES

TA was initially an exciting research tool whose potential therapeutic applications tempted the clinician prematurely. A labor intensive procedure, expensive, minimally invasive, and with low attending morbidity and mortality, did not escape scrutiny for long. As the procedure gained popularity and started to be used in diseases that afflict relatively large segments of the population, it raised concerns in the private and public health insurance sectors. Typically, health insurance contracts with third party payers and government supported programs (Medicare, Medicaid) include a clause that excludes reimbursement for medical treatments that are considered experimental. The intent of the clause is to preclude the widespread utilization of therapeutic modalities which may not prove to be beneficial to patients, but which may increase the cost of providing health insurance. TA was deemed to be an experimental procedure by some health insurance companies in the United States.

No reimbursement for TA has become standard practice in some states where the treatment is considered experimental in nature. This is particularly so in the case of rheumatoid arthritis, multiple sclerosis, and lupus erythematosus. This practice is defensible since at the present time adequate controlled trials are lacking or are equivocal regarding the benefits of TA in those disorders. Since the number of patients with those diseases is large, the potential costs are astronomic and surely would necessitate increased rates. It is very doubtful that third party payers could bear the cost of a widespread and indiscriminate use of TA in those diseases. Unless well-documented evidence of the benefit of TA is forthcoming, the state of affairs is not likely to change.

The US government through the National Center for Health Technology (NCHT) has begun assessing Medicare coverage of TA. In June of 1980, NCHT announced the beginning of a scientific evaluation of the clinical safety and effectiveness of plasma exchange for the treatment of rheumatoid arthritis (3). Based on that evaluation, NCHT was to make a recommendation to assist the Health Care Financing Administration (HCFA) in establishing Medicare coverage. In June of 1981, the same office announced that it was conducting an evaluation of safety and clinical effectiveness of apheresis for the treatment of Goodpasture's syndrome, systemic lupus erythematosus, membranous and proliferative glomerulonephritis, multiple sclerosis, potentially life-threatening complications of rheumatic diseases (rheumatoid arthritis, systemic lupus erythematosus, polymyositis/dermatomyositis, and progressive systemic sclerosis), and thrombotic thrombocytopenic purpura (4). More recently, HCFA has asked the Public Health Service to conduct an assessment of the treatment of pruritus of cholestatic liver disease by plasma perfusion of a charcoal filter and to make a recommendation concerning its coverage by Medicare. In Canada, in December of 1980, the Canadian National Plasma Exchange Study Group met for the first time with the purpose of establishing prospective clinical trials and to provide a forum for exchange of information (5). This group is supported by the Department of Health and Welfare of the Canadian government.

INTERNAL PRESSURES

TA was originally regarded as an esoteric technique typically available only in major research or in tertiary care centers. Currently, it is regarded by many physicians as an essential part of initial care in diseases such as Goodpasture's syndrome, hyperviscosity syndrome, myasthenia gravis, and thrombotic thrombocytopenic purpura. TA is available through most regional blood centers, tertiary care centers, and major general hospitals in the USA and Canada. Although in widespread use, a scientific assessment of the therapeutic effect of TA has lagged behind the dramatic increased use of the procedure. The scientific merits of TA, particularly of an intermediate technology such as plasma exchange, are being examined by a number of medical societies including the World Health Organization (WHO), American Association of Blood Banks (AABB), American Medical Association (AMA), American Red Cross (ARC), and physician subspecialty groups. Additionally, individuals working in the field of apheresis have organized two groups, the American Society for Apheresis and the Society of Hemopheresis Specialists, partially to stimulate scientific assessment of TA.

WHO has sponsored conferences to evaluate the merits of plasma exchange. AABB has had a standing committee on pheresis since 1978 and the inspection report form used in its Inspection and Accreditation Program includes 10 questions pertaining to protocols, records of procedures, informed consent forms, and care of reactions. The standards of AABB for blood banks and transfusion service centers establish minimum performance guidelines pertaining to therapeutic plasmapheresis and cytapheresis to be followed by member blood banks (6). The AMA has recently formed an Apheresis Committee charged with evaluating scientific merit of TA. ARC is planning to form a TA committee in the near future. Among the subspecialty groups, the American Rheumatism Association has formed an Apheresis Committee to begin functions in July 1982, and the Arthritis Foundation (AF) has issued an apheresis statement.

The AF's statement considers TA "experimental" in the treatment of rheumatic disease and to be used in a planned, well-designed study with protocols approved by peer groups. TA is not to be considered for patients in whom conventional therapy is effective or not tried; however, it leaves the door open for the use of TA in life-threatening complications of rheumatoid arthritis such as vasculitis with or without cryoglobulinemia or hyperviscosity syndrome. Likewise, life-threatening complications of systemic lupus erythematosus and polymyositis in selected patients who fail conventional therapy may be treated with TA. The AF suggests that agencies responsible for third party payment of bills may consider paying for apheresis carried out as part of an experimental study (7). A new society, the American Society for Apheresis (ASFA), officially inaugurated in October 1981, has as one of its purposes for corporation the promotion of controlled studies in apheresis and the acquisition of information concerning the cost–benefit ratio of apheresis and its various applications. Additionally, ASFA intends to serve as a resource to assist accreditation and regulatory agencies in the formulation of standards and regulations in the field of apheresis.

CURRENT UTILIZATION OF THERAPEUTIC APHERESIS

The high cost of TA coupled with a paucity of controlled studies that assess therapeutic effectiveness of TA, have forced centers practicing this form of treatment to develop guidelines for its rational use. This task has not been easy, particularly due to the lack of sufficient data on which to base guidelines. Such guidelines are bound to vary from institution to institution. For instance, the Mayo Clinic Apheresis Laboratory, in operation since 1973, currently recognizes several clinical indications for TA. Therapeutic plasma exchange is used in the conditions indicated in Table 1. Therapeutic cytapheresis is utilized to treat the conditions listed in Table 2.

In the absence of a national registry of TA in the USA, it becomes extremely difficult to determine volumes of TA performed and diseases treated. In 1980, 263 institutional members of AABB performed 18,448 TA procedures. Three types of institutions comprise the total of reporting facilities. Hospital-based blood banks and transfusion services performed 10,930 or 59% of the total, whereas the remaining 41% was performed by blood banks that are mainly collecting facilities or blood banks that depend on collecting facilities for their entire blood supply. These

TABLE 1. *Clinical applications of plasma exchange*

Hyperviscosity syndrome
TTP
Life-threatening complications of ITP, cryoglobulinemia, and idio-pathic factor VIII inhibitor
Myasthenia gravis; acute, nonresponsive to coventional therapy
Refsum's disease
Goodpasture's syndrome
Life-threatening complications of rheumatoid arthritis, systemic lupus erythematosus, scleroderma, polymyositis, and dermato-myositis
Familial homozygous hypercholesterolemia

TABLE 2. *Clinical applications of cytapheresis*

Blastapheresis:	Blast crisis of nonlymphocytic leukemia ($>$100,000/mm^3 blasts)
Plateletapheresis:	Thrombocytosis ($>$1,000,000/mm^3 platelet count in symptomatic patients)

data from AABB do not include the great majority of ARC centers and some large tertiary care facilities known to perform a large volume of TA. ARC centers treated 2,601 patients from July 1980 to July 1981 with TA. In 1981, 3,296 TA procedures were performed in Canada.

CONTROLLED TRIALS

Since the initiation of TA, there has been a clamor for controlled trials. Since pilot studies have begun yielding meaningful information pertaining to the volume of plasma exchange, hemostasis alterations, the frequency of therapy, and other parameters that should be followed, the tendency has been to apply the scientific method to TA. Controlled trials on rheumatoid arthritis, myasthenia gravis, scleroderma, and renal allograft rejection have been completed. A number of trials are still in progress, including some studies being completed on plasma exchange in rheumatoid arthritis (Ontario, Canada) and lymphaplasmapheresis in the same disease (Los Angeles, CA). Two controlled trials of plasma exchange on Rh hemolytic disease and thrombotic thrombocytopenic purpura are commencing in Canada. Also commenced is a multicenter, randomized, controlled trial of plasma exchange in the management of severe lupus nephritis in the US. A single-center trial on lupus nephritis is under way in Canada.

In the US, the treatment of Guillain–Barré syndrome by plasma exchange is being studied in a controlled, multicenter fashion. Multiple sclerosis will be the subject of a randomized controlled trial of TA, to be started by multiple centers. The last two studies use a protocol that incorporates carefully matched cohorts of patients randomly assigned to groups to be treated with TA or with conventional therapy. The Mayo Clinic Apheresis Laboratory is carrying out two controlled trials that involve as a control a group of patients who are treated with "sham apheresis," either plasma exchange or lymphapheresis. The studies are double-blinded and hope to assess the therapeutic effects of plasma exchange on Guillain–Barré syndrome and of lymphapheresis on rheumatoid arthritis, as well as to determine the placebo effect of TA. The placebo effect has recently been demonstrated in a controlled study of plasma exchange on scleroderma (8). We are also studying the effect of plasma exchange on acute renal failure secondary to multiple myeloma in a randomized study that does not involve "sham apheresis." The National Institutes of Health have controlled trials of TA on schizophrenia, lupus nephritis, and multiple sclerosis.

NEW TECHNIQUES

Methodology for the removal of selected plasma constituents is being investigated in North America. The selective removal of plasma components whose presence is associated with a disease process can now be accomplished by physical or chemical means with either on-line or off-line systems. Studies on the plasma perfusion over affinity columns for the removal of bile acids, low-density lipoproteins, IgG and immune complexes, DNA antibodies, and A and B isoagglutinins have been published (9). Systems based on extracorporeal perfusion of plasma over sorbents embedded in membrane filtration systems have been used in the treatment of human and canine malignancies. There is also a system for on-line separation of macromolecules by membrane filtration and cryoprecipitation. These systems, still in the experimental phase, promise to provide some alternatives to plasma exchange.

As more selective techniques for the removal of plasma constituents or cells from whole blood become available, we will have made significant progress toward the goal of removing an undesirable component of blood and returning the remainder to the patient. This approach is likely to become more widely used, if in fact it proves to be less expensive, more efficient, and safe. In the meantime, TA needs to be assessed critically by those requesting it as well as by those performing it. It is incumbent on those of us performing TA to provide proof of its efficacy via randomized trials. TA has ushered in a novel and exciting era of medicine. Let us hope that the interaction of internal and external forces will help in defining the proper niche of TA in modern medicine.

REFERENCES

1. Pineda, A. A., Brzica, S. M., and Taswell, H. F. (1977): Continuous and semicontinuous flow blood centrifugation systems. Therapeutic applications with plasma-, platelet-, lympha-, and eosinapheresis. *Transfusion*, 17:407.
2. Taft, E. G. (1979): Plasma exchange transfusion: The concept of dose. *Proc. First Annual Apheresis Symp.*, American Red Cross Blood Services, Mid-America Region, p. 25.
3. National Center for Health Care Technology (1980): Scientific evaluation of medical technology. *Federal Register*, 45:41,222.
4. National Center for Health Care Technology (1981): Evaluation of medical technology. *Federal Register*, 46:31770.
5. Rock, G. (1981): A forum for information. Plasma therapy. *Plasma Therapy Trans. Tech.*, 2:51.
6. American Association of Blood Banks (1981): Standards for blood banks and transfusion services, 10th edition.
7. McDuffie, F. C. (1981): Recommendations of the Arthritis Foundation and the American Association on Plasmapheresis in Rheumatic Diseases. Atlanta, Georgia.
8. McCune, M. A., Pineda, A. A., Winkelmann, R. K., and Osmundson, P. J. (1980): Controlled study of the therapeutic effect of plasma exchange on scleroderma. *Transfusion*, 20:649.
9. Pineda, A. A., and Taswell, H. F. (1981): Selective plasma component removal: Alternatives to plasma exchange. *Artif. Organs*, 5:234.

Plasmapheresis, edited by Y. Nosé, P. S. Malchesky, J. W. Smith, and R. S. Krakauer. Raven Press, New York © 1983.

Medicare Coverage of Therapeutic Apheresis

Stephen P. Heyse

Office of Program Planning and Evaluation, National Institute of Arthritis, Diabetes, and Digestive and Kidney Diseases, National Institutes of Health, Bethesda, Maryland 20205

The policy of third party payers covering therapeutic apheresis varies from payer to payer, from disease to disease, and from locale to locale. I will not attempt in this chapter to review the current status of coverage of therapeutic apheresis because, for the most part, I do not know what it is. Instead I will review the process used by the Public Health Service (PHS) in developing its recommendations to the Health Care Financing Administration (HCFA) regarding Medicare coverage, and present the issue of therapeutic apheresis as an example of how the process works.

Since the enactment of Title XVIII of the Social Security Act which authorized the Medicare program, the administrators of that program have turned to the PHS for advice when there were questions of the reasonableness and/or necessity of various medical procedures or treatments. Over the years, various components of the PHS have been responsible for developing the PHS recommendations. Most recently, this function had been performed by the National Center for Health Care Technology (NCHCT). When NCHCT ceased to exist in 1981, the Office of Health Research, Statistics, and Technology (OHRST) assumed the function.

When NCHCT took on the function, there was a backlog of nearly 60 issues which were awaiting review and assessments. In order to deal with this backlog and incoming new issues (which arose at a rate of approximately 4 to 5 per month), NCHCT developed and implemented an assessment process which has been praised by most who have had contact with it. The process is based on an overriding desire to be fair and open so that all interested parties could contribute information and advice. Toward this end, assistance with these assessments is requested from the public through announcements published in the *Federal Register* and in the publications of the appropriate medical specialty societies and other groups which might have an interest in the technology under assessment. The American Medical Association, the American College of Physicians, and the Council of Medical Specialty Societies are always notified. By and large, the responses to these requests have been timely and thorough, reflecting an awareness of the importance of these assessments. Almost invariably, expressions of thanks for having been asked to participate are given.

Other sources of information and advice are used, too. These include the agencies of the PHS (National Institutes of Health; Food and Drug Administration; Centers for Disease Control; Alcohol, Drug Abuse, and Mental Health Administration; Health Services Administration; and Health Resources Administration), other Federal departments, and the Veterans Administration.

When all the responses have been received and a review of the medical literature completed, the information is synthesized into a draft assessment which is reviewed by the appropriate PHS agencies (typically NIH and FDA). After the final corrections are made, a recommendation regarding coverage by the Medicare program is made based on the assessment. These recommendations can be for coverage without restrictions, coverage with certain restrictions, or noncoverage.

Section 1862(a) of the Medicare law excludes from payment items and services that are "not reasonable and necessary" for diagnosis or treatment. This section has never had regulations or guidelines promulgated for it. Traditionally, "reasonable and necessary" have been equated with "safe and effective" and with general acceptance by the medical profession. The National Council on Health Care Technology developed some guidelines for determining reimbursement of medical technologies. These guidelines were used by NCHCT and later by OHRST in developing the PHS recommendations to HCFA. The guidelines describe different levels of evidence of safety and effectiveness and indicate the level of evidence necessary for different circumstances. For example, if a procedure is considered controversial, a higher level of evidence would be necessary than if it were not controversial.

New medical technologies are usually considered experimental until their safety and effectiveness have been demonstrated, and as such are usually not covered by Medicare. The transition of a technology from the experimental category into something considered generally accepted and nonexperimental is not usually clear-cut. This is an area where the opinions of the appropriate specialty societies have been very helpful. The assessments are never considered final and, if new information becomes available which warrants a reassessment, the issue can be reexamined.

The issue of apheresis was brought to the attention of NCHCT approximately 2 years ago when HCFA requested advice about coverage for its use in treating a lengthy list of diseases. At the same time, they requested that NCHCT assess plasmapheresis for rheumatoid arthritis and review Medicare's policy of covering plasma exchange for myasthenia gravis, plasmapheresis for hyperviscosity syndromes and macroglobulinemia associated with diseases such as Waldenstrom's macroglobulinemia and multiple myeloma, and leukocytapheresis for severe leukocytosis in leukemia. PHS advised HCFA that coverage of those indications already covered appeared appropriate, and recommended that coverage be continued. The assessment of plasmapheresis (later expanded to include other forms of apheresis) for rheumatoid arthritis was initiated by requesting advice and information from NIH and FDA, the American Rheumatism Association, the American Medical Association, and by publishing an announcement in the *Federal Register*. Based on all their advice and a review of the medical literature, it was concluded, as of May 1981, that apheresis was an experimental therapy for rheumatoid arthritis, with the possible exception of treatment for life-threatening complications such as rheumatoid vasculitis, hyperviscosity states, and severe cryoglobulinemia. It was recommended that Medicare not cover apheresis for rheumatoid arthritis unless these severe, life-threatening complications were present and unresponsive to more conventional therapies. HCFA indicated that a more thorough review of apheresis for the life-threatening complications of rheumatoid arthritis was necessary and requested that the issue be reassessed. In the meantime, the original list of additional indications had been refined to include apheresis for systemic lupus erythematosus, Goodpasture's syndrome, membranous and proliferative glomerulonephritis, thrombotic thrombocytopenic purpura, and multiple sclerosis. These indications were chosen because it was felt that there might be sufficient information available regarding the application of apheresis in their treatment to permit an assessment. The assessments for these indications are still in process. Some are in draft and others are yet to be drafted.

NCHCT ceased to function last Fall because no funds were appropriated for it in the current Federal budget. The functions of NCHCT were redistributed to other agencies of the PHS. The coverage function was shifted to OHRST where it currently resides. However, OHRST is an office which is expected to be abolished at the end of the current fiscal year (September 30, 1982). Where the coverage function will be transferred is not clear. Some have suggested that NIH should handle these issues; however, NIH would strongly resist such a move because it would not be an appropriate function for it to assume. Another possibility would be to have HCFA perform the function itself. Concern over the obvious conflict of interest makes such a move unlikely. The Office of the Assistant Secretary for Health is a logical placement of this function since it requires coordination of different agencies of the PHS. Or perhaps the private sector will be called on to perform these assessments. Organizations such as the American Medical Association, the American College of Physicians, and the Council of Medical Specialty Societies may be able to assume this function. There has also been discussion of establishing an institute outside the Federal government to deal with these issues and other issues related to health care technology assessment. Interest for such an institute has come from third party payers of medical insurance who need a source of advice about the rapidly developing medical technologies. The health insurers have, of course, not been bound by the PHS assessments, but many have relied upon NCHCT and OHRST for this advice in the past.

Where does all this leave the issue of therapeutic apheresis for the indications under review and others that will need assessment or reassessment? Presently, OHRST has two professionals assigned to the coverage function. They do not have any support staff assigned to them. This lack of resources has slowed progress in these and other assessments. Hopefully the assessments already in progress can be completed before OHRST ceases to exist.

Plasmapheresis, edited by Y. Nosé, P. S. Malchesky, J. W. Smith, and R. S. Krakauer. Raven Press, New York © 1983.

Concepts of Blood Purification Through History

Olgierd Lindan

International Center for Artificial Organs and Transplantation, Cleveland, Ohio 44106

Throughout human history, there has been an intuitive belief that impurities or poisons in the body cause disease. The priests of ancient Egypt, the healers of classical Greece and imperial Rome, the learned doctors of feudal Europe, all took for granted the necessity of cleansing the body of sick patients in order to get rid of the foul and noxious matter. Thus for 3,000 years of our Western civilization, the sick were required to sweat; to drink copious amounts of potions to rinse their bodies; to take emetics, purgatives, and enemas to cleanse their bowels; and, finally, they were bled. The practice of bloodletting was based on a simple logical analogy: "You must first draw out the old and stagnant water from a drinking well in order to allow the fresh spring water to flow in."

It is both horrifying and puzzling to us nowadays that so-called "Heroic Medicine," based empirically on purging and bloodletting, could have persisted for 3,000 years until the middle of the last century. Bloodletting was considered as a panacea for most ailments, although there were occasional dissenters to its unrestrained use. Yet the majority of the patients seemed to agree with their physicians, that the treatment—in order to be effective—had to be unpleasant. It was not until the middle of the last century (a mere 100 years ago) that the students in medical schools rather suddenly ceased to be instructed in the great art of venesection.

With the advent of the artificial kidney, blood and plasma exchange, and now plasmapheresis, the ancient concept of body and blood purification has been dramatically revived during our lifetime. All of these new procedures are now based on a scientific effort to understand what we are really doing. But let us keep in mind that some of our present-day ministrations are still empirical, since we assume that some patients get better after "XYZ" substances are removed from their blood, although still we do not know exactly what some of these XYZ substances are made of. History teaches us that any new or rediscovered medical concept, when enthusiastically accepted, carries with it a danger of indiscriminate overuse. Only with time does a balanced evaluation become possible.

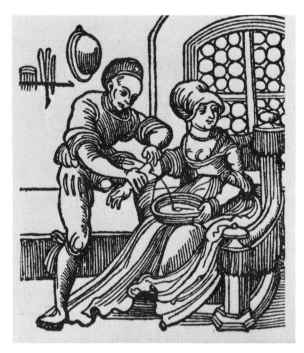

FIG. 1. Phlebotomy, 1520. (From Davis and Appel, ref. 1, with permission.)

Although this volume is a compilation of research into the physicochemical intricacies of plasmapheresis, this chapter presents a glimpse of the lighter side of human endeavors to purify the body and the blood.

The Renaissance woodcut reproduced in Fig. 1 demonstrates that in 1520, bloodletting by venesection was done both elegantly and expertly. Not one drop of blood was allowed to fall on the patient's clothing or on the floor. Obviously, good training and continuous practice were required.

Sometimes bloodletting was done by scarification (Fig. 2)—a messy procedure in itself—and then the patient stood in a tub. The actual cutting of the flesh was done by the surgeon-barber. The elegantly dressed physician supervised the procedure and did not get his hands soiled.

There were times when bloodletting was even fashionable, and was applied to the healthy and wealthy (1) (Fig. 3). The well-to-do Englishman in the 17th–18th century, who could afford to be on a health maintenance program, was subjected to the following routine procedures: (a) he was given a strong emetic once a month; (b) he was adequately purged every week; and (c) he was bled twice a year, once in the spring, and once again in the fall.

Botallus, a medical authority of the 17th century on bloodletting, was of the opinion that: "The more foul water you draw from a well, the more pure water takes its place." So, King Louis XIII of France (1601–1643) who could of course

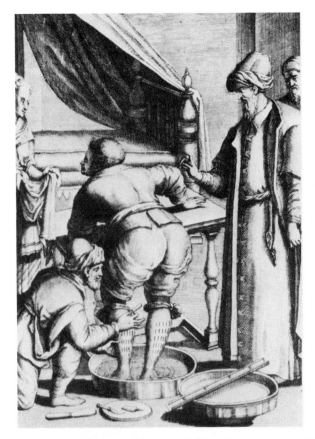

FIG. 2. Bloodletting by scarification, 1719. (From Davis and Appel, ref. 1, with permission.)

avail himself of the best medical talent, was bled 47 times within one year (2). Presumably, the king was bled so often because he was sick, and, in the opinion of his doctors, he needed it. Yet on the other hand, he must have been an unusually resilient man to have survived such a treatment.

The epitaph on the tombstone of Dr. John Coakley Lettsom, a Quaker practitioner in the 18th century, demonstrates that some of the practitioners of bloodletting had good insight into the real value of their procedures (3):

> When patients sick to me apply,
> I purges, bleeds and sweats 'em:
> If after that they choose to die,
> What's that to me? I Lettsom.

It can easily be understood that the bowels were always considered to be a source of impurities in the body and in the blood. Therefore the use of enemas was common, especially in the Middle Ages. The giving of enemas was even the subject of art and humor, as shown in Figs. 4–6.

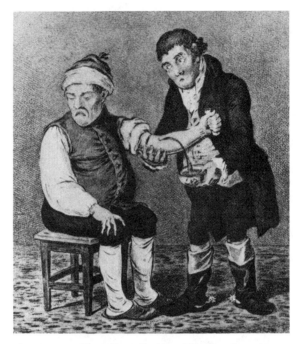

FIG. 3.   Phlebotomy, 1804. (From Davis and Appel, ref. 1, with permission.)

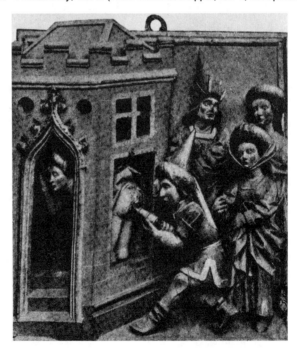

FIG. 4.   Enema by piston syringe, 15th century. (From Brockbank, ref. 4, with permission.)

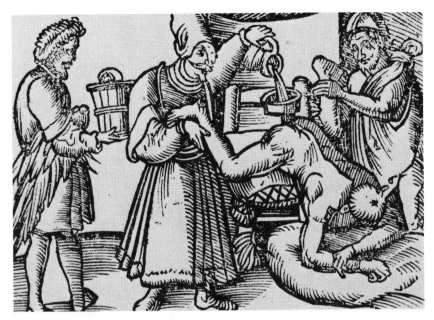

FIG. 5. The Vartomans enema, 1516. (From Brockbank, ref. 4, with permission.)

The medieval, aristocratic lady shown in the wood carving (Fig. 4) looks distressed but not embarrassed, as modesty and decorum for the procedure are properly maintained. There are two ladies-in-waiting and a medical consultant who, please note, bears an expression of professional detachment as he awaits completion of the procedure.

On the other hand, the picture of the Vartomans enema of 1516 (Fig. 5) shows a more straightforward, almost rabelaisian, procedure applied to the poor man.

The charming picture by a Dutch painter, Jan Steen (Fig. 6), shows beautifully the fear and embarrassment of the modest lady, and the reassuring attitude of her attendants. You can almost hear them saying to her: "It won't hurt you." Notice a young man to the left, trying to satisfy his sinful curiosity.

In parallel to the orthodox, unpleasant, and sometimes dangerous procedures for blood and body purification there has always been a popular desire for more simple and painless procedures. This desire has been well exploited by the clever entrepreneur, eager to make easy money. Figure 7 shows one of the more recent medical quack devices which was supposed to purify blood. This Magneto-Galvanic medallion of A. M. Richardson, made of 3 metals, possibly nickel, brass, and lead, was not only worn as jewelry but also guaranteed the wearer vigor and beauty. In addition, it purified the blood, as noted in the advertisement for the medallion presented in Fig. 8. It's amazing that this medallion was actually patented in the United States and in Canada in 1880. Such medallions, however, are extremely rare nowadays.

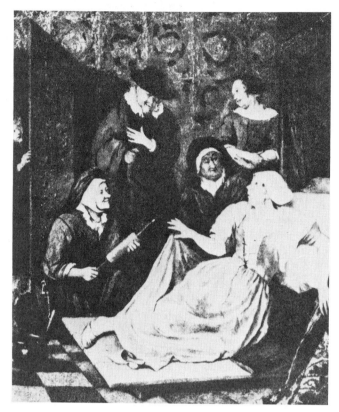

FIG. 6. Administration of a clyster, 17th century. (From Brockbank, ref. 4, with permission.)

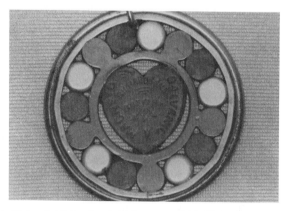

FIG. 7. Magneto-Galvanic Richardson's Battery, ca. 1880. (From the "Historical Collection of Electro-Medical and Quack Devices" of Olgierd Lindan, Cleveland, Ohio.)

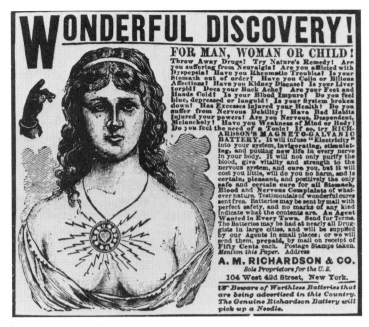

FIG. 8. Enumeration of the benefits to be derived from wearing the Magneto-Galvanic Battery of Dr. Richardson. (From the "Historical Collection of Electro-Medical and Quack Devices" of Olgierd Lindan, Cleveland, Ohio.)

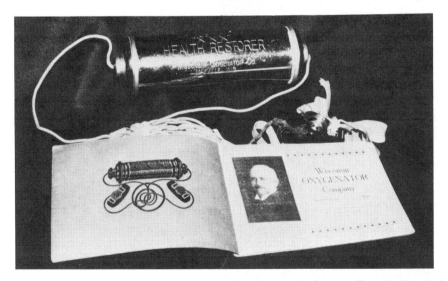

FIG. 9. A later model of the "oxygenator" invented by Dr. Hercules Sanche. (From the Historical Collection of Electro-Medical and Quack Devices" of Olgierd Lindan, Cleveland, Ohio.)

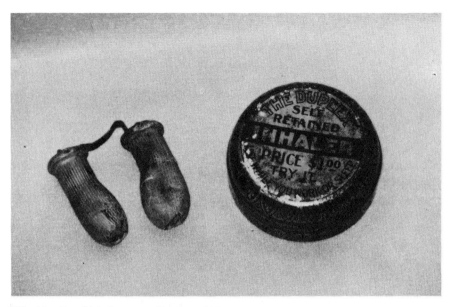

FIG. 10. Nasal inhalers to purify air and blood. (From the "Historical Collection of Electro-Medical and Quack Devices" of Olgierd Lindan, Cleveland, Ohio.)

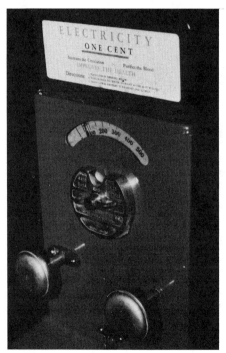

FIG. 11. Penny arcade machine of 1925 to improve circulation and purify blood. (From the "Historical Collection of Electro-Medical and Quack Devices" of Olgierd Lindan, Cleveland, Ohio.)

The United States Post Office tried in vain to stop the interstate commerce of the so-called "oxygenator" (Fig. 9), which was conceived, manufactured, and sold as a "health restorer" by a Dr. Hercules Sanche until 1920. The device consisted basically of a piece of pipe with one or two wires attached to it. It worked very simply. The oxygenator was put into a pot filled with water and the wire was attached to the ankle of the gullible purchaser. Dr. Hercules Sanche claimed that the body was thereby oxygenated and purified during the night while the person was asleep. When the oxygenator had two wires, one was for the husband's ankle, the other was for the wife's ankle. Thousands of these oxygenators were sold under different names, but only a few survived to this day.

There were also special inhalers filled with medicated paste (Fig. 10). They had to be inserted into the nostrils and worn both at work and at home. They were supposed to purify both the inspired air and the blood.

Finally, if you went to an amusement arcade in 1925, you could drop a penny into the slot of the machine shown on Fig. 11, grasp the two metal knobs with your hands, and feel a faradic shock going through your arms. By turning the right handle clockwise you could increase the current. As you can read on the top of the machine, this treatment—for only one penny—increased your circulation and purified your blood.

Exaggerated and deceitful advertising in the health field is still with us, unfortunately, with commercial television and some magazines offering far too many examples.

The concept of blood purification, as we have seen, has had many aspects during the history of mankind. We must realize that without understanding the history of the social and mystic forces which govern the attitudes and beliefs of both the patients and the healers (to whom the sick must turn for help in times of distress), we cannot make much progress in the healing art.

ACKNOWLEDGMENT

This work was supported in part by the Minwendam Medical Research Foundation, 1010 Washington Blvd., Stamford, Connecticut 06901.

REFERENCES

1. Davis, A., and Appel, T. (1979): Bloodletting instruments in the National Museum of History and Technology. In: *Smithsonian Studies in History & Technology*, No. 41. Smithsonian Institution Press, Washington, D.C.
2. Stern, H. (1915): Theory and practice of bloodletting. Rebman, New York.
3. Garrison, F. M. (1913): The history of bloodletting. *N.Y. Med. J.*, March 8, p. 500.
4. Brockbank, W. (1954): *Therapeutic Arts*. Heinemann, London.
5. The medical quack devices described here are from the "Historical Collection of Electro-Medical and Quack Devices" of Olgierd Lindan, Cleveland, Ohio 44121.

Plasmapheresis, edited by Y. Nosé, P. S. Malchesky, J. W. Smith, and R. S. Krakauer. Raven Press, New York © 1983.

Plasma Exchange and Immunosuppressive Drugs in the Treatment of Non-Antibody Mediated Glomerulonephritis

C. D. Pusey, C. M. Lockwood, and D. K. Peters

Department of Medicine, Royal Postgraduate Medical School, Hammersmith Hospital, London W12 OHS, United Kingdom

The clinical syndrome of rapidly progressive glomerulonephritis (RPGN) is usually accompanied by the histological appearances of focal necrotizing glomerulonephritis with a high proportion of crescents. A minority of cases are due to autoantibodies to the glomerular basement membrane (GBM) (1), but the majority are associated with systemic vasculitides such as Wegener's granulomatosis, polyarteritis, systemic lupus erythematosus, Henoch–Schonlein purpura, and mixed essential cryoglubulinemia. Some patients develop idiopathic crescentic nephritis as an isolated disease. In many of these conditions there is evidence for the pathogenetic role of immune complex deposition in the glomerulus (2), although this has been debated.

Plasma exchange was introduced into the management of anti-GBM disease in view of the lack of success of immunosuppressive drugs alone. The effectiveness of plasma exchange in this condition (3) led to its application in other forms of RPGN, where immune complexes were thought to be important (4). Possible mechanisms of action of plasma exchange in non-antibody mediated glomerulonephritis include the removal of circulating immune complexes pending the effects of cytotoxic drugs on the immune response, depletion of humoral mediators of inflammation such as complement components and fibrinogen, and improvement in reticulophagocytic function.

PATIENTS

Between 1974 and 1982, 41 patients (29 male and 12 female) ranging in age from 16 to 71 years were treated. The clinical diagnosis was Wegener's granulomatosis in 23 patients, polyarteritis in 14, and idiopathic RPGN in 4. Although patients with systemic lupus erythematosus, Henoch–Schonlein purpura, cryoglobulinemia, and other forms of immune complex nephritis have been treated with a similar regimen, they were excluded from this analysis in view of the variable natural history and response to conventional therapy. Focal necrotizing glomerulonephritis

59

with crescents was confirmed on renal biopsy in 40/41 cases, and in 1 case the initial biopsy was unsuccessful, although a subsequent specimen revealed evidence of crescentic nephritis. Circulating immune complexes were demonstrated in 19/35 cases.

MANAGEMENT

Daily 3–4-liter plasma exchanges for plasma protein fraction were performed (depending upon the weight of the patient), using a cell separator (Haemonetics Model 30). Fresh frozen plasma was used only when clinically indicated, for example, within 48 hr of renal biopsy or surgical operation, and in the presence of active pulmonary hemorrhage. Vascular access was originally achieved by the use of arteriovenous shunts, but since the appreciation of the importance of infection at these sites, venipuncture of antecubital veins or femoral vein catheterization has been preferred. The duration of plasma exchange was determined by the clinical response, and was performed for a mean of 7 days.

Drug therapy consisted of prednisolone 60 mg/day, reducing to 20 mg/day by 4 weeks, and more slowly thereafter; cyclophosphamide 3 mg/kg/day; and azathioprine 1 mg/kg/day. In patients over 55 years, cyclophosphamide dosage was reduced to 2 mg/kg/day and azathioprine was omitted because of their increased susceptibility to bone marrow toxicity. Cytotoxics were temporarily withdrawn if leukopenia ($<4.0 \times 10^9$/liter) or infection developed. All patients normally received cytotoxics for 8 weeks, and long-term maintenance therapy at a lower dose was frequently required, especially in Wegener's granulomatosis.

Disease activity in those patients with systemic vasculitis was assessed by daily clinical examination. Renal disease was monitored by regular urine microscopy (looking particularly for red cell casts) and serial measurements of plasma creatinine and creatinine clearance. Patients with associated pulmonary vasculitis were also followed by regular chest radiographs and by measurement of the corrected carbon monoxide transfer factor (KCO) (5). Circulating immune complexes were measured by solid phase Clq and rheumatoid factor binding assays (6).

RESULTS

Although circulating immune complexes were present in 19/35 patients at presentation, their levels correlated poorly with disease activity. Treatment with the plasma exchange regimen led to a rapid fall in immune complexes in all patients, and in 10/15 cases who were more intensively studied, assays remained consistently negative after stopping plasma exchange.

The effect of treatment on renal function is summarized in Table 1. Of 19 oliguric or dialysis-dependent patients, 13 recovered renal function, 1 remained on dialysis, and 5 died without response. Of 9 patients whose initial plasma creatinine was >600 μmoles/liter, 7 recovered renal function (although 1 later died), 1 proceeded to dialysis and 1 died without response. Of 13 patients with plasma creatinine <600

TABLE 1. *Outcome of treatment for immune complex RPGN (41 patients)*

Presentation	N	Outcome		
		Improved	No response	Death
Oligoanuric	19	13	6	5
Creatinine > 600 μmoles/liter	9	7	2	2
Creatinine < 600 μmoles/liter	13	12	1	0

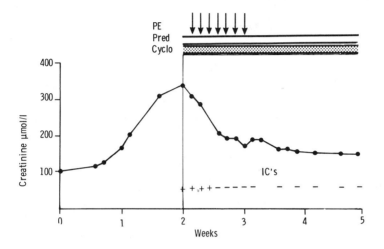

FIG. 1. Response of plasma creatinine and immune complexes (IC) to the plasma exchange (PE) regimen in a patient (No. 501457) with RPGN related to polyarteritis. Pred, prednisolone; Cyclo, cyclophosphamide.

μmoles/liter, 12 showed an improvement in renal function and 1 became dialysis dependent. The course of a patient with RPGN related to polyarteritis is shown in Fig. 1.

Although not amenable to such detailed analysis, many patients with extrarenal manifestations of disease activity, for example, pulmonary hemorrhage, cerebral vasculitis, or digital ischemia, also showed a dramatic improvement in those features. Relapses in disease activity were found to be related to intercurrent infection in 11/18 episodes, in cases associated with Wegener's granulomatosis (7).

Long-term follow-up of the surviving patients who recovered renal function revealed that only 3/21 subsequently deteriorated (Fig. 2). One patient who initially failed to respond became independent of dialysis, and 2 others were maintained on regular dialysis with no evidence of disease activity. Of the 13 cases who died, 7 did so during their initial hospital admission (3 of pulmonary disease, 3 of infection, and 1 of uncontrolled vasculitis), and 6 died after discharge (2 of infection, 2 of untreated renal failure, 1 of a cerebrovascular accident, and 1 of myocardial infarction following renal transplantation).

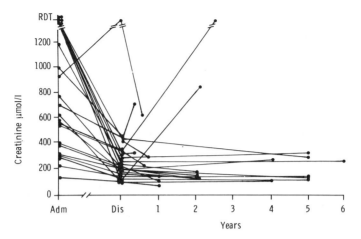

FIG. 2. Renal function on follow-up of 22 patients with non-antibody mediated glomerulonephritis who responded to treatment with the plasma exchange regimen. Adm, admission; Dis, discharge.

DISCUSSION

Assessment of the effects of the plasma exchange regimen on the underlying immunopathological process is more difficult in non-antibody mediated RPGN than in nephritis due to anti-GBM antibodies, where circulating levels of the pathogenetic autoantibody can readily be measured. These antibody levels correlate with disease activity in general, and provide a useful guide to therapy (8), despite our observation that increased allergic tissue injury may result from a variety of other factors, such as infection. Although circulating immune complexes were detected in more than half of our patients, their concentration correlated poorly with disease activity, and their pathogenicity remains unproven. Any therapeutic benefit of plasma exchange could be due to effects other than the removal of immune complexes, for example, depletion of inflammatory mediators or improvement in reticulophagocytic function (9).

The sustained improvement in renal function in two-thirds of the oliguric or dialysis-dependent patients contrasts with our experience in anti-GBM nephritis (8), in which none of 22 oliguric cases have improved. It is therefore worth treating the non-antibody mediated group aggressively, even when presenting with advanced renal failure. The duration of dialysis before starting treatment is relevant, however, as only 1 patient who improved had been on dialysis for more than 5 days. Their recovery occurred within 26 days (mean 11 days), making it unlikely that continuation of plasma exchange for longer periods would be of benefit.

As in anti-GBM nephritis (10), relapses in disease activity during the initial admission were often related to intercurrent infection. Although the cause of this phenomenon remains unknown, an increased load of immune complexes or a nonspecific activation of inflammatory mediator systems are possible mechanisms.

Many of these infections occurred at the site of indwelling arteriovenous shunts, and the frequency of the problem has been greatly reduced by the use of antecubital venipuncture or femoral vein catheterization whenever possible.

Increasing disease activity after discharge from hospital was frequently related to reduction in drug therapy. Although cytotoxic drugs can safely be stopped after 8 weeks in anti-GBM disease, the same is not true of RPGN associated with systemic vasculitis. Azathioprine was most commonly used for maintenance therapy, in view of its lower toxicity, but some patients with Wegener's granulomatosis required long-term cyclophosphamide.

The role of plasma exchange in our treatment regimen remains unclear. Although there are many reports of the benefit of treatment with plasma exchange combined with immunosuppressive drugs (4,11), it is clear that some patients may respond to drug therapy alone (12). There is a lack of controlled trials to clarify this problem, and since 1977 we have been conducting a prospective controlled trial of plasma exchange combined with drugs compared with drugs alone. Patients with the diagnoses described above have been randomly allocated into two treatment groups, stratified for renal function; one group received the immunosuppressive drug regimen and the other group received the same drugs combined with at least 5 daily 4-liter plasma exchanges.

Although it is too early to describe the results in full, a preliminary analysis reveals that nonoliguric patients appear to show a good initial response in both treatment groups, whereas oliguric patients may benefit from the addition of plasma exchange. The immediate effect of plasma exchange may be important in preventing irreversible renal damage in those cases with advanced disease, and we await the long-term results of the trial with interest.

Despite the lack of information concerning the mechanism of action of plasma exchange, or indeed of its role in the immunosuppressive treatment regimen, many patients who would have developed end stage renal failure have now been successfully treated. Further basic research and clinical trials are clearly required before the use of plasma exchange in non-antibody mediated glomerulonephritis can be fully established.

ACKNOWLEDGMENTS

We would like to thank Miss S. Gibbons, Miss B. Roberts, and Miss G. Fox for performing the plasma exchanges, and Miss S. Goodwin for excellent secretarial assistance.

REFERENCES

1. Wilson, C. B., and Dixon, F. J. (1973): Antiglomerular basement membrane antibody-induced glomerulonephritis. *Kidney Int.*, 3:74.
2. McCluskey, R. J., and Bhan, A. K. (1981): Immune complexes and renal disease. *Clin. Immunol. Allergy*, 1:397.
3. Lockwood, C. M., Rees, A. J., Pearson, T. A., Evans, D. J., Peters, D. K., and Wilson, C. B. (1976): Immunosuppression and plasma exchange in the treatment of Goodpasture's syndrome. *Lancet*, i:711.

4. Lockwood, C. M., Pusey, C. D., Rees, A. J., and Peters, D. K. (1981): Plasma exchange in the treatment of immune complex disease. *Clin. Immunol. Allergy*, 1:433.
5. Ewan, P. W., Jones, H. A., Rhodes, C. G., and Hughes, J. M. B. (1976): Detection of pulmonary haemorrhage with carbon monoxide uptake. *N. Engl. J. Med.*, 195:1391.
6. Pussell, B. A., Lockwood, C. M., Scott, D. M., Pinching, A. J., and Peters, D. K. (1978): Value of immune complex assays in diagnosis and management. *Lancet*, ii:359.
7. Pinching, A. J., Rees, A. J., Pussell, B. A., Lockwood, C. M., Mitchison, R. S., and Peters, D. K. (1980): Relapses in Wegener's granulomatosis: The role of infection. *Br. Med. J.*, ii:836.
8. Pusey, C. D. (1982): Glomerulonephritis due to autoantibodies to the glomerular basement membrane: Treatment with plasma exchange. *Med. Grand Round*, 1:67.
9. Lockwood, C. M., Worlledge, S., Nicholas, A., Cotton, C., and Peters, D. K. (1979): Reversal of impaired splenic function in patients with nephritis or vasculitis (or both) by plasma exchange. *N. Engl. J. Med.*, 300:524.
10. Rees, A. J., Lockwood, C. M., and Peters, D. K. (1977): Enhanced allergic tissue injury in Goodpasture's syndrome by intercurrent infection. *Br. Med. J.*, ii:723.
11. McKenzie, P. E., Taylor, A. E., Woodroffe, A. J., Seymour, A. E., Chan, Y. L., and Clarkson, A. R. (1979): Plasmapheresis in glomerulonephritis. *Clin. Nephrol.*, 12:97.
12. Fauci, A. S., Haynes, B. F., and Katz, P. (1978): The spectrum of vasculitis. Clinical, pathologic, immunologic and therapeutic considerations. *Ann. Int. Med.*, 89:660.

Plasmapheresis, edited by Y. Nosé, P. S. Malchesky, J. W. Smith, and R. S. Krakauer. Raven Press, New York © 1983.

Substitution Therapy in Plasma Exchange

R. Ben Dawson, Alberto C. Seiguer, Bennett B. Edelman, Peter J. Kragel, Eva H. Schwartz, Florence E. Metrinko, Valerie A. McCahon, and Rouben M. JiJi

Apheresis Center, Blood Transfusion Labs, University of Maryland Hospital, Baltimore, Maryland 21201

In 1914 plasmapheresis was first performed and proposed as an economical step in the production of therapeutic products (1). In the same year, the safety of citrate for intravenous infusion was demonstrated (2). Plasmapheresis became established in the U.S. for the manufacture of therapeutic products (3) in 1959, and the introduction of a continuous flow centrifuge in 1969 marked the beginning of the current era of therapy by plasma exchange (4).

There appears to be a common pattern to emerging technologies which is illustrated by these two fields. First, a perceived need for a product or procedure is realized. The technology becomes available and then application begins. After a sufficient amount of experience, potential or actual problems become obvious, necessitating reappraisal and, at times, intensive investigation.

For therapeutic products, plasmapheresis is performed by replacing some of the 1-liter volume of plasma removed per week with saline. This two times a week removal of 500 ml of plasma is an upper limit; for example, for production of albumin, antihemolytic factor, and rhesus immunoglobulin. The limit is reduced to a once-weekly 500-ml plasma donation for hepatitis vaccine source material, since subjects may have abnormal liver function. These restrictions on the maximum rates of plasma donation are based in large part on the known ability of the normal liver to synthesize albumin. Since only one-third of the liver is normally involved in synthesis of albumin at any one time, and a 50-liter per year plasmapheresis donor requires about a one-third increase in synthesis to maintain a normal plasma level of about 3.5 g/dl, the reserve capacity would seem to be available. Also, it is known that albumin synthesis begins almost immediately after someone who has been starved is re-fed. Further, the time for delivery of synthesized albumin is also short, about 20 min (5).

Although this knowledge was sufficient for initiating the US plasmapheresis program for manufacture of therapeutic products, when experience was gathered it became necessary to validate the predictions and indeed the observations that such an intensive practice was without harm. Two studies have served this purpose. In the first, data from almost 900 commercial plasmapheresis donors giving for more than 2 years (range 6 months to 6 years) led to the conclusion that even in individuals being plasmapheresed for the maximum permissible yield, plasma protein concentrations generally stay within the normal range. However, 7–8% of donors acquired an abnormality in the levels of some plasma proteins. Further, individuals in plasmapheresis for an average of more than 3½ years established equilibrium at a level lower though normal, than when they started (6). In the second study, long-term (6–14 year) plasmapheresis donors from several centers giving 40–60 liters per year maintained normal albumin levels (7). In another study, on a small group of donors giving more than 40 liters per year over 5 years, normal but significantly lower albumin levels were seen after each year compared with the prepheresis value. However, values for years 4 and 5 were not significantly different from the 2-year values. These data also suggested a new steady state at a lower level, but with values still within the normal ranges (8). These and other studies have led to the definition of three levels of plasmapheresis; first level, one or two donations per year; second level, a quantity and frequency of donation such as to allow both serum levels and synthesis rates of serum proteins to return to normal before subsequent collection; and the third level, allowing 50–60 liters of plasma removal per year for each donor, recognizing that although plasma protein levels change from the initial values, they remain within accepted normal ranges, and that the rates of plasma protein synthesis may not have returned to normal for any subsequent collection (9).

Paralleling the above developments and our improved understanding of the events taking place in the person undergoing plasmapheresis for production of therapeutics, there have been several useful studies on protein and hemostatic changes during plasma exchange of various intensities (10–12). These findings and others will be considered below since they provide essential data on the various modes of replacement that may be necessary, from normal saline through coagulation factor substitutions. It is clear from some of our experiences and others that fresh frozen plasma (FFP), and indeed sometimes platelet concentrates, need to be substituted. The subject of replacement and substitution is diverse, but not so large as the number of disease situations. What will be attempted below is a synthesis based on the data that we view as representative of the major, useful studies in the literature. This will be an approach toward guidelines which, of course, must be written by and have the authority of a larger group of experts from a variety of experienced centers.

Parenthetically, because of inadequate data, we cannot yet address such questions as what effect albumin replacement has upon the rate of endogenous synthesis and the release of this important protein. And we can only infer the result of substituting FFP for albumin and thus the effect that exogenous fibrinogen might have on the synthetic rate of this plasma protein. Further, in contrast to plasmapheresis for therapeutic products, in which the rate of removal has been limited by the ability of normal individuals to increase synthetic rates, plasma exchange often obviates this limitation by supplying as replacement at least albumin, and at times, other normal plasma proteins, to maintain functional homeostatic and hemostatic concentrations. The effects of such replacement and substitution regimens for the removal of large amounts of plasma, usually containing only one unwanted protein or complex, are virtually unknown. Although the emergence of specific absorptive columns and related technologies will help us bypass this problem in the not too distant future, it will remain a perplexing set of unknowns demanding imaginative approaches.

MATERIALS AND METHODS

Six patients admitted to the hematology and neurology services at the University of Maryland Hospital were subjected to 26 1-plasma volume exchanges over 2 months. Plasma volume was taken from the standard table (13) using the same-day measured body weight and hematocrit. One exception was an extremely obese patient for whom a blood volume estimate based on kilograms of body weight and hematocrit was used (14), adjusted downward by 20% as a compromise to the suggestions made for reduction which range from 10 to 50% (15).

Plasma exchange was carried out by continuous flow centrifugation using the IBM 2997 Blood Cell Separator (International Business Machines, Princeton, NJ) (16). Terumo "back eye" needles were used for bleeding into ACD formula A at a ratio of 13:1. The blood flow rate was 40–50 ml/min and separation was at 1,600–2,000 rpm.

Replacement of plasma removed was attempted simultaneously on a volume per volume basis. Replacement fluids consisted of 10 to 50% normal saline solution (NSS) and the remainder colloid (17). Colloids were PPF (plasma protein fraction, 5%; Cutter Labs, Berkeley, CA for ANRC) except for the special indications described under results for which 5% albumin (American National Red Cross, Washington, DC), FFP, or platelet concentrates were used.

PATIENTS

Three of the patients were exchanged for immune or idiopathic thrombocytopenic purpura (ITP) unresponsive to the usual therapeutic modalities. Two patients with autoimmune hemolytic anemia, one chronic and one acute and life-threatening, were not responding to other usual therapies. The sixth patient, who had a nearly life-long history of myasthenia gravis, was finding it increasingly difficult to perform her work as a clerk–typist while being treated with high, frequent doses of anti-cholinesterase drugs.

Patient 1 underwent exchange for persistent, proven hydrochlorothiazide-induced thrombocytopenic purpura, with increased bone marrow megakaryocyte numbers and activity. One plasma volume was exchanged for saline and 5% albumin. Because the patient had a long history of aplastic anemia with many febrile transfusion reactions, the colloid chosen for replacement was 5% albumin rather than PPF. No reactions or untoward effects associated with the exchange occurred.

Patient 2 had idiopathic thrombocytopenic purpura which had been unresponsive to high steroid doses during this exacerbation. She previously had splenectomy, and had hereditary hemophilia A trait with Factor VIII levels averaging 40% of normal. For this reason, her replacement colloid consisted of one-half FFP. Two exchanges of one plasma volume were carried out on successive days. PT (prothrombin time) and PTT (partial thromboplastin time) were normal before and after the first exchange.

Patient 3 had symptomatic ITP which was unresponsive to increased steroid dose on this admission. Her ITP was of 10 years duration; 9 years previous the diagnosis of systemic lupus erythematosus had been made. Her thrombocytopenia was severe enough (platelet counts of 3,000–7,000) to warrant the use of FFP, thus avoiding hypofibrinogenemia which would impair hemostasis. Separations were carried out at higher centrifuge speeds (2,000 vs 1,600 rpm) for all patients with thrombocytopenia in order to minimize platelet loss.

Patient 4 had cold agglutinin hemolytic anemia which had become symptomatic with hemoglobin less than 10 g/dl just prior to this admission. Four exchanges of 1 plasma volume each were carried out over 11 days using NSS and PPF as replacement fluids. Fluids and red cells returned to the patient were warmed to 37°C to minimize hemolysis.

Patient 5 had an acute autoimmune hemolytic anemia which developed within the 3 weeks following uneventful coronary artery bypass surgery. Upon admission, the anemia was severe (Hgb = 7.4 g/dl). The patient was splenectomized on the third hospital day (thrombosis was demonstrated). She subsequently developed a stroke-like syndrome, acute renal failure, and gangrene of the distal portions of most toes. Exchanges of 1 plasma volume each were carried out at 1–3-day intervals for 2 weeks. Colloid replacement was part PPF, but mostly FFP, in amounts calculated to prevent further prolongation of her PTT. Plasma fibrinogen values were never below 200 mg%. Also, on numerous determinations fibrin split products were not elevated. Heparin was not administered, as the dialysis for renal failure was carried out by the peritoneal route.

Patient 6, with signs of myasthenia gravis since age 2 and a diagnosis since age 5, was admitted for an elective course of exchanges of 1 plasma volume each. This was an attempt for her to continue useful employment as a clerk–typist in a community hospital laboratory. In spite of high, frequent doses of anticholinesterase drugs, she had recently begun to have serious difficulty typing and climbing the steps of the city buses to get to work. Plasma exchanges were carried out using NSS and PPF as replacement fluids.

RESULTS AND DISCUSSION

The 6 patients who underwent up to eight exchanges of 1 plasma volume each, had a variety of needs for replacement fluids, mostly because of their complicating diagnoses and diseases, some of which were unrelated to their being accepted for therapy by plasma exchange. Because plasma removal was planned to exceed 1,000 ml/week, colloid replacement was given on a volume per volume basis in excess of that amount. In other words, for up to 1,000 ml/week, saline could be used, but for the amount of plasma removal in excess of 1,000 ml, an equal amount of colloid was replaced. The type of colloid chosen was PPF, because 5% albumin is not as readily available in our area. In patient 1, 5% albumin was substituted for PPF because of the history of multiple transfusion reactions. In patients 2, 3, and 5, FFP was substituted for PPF to provide active plasma coagulation factors in amounts calculated to avoid seriously low levels that would be associated with impaired hemostasis. In patient 5, platelet concentrates were used in addition to FFP for four of the exchanges for the same reason—that is, to protect hemostasis. Substitution in this report refers to the use of human blood products or components instead of PPF and does not refer to artificial plasma substitutes. In our standard replacement therapy with PPF or in substitution replacement with albumin, FFP, or platelet concentrates, the plasma albumin level in the patient is not being critically diluted by these substitutions.

Maintenance of an adequate plasma albumin level is important. It is clear that a patient with normal liver function will maintain the needed plasma albumin level without colloid replacement if no more than 1,000 ml of plasma is removed from the patient per week (9). Indeed, at least one country is incorporating this limitation into its guidelines for cytapheresis procedures (13). Since no such limitation or government guidelines are being generally proposed for plasma exchange, a safe, low level for albumin needs to be discussed. The lower limit of normal is usually given as 3.5 g/dl. In discussing the minimum levels to be maintained in transfusion therapy for trauma in the context of colloid versus crystalloid resuscitation, there is agreement that the critical level is 2.5 g/dl (18,19). Since 2.5 is 70% of 3.5, this is in agreement with the conclusion that a 30% reduction may lead to edema (20). This latter group especially suggests pulmonary edema as a potential clinical manifestation of the 30% reduction in albumin, but impressive arguments have recently been made against this possibility if the lungs are normal (19). However, peripheral edema is a likely event when colloid is underutilized in fluid resuscitation (18,21,22) and probably also in high volume plasma exchange. In areas where the lower limit of normal is 4.5 g/dl, the low safe level is given as 3.0 g/dl albumin or 5.2 g/dl total serum protein (22).

For partial plasmapheresis a common practice is to replace entirely with normal saline (0.9% sodium chloride) (23). Another experienced group agrees that plasmapheresis of 1,500 ml every other week or so, as for hyperviscosity, requires no colloid and that saline alone suffices for replacement. A common replacement regimen for total plasma exchange consisting of 5% of the body weight in kilograms uses ¾ NSS and ¼ PPF (23). Since normal plasma albumin has a lower limit of 3.5 g/dl, albumin and PPF are slightly concentrated with albumin levels of 4.9 and 4.4, respectively. There is general agreement that 1 plasma volume exchanges, two or three times a week, will need some colloid and that an exchange of 1 plasma volume generally reduces plasma components to about 35% of their original values, not depleting coagulation factors dangerously (17). However, for occasional or infrequent exchanges, this suggests the possibility of using crystalloid alone, perhaps a modified Ringer's such as Plasma-Lyte (Travenol Labs, Inc., Deerfield, IL) containing magnesium instead of calcium, in replacement volumes that are enough in excess of the plasma removed to prevent hypotension. This notion of extra volume replacement with crystalloid has not to our knowledge been explored satisfactorily in plasma exchange, but it is an intriguing and feasible possibility especially in view of the high cost of colloid.

In routine exchanges of 1 plasma volume to 3 liters, a common and satisfactory approach to replacement is to use 500 ml of NSS at first, and then use 5% albumin or PPF for the rest of the volume replacement (17). These workers earlier used up to 1,000 of NSS at the beginning of the procedure followed by replacement of the rest of the volume with albumin or PPF which was diluted to half-strength with NSS. The earlier procedure was abandoned in favor of more than doubling the amount of colloid used because of too frequent patient reactions. Our experience was similar; that is, in early procedures we used 800–1,000 ml of NSS initially, followed by colloid. But because of the frequency of hypotensive patient reactions we reduced the initial normal saline to 300–500 ml, and found that reactions became rare and were limited mostly to transient episodes of perioral parethesias caused by citrate.

Although the efficiency of the exchange for reducing the levels of some plasma constituents is decreased with an enlarged plasma volume, it seems reasonable to suggest that infusion of crystalloid in a greater rate than removal of plasma may allow satisfactory plasma exchanges to be carried out with very little use of colloid. Whether reducing colloid is a goal or not, there is apparently a great reluctance to leave the patient with a positive fluid balance. With adequate renal function a positive balance should not be harmful. Planning for a positive balance by using excess crystalloid may not enlarge the plasma volume, since crystalloid loss from the vascular space is rapid and results in a two- to threefold greater volume requirement, compared with colloid (18,21). In hemodilution for cardiac surgery, crystalloid is commonly used in twofold excess volume. Among the variables that theoretically increase the efficiency of a plasma exchange are reduced initial plasma volume, low albumin concentrations during the procedure, and brief and tightly spaced sessions (24).

Considering the data and experience reviewed above, a regimen for fluid replacement during routine plasma exchange of 1 patient plasma volume up to 3 liters of plasma removed can be proposed. Initial replacement would consist of crystalloid alone, perhaps 300–500 ml equivolume, then in excess volume of around twofold, until patient's plasma albumin reaches a level of 2.5 g/dl or total serum protein reaches 5.2 g/dl, the critical thresholds. From this point on, the decision will have to be made whether to continue only crystalloid, which will now surely have to be at a rate of infusion in excess of the rate of plasma removal, or to use equivolume supplementation of crystalloid with an amount of 5% albumin or 5% PPF calculated to maintain the minimal critical levels in the patient of 2.5 g/dl albumin or 5.2 g/dl total protein (21). In the former case, with continuation of crystalloid in excess volume it will be necessary to reconstitute the patient near the end of the procedure to critical colloid levels of 2.5 g/dl albumin or 5.2 g/dl total protein as termination values. If the excess crystalloid option has been followed throughout, reconstitution with 25% albumin would seem to be worthy of consideration (21,22). In any case, it must be kept in mind that increases in serum albumin beyond the normal level of 3.5 to 5 g/dl depress synthesis and enhance catabolism (22).

Since the citrate anticoagulant used in most procedures is the cause of the commonest patient reactions to plasma exchange, some consideration of additional sources will be useful. Citrate reactions are usually only bothersome, but they do alarm patients, and sometimes considerably delay restarting procedures, wasting valuable time; rarely, however, are they severe and life-threatening. Normal plasma citrate levels are 0.1–0.2 mM/liter. Levels in FFP are the highest among fluids in common use at 17.4 or nearly 200 times normal plasma levels. The next highest citrate levels are in PPF, at 9.6 or approximately 100 times the normal plasma levels. The lowest levels in "isotonic" colloids discussed here are in the 5% albumin at 4.4 (22). An appealing feature of 25% albumin is that upon dilution, either *in vitro* in crystalloid or *in vivo* with infusion, its concentration of citrate will be reduced 10 times if it is used to effect a final plasma concentration of 2.5 g/dl.

In addition to the above considerations of the composition of the commonly used colloids for replacement in the US, another concern is the difference in cost. In our region, 5% albumin and PPF are provided by the major supplier at equal costs. This curious arbitrary or economic manipulation is unfortunate because of the known 20% lower cost for manufacturing PPF. There is no longer any reason to avoid using PPF because of the hypotensive reactions that occurred some years ago from

TABLE 1. *Summary of data obtained on coagulation factor and platelet depletion and recovery with plasma exchange*

Effects on coagulation tests: 4-liter plasma exchange, 5% albumin or PPF[a]							
PT	PTT	F	VIII	V	IX	AT 111	PLT
Pre							
12	33	185	100	100	125	28	240K
Post							
18	68	60	50	50	95	12	161K
4 hr							
15	38	95	90	75	100	18	(−33%)
24 hr							
		150	100	100		22	

Pre: PT 12, PTT 33, F 185, VIII 100, V 100, IX 125, AT 111 28, PLT 240K
Post: PT 18, PTT 68, F 60, VIII 50, V 50, IX 95, AT 111 12, PLT 161K
4 hr: PT 15, PTT 38, F 95, VIII 90, V 75, IX 100, AT 111 18, PLT (−33%)
24 hr: F 150, VIII 100, V 100, AT 111 22

Platelet count after 1.3–2.1 plasma volume exchanges (% change from 150K–450K)						
Hr after exchange	0	24	48	72	96	110	168
% Change	−30	−20	−10	−5	−3	100	+5

Fibrinogen remaining after exchange[b]					
Plasma volume exchanged	0.5	1	1.5	2	2.5
% Remaining	62	40	25	15	10

Fibrinogen recovery after 1.3 plasma volume exchange					
Hr after exchange	0	24	48	72	96
% Change	−66	−38	−15	−5	+10

[a]Data from Flaum et al., ref. 11.
[b]Data from Chopek and McCullough, ref. 12.

the change in a manufacturing process that has long since been corrected. PPF is currently as safe as albumin and should have a price advantage in addition to its ready availability. A greater difference is possible with the use of FFP rather than albumin, which can save as much as 60% in the cost of an exchange of 3 liters of plasma. However, the risk of hepatitis in this substitution seems to have been realized (25). Further, hemostasis is adequate without FFP in some uncomplicated patients with 4-liter exchanges (11). Besides the safety of 5% albumin and 5% PPF, they both cause plasma volume expansion when used in isovolumetric exchanges. Plasma expansion was not seen when using FFP replacement (12). This may be because the albumin concentration in FFP is normal with respect to a physiologic, oncotic effect, but osmotically hypertonic in albumin and PPF.

The subject of coagulation factor and platelet depletion and recovery with plasma exchange is complex, but useful data are available (10–12). With exchanges of 1–2 plasma volumes, platelet loss is one-third (11,12) and Factors V and VIII are one-half (11), but fibrinogen can decrease to 15% (12). Table 1 summarizes useful approximations of the published graphs.

REFERENCES

1. Abel, J. J., Rountree, L. G., and Turner, B. B. (1914): Plasma removal with return of corpuscles. *J. Pharm. Exp. Ther.*, 5:625.
2. Hustin, A. (1914): Principe d'une nouvelle methode de transfusion muquesuse. *J. Med. Brux.*, 2:436.
3. Crispen, J. F. (1978): Medical ethics and the morality of plasmapheresis. *Plasma Forum*, 1:39.
4. Bruckner, C. D., Clift, R., and Thomas, E. D. (1969): Plasma exchange with NCI-IBM Blood Cell Separator. *Rev. Fr. Clin. Biol.*, 14:803.
5. Swisher, S. (1979): Plasmapheresis, a medical viewpoint. *Plasma Forum*, 1:67.
6. Ascari, W. Q. (1979): Effects on protein components during plasmapheresis of 6 months to 6 years. *Plasma Forum*, 2:119.
7. Dawson, R. B., Crispen, J. F., Ascari, W. Q., Sohmer, P. R., and Miller, R. M. (1979): Laboratory profiles on donors participating in long-term plasmapheresis programs. *Plasma Forum*, 2:141.
8. Dawson, R. B., Crispen, J. F., Gorsuch, C. D., Bilenki, L. A., and Miller, R. M. (1980): Laboratory findings on long-term plasmapheresis donors; protein levels. *Plasma Forum*, 3:209.
9. World Health Organization (1981): The collection, fractionation, quality control, and uses of blood and blood products, WHO, Geneva, 1981, p. 10.
10. Bayer, W. L., Farrales, F. B., Summers, T., and Belcher, C. (1975): Coagulation studies after plasma exchange with plasma protein fraction and lactated Ringer's solution. In: *Leukocytes: Separation, Collection and Transfusion*, edited by J. M. Goldman and R. M. Lowenthal, p. 551. Academic Press, London.
11. Flaum, M. A., Cuneo, R. A., Appelbaum, F. R., Deisseroth, A. B., Engel, W. K., and Gralnick, H. R. (1979): The hemostatic imbalance of plasma exchange transfusion. *Blood*, 54:694.
12. Chopek, M., and McCullough, J. (1980): Protein and biochemical changes during plasma exchange. In: *Therapeutic Hemapheresis: A Technical Workshop*, edited by E. M. Berkman and J. Umlas, p. 13. AABB, Washington, D.C.
13. Mollison, P. L. (1979): *Blood Transfusion in Clinical Medicine*, 6th edition. Blackwell, Oxford, p. 137.
14. Williams, W. J., Beutler, E., Erslev, A. J., and Rundles, R. W., Editors (1977): *Hematology*, 2nd edition, McGraw-Hill, New York, p. 239.
15. Albert, S. N. (1971): *Blood Volume and Extracellular Fluid Volume*, 2nd edition. Charles C Thomas, Springfield, Illinois, p. 65.
16. Hester, J. P., Kellog, R. M., Mulzet, A. P., Kruger, V. R., McCredie, K. M., and Freireich,

E. J. (1979): Principles of blood separation and component extraction in a disposable continuous-flow single-stage channel. *Blood*, 54:254.

17. Heustis, V. W., and Thomas, S. F. (1980): Presently available plasmapheresis techniques. In: *Therapeutic Hemapheresis, A Technical Workshop*. AABB, Washington, D.C.

18. Dawson, R. B., and Cowley, R. A. (1982): Crystalloid versus colloid in initial resuscitation of trauma patients. In: *Controversies in Trauma Management, Clinics in Emergency Medicine (in press)*.

19. Traunbaugh, R. S., and Lewis, R. (1982): Crystalloid versus colloid in the initial fluid resuscitation of the trauma patient. In: *Controversies in Trauma Management, Clinics in Emergency Medicine (in press)*.

20. Seiler, F. R., Karges, H., Geursen, R., and Sedlacek, H. H. (1981): Possibilities, problems and hazards with blood plasma substitution therapy. In: *Plasma Exchange Therapy*, edited by H. Bordberg and P. Reuther, p. 37. International Symposium, Wiesbaden, Thieme-Stratton, New York.

21. Tullis, J. L. (1977): Albumin, background and use: Guidelines for clinical use. *J.A.M.A.*, 237:4–5, 355–360, 460–463.

22. O'Riordan, J. P., Aebischer, M., Darnborough, J., and Thoren, L. (1978): The Indications for the Use of Albumin, Plasma Protein Solutions and Plasma Substitutes. European Public Health Committee, Council of European Coordinative Research and Blood Transfusion, 1976 program, Strasbourg, pp. 40–51.

23. Mielke, C. H., and Mielke, M. R. (1981): Technical and therapeutic application of plasma exchange. In: *Apheresis: Development, Application, and Collection Procedures*, edited by C. H. Mielke, pp. 123–145. Allen R. Liss, New York.

24. Lundsgaard-Hansen, P., Riedwyl, H., and Deubelbeiss, K. (1981): Computer simulation of therapeutic plasma exchange. In: *Plasma Exchange Therapy*, edited by H. Bordberg and P. Reuther, p. 53. International Symposium, Wiesbadden, 1980. Thieme-Stratton, New York.

25. Patten, E. (1980): Therapeutic pheresis, organization of a hospital program. In: *Therapeutic Hemapheresis, A Technical Workshop*, edited by E. M. Berkman and J. Umlas, p. 121. AABB, Washington, D.C.

Plasmapheresis, edited by Y. Nosé, P. S.
Malchesky, J. W. Smith, and R. S. Krakauer.
Raven Press, New York © 1983.

Centrifugal Apheresis Techniques

G. Rock

*Canadian Red Cross, Blood Transfusion Service, Ottawa Centre and Department of
Medicine, University of Ottawa, Ottawa, Ontario K1S 3E2 Canada*

Large volume plasma exchange has been made possible by the development of machines which were originally intended for the collection of white blood cells for support of septic patients. These machines utilize the principle of centrifugation to separate whole blood into its various components, permitting the selective collection of various cellular populations and/or plasma. Whole blood is drawn from a donor, anticoagulated, and directed into a centrifuge where separation of the constituents takes place. The component in question is then selectively removed and directed into a collection bag and the rest of the blood components are returned to the donor. This usually involves a two-arm venipuncture technique, one arm used for removal and the other for return of the blood. Centrifugal apheresis therefore requires a considerable extracellular volume to fill the centrifugation device and the connecting tubes. At present there are two types of centrifugation devices: (a) *continuous*— IBM, Fenwal (Aminco and Celltrifuge II); and (b) *discontinuous*—Haemonetics Model 30, Haemonetics V 50. While operating on a similar principle, these machines differ somewhat in performance and will therefore be described in detail.

FENWAL CS-3000 CELL SEPARATOR

The Fenwal CS-3000 is a continuous flow cell separator developed by Fenwal Laboratories Inc., a division of Travenol Laboratories, Inc., Deerfield, Illinois. The machine was first marketed in the United States in 1979 and in Canada and Europe in 1981.

This cell separator does not involve use of a rotating seal, and in this respect differs from the IBM-2997 Continuous Cell Separator. The resultant continuous flow, closed system is thought to reduce the potential risk of contamination or leaks during cell or plasma collection. Whole blood is withdrawn from the donor through a multiple lumen tubing and is pumped into a separation container. During centrifugation blood in the separation container separates into component rich plasma and red cells. The component rich plasma is pumped into a collection container in which separation into plasma and cell components occurs. The desired product, either plasma or cells, is harvested using specific computer programs which have been developed and stored in the solid state memory of the cell separator. This separator is a highly automated instrument although it may be operated in the manual mode. A microcomputer monitors instrument operation, and donor/patient safety alarms are present in either the automated or manual modes of operation.

Standard operating protocols are available from the manufacturer for the following procedures: cell collection and cell depletion (granulocytes, platelets, lymphocytes), plasma exchange, and plasma collection (500 ml plasma may be obtained in combination with granulocyte or platelet collection).

Machine Characteristics

Physical characteristics are width, 60.9 cm; depth, 97.8 cm; height, 142.2 cm; and weight, 316 kg.

Advantages are (a) the setup is fast and easy, requiring only 10 min for trained personnel to set up this machine, and (b) the collection procedures, including automatic prime and line irrigation, and programed.

Disadvantages are (a) there is a high extracorporeal volume which differs for each procedure as indicated: plasma exchange, 440 ml; leukapheresis, 440 ml; plateletpheresis, 347 ml. (b) The CS-3000 is not easily transported. (c) Platelet rich plasma in the collection bag at the end of the plasma exchange must be agitated manually if the platelets are to be returned to the patient. The manufacturer recommends the return of platelets, as otherwise the patient's platelet count is decreased by 15 to 35%. (d) The anticoagulant must constantly be observed to be sure it is flowing, and the number of drops/minute must be manually counted to calculate anticoagulant:whole blood ratio. (e) Two venipunctures are required. Antecubital veins are preferred due to negative pressure in the return line when the centrifuge first starts. During plasma exchange replacement fluids are returned by gravity flow and large diameter needles are required to parallel the whole blood withdrawal rate. (f) The pumps are noisier than other cell separators.

Safety features include detectors for monitoring excess pressure in return and access lines, blocked lines, low level of anticoagulant, overheating, overspeed, unbalanced centrifuge, and humidity in the centrifuge. There is also a code to alert the operator if the safety sensors are not activated.

This machine is very new; therefore the actual potential has not yet been tested. It is conceivable that the introduction of new software programs will make it possible to selectively collect subpopulations of cells and make combined exchange-cell procedures easier.

IBM-2997 CELL SEPARATOR

The IBM-2997 Continuous Flow Cell Separator was developed by International Business Machines Corporation, Princeton, New Jersey and was first marketed in the United States in November 1977. This cell separator became available in Canada and Europe in June 1980.

The principle of this machine depends on the separation of blood into plasma and cellular components as the blood is centrifuged in a separation channel. Whole blood withdrawn from the donor/patient passes through a rotating face seal into the separation channel and is separated into plasma and cell components. Three exit ports allow collection of separated components from different radial positions in the collection chamber of the separation channel. Separation is done at 1,600 rpm.

Standard operating protocols are available from the manufacturer for the following procedures: cell collection (granulocytes, platelets, granulocyte/platelets, lymphocytes, neocytes), cell depletion (granulocytes, platelets, lymphocytes), plasma exchange, and red cell exchange.

Machine Characteristics

Physical characteristics are width, 101.6 cm; depth, 73 cm; height, 78.7 cm; and weight, 263 kg.

Advantages are (a) the extracorporeal volume is low, although this differs for each procedure: plasma exchange, 280 ml; leukapheresis, 280 ml; plateletpheresis, 150 ml. (b) Plasma exchange is fast: with a donor blood flow rate of 40–60 ml/min it takes 2 hr for a 3-liter exchange.

Disadvantages are (a) the setup and priming time is long and complex. The average setup time for a trained nurse is 40 min. (b) The machine is operator dependent. This is especially true for plateletpheresis procedures using the dual stage channel when constant operator observation is required to prevent red cell contamination and to achieve good yields. (c) The alarm is loud and sometimes provokes anxiety in nervous or first-time donors. (d) The separator is not easily transported. The machine must be set up by service personnel if moved any distance. This may take up to 4 hr. (e) There is an increased frequency of citrate toxicity during plateletpheresis collections. The anticoagulant:whole blood ratio is deliberately decreased during platelet collections using the Dual Stage Channel, and varies between 1:6 and 1:8 depending on the donor circulating blood volume and hematocrit. The calculated ratio is maintained until the donor experiences hypocalcemic symptoms continuously, for example, circumoral tingling, and the ratio is then increased. (f) Two venipunctures are always required.

Safety features include detectors for monitoring occluded veins, blocked veins, air in the lines, anticoagulant ratio limits, low intravenous fluid, and overheating or overspeed of the centrifuge.

The circuit breakers are poorly positioned at the front of the machine where the operator sits and therefore the circuits can easily be inadvertantly turned off.

HAEMONETICS 30/HAEMONETICS 30-S CELL SEPARATOR

The Haemonetics Model 30 and 30-S are discontinuous cell separators developed by Haemonetics Corporation, Braintree, Massachusetts. The separator was first marketed in the United States in 1973 and in Canada and Europe in 1975.

The most important component of this separator is a disposable plastic bowl in which blood is separated into plasma and cell components. Donor whole blood flows into a small pouch by gravity flow and is pumped from this pouch into the disposable centrifuge bowl via a rotating seal. Separation of blood into cell-free plasma, platelet or white cell concentrations, and packed red cells is possible; any or all of the first three components can be retained in sterile bags while returning red cells to the donor/patient. By repeating the cycle, several units of one or more cell components can be isolated. The Haemonetics 30 or 30-S Cell Separator is completely operator dependent.

These machines are used to collect cell concentrates including granulocytes, platelet, or granulocyte/platelet as well as for plasma exchange of patients.

Standard operating protocols are available from the manufacturer for the following procedures: cell collection (granulocytes, platelets, granulocyte-platelet concentrates, lymphocytes), cell depletion (granulocytes, platelets, lymphocytes), plasma exchange, plasma collection, and red cell exchange.

Machine Characteristics

Physical characteristics of the H30 are width, 38 cm; height, 208 cm; depth, 81 cm; and weight, 134 kg. Physical characteristics of the H30-S are width, 38 cm; height, 127 cm; depth, 81 cm; and weight, 125 kg.

Advantages are (a) the machine is easily transported. (b) The procedure can be completed through one venipuncture. (c) Donors/patients with small veins bleed better with gravity flow such as is possible with the H30-S rather than with negative pressure withdrawal of donor blood as seen with other machines. (d) Routine maintenance can be performed by trained operators. (e) This machine has proven reliability and durability—some machines are 8 years old; (f) Gravity flow reinfusion minimizes the risk of air embolism.

Disadvantages are (a) plasma exchange is slow; for example, a 3-liter exchange will take approximately 3–3½ hr with a donor blood flow rate of 40–60 ml/min. By comparison, the equivalent time for the IBM-2997 and Fenwal CS-3000 cell separators is 2 hr. (b) There is a large extracorporeal volume; for example, using the small bowl (225 ml) during a granulocyte collection, a 70-kg adult with a hematocrit of 45% would have a total extracorporeal volume of 475 ml per pass compared with 280 ml for the same individual during a leukapheresis procedure on the IBM-2997 cell separator.

TABLE 1. *Bleed rates and anticoagulant ratios*

Machine	Plasma exchange			Bleed rate (ml/min)
	Anticoagulant	WB: Anticoagulant	rpms	
IBM-2997	ACD-A	13:1	1,600	50–60
Fenwal CS-3000	ACD-A	13:1	1,400	40–50
Haemonetics 50	4% Na citrate solution	14:1	5,600	60–80
Haemonetics 30	ACD-A	8:1	4,800	60–80

TABLE 2. *Anticoagulant used per liter and collection time per liter*

Machine	Plasma exchange		Time/liter (min)
	Bleed rate (ml/min)	Anticoagulant used/liter (ml)	
IBM-2997	50	125	40
Fenwal CS-3000	50	120	34
Haemonetics 50	70–80	110	50

TABLE 3. *Constituents of the plasma removed during operation*

Machine	WBC ($\times 10^3/\mu l$)	Platelets ($\times 10^3/\mu l$)	Hct (%)	Platelets ($\times 10^{10}$)
IBM-2997[a]	<0.5	76.0 ± 59.0	<1	2.94 ± 2.3
Fenwal CS-3000[b]	<0.5	155 ± 51.0	<1	6.36 ± 2.4
Haemonetics 50[c]	<0.5	103 ± 47.5	<1	5.17 ± 2.4

[a]$N = 12.$
[b]$N = 6.$
[c]$N = 10.$

Safety features include (a) the pump stops automatically when there is excess pressure in the lines. (b) The machine shuts down automatically when the centrifuge overheats or overspeeds. (c) A cover interlock switch shuts down the centrifuge when the centrifuge cover is opened. (d) There are internal electrical sensors to prevent electrical shocks. There are no safety alarms on this machine.

We have used all these machines during plasma exchange procedures and report in Tables 1–3 our experience using these machines for treatment of various patients.

SUMMARY

Plasma exchange can be carried out using any of the various centrifugation devices. The advantage of using centrifugation rather than filtration techniques is the instrument's flexibility, which permits therapeutic removal of cells as well as plasma. The relative disadvantage, compared with filtration, is that higher flow rates can be maintained with many of the filtration techniques.

Plasmapheresis, edited by Y. Nosé, P. S.
Malchesky, J. W. Smith, and R. S. Krakauer.
Raven Press, New York © 1983.

Membrane Plasma Separation

P. S. Malchesky, A. Sueoka, S. Matsubara, J. Wojcicki,
and Y. Nosé

Department of Artificial Organs, Cleveland Clinic Foundation, Cleveland, Ohio 44106

Plasma separation from whole blood is performed routinely. Several million liters of plasma are collected annually in the United States for use in transfusion and in the production of plasma products (1). Within the past several years there has been reasonable success with plasma exchange for the treatment of various clinical disorders. This success has stimulated various clinicians and researchers to investigate plasma exchange in the treatment of a wide range of clinical disorders. The list of diseases treated encompasses nearly all phases of medical practice (2). Consideration of the increased factor or abnormality associated with various immunological diseases treated by plasmapheresis indicates that these molecules are of high molecular weight, and greater than the size of albumin which is the common replacement fluid (2). It is for this reason that plasmapheresis could be beneficial. When the plasma is separated from the whole blood and removed, the macromolecules are also removed. Therapeutic plasma exchange is still in a relatively early stage of development and controlled clinical trials are lacking in most instances. The majority of clinical trials to date have employed on-line centrifugal techniques.

CENTRIFUGAL VERSUS MEMBRANE SEPARATION

Centrifugal plasma exchange is a simple technique to apply clinically. It may be done manually or with automated equipment. With the use of automated equipment, blood is withdrawn from the patient into a bowl or collection bag, the plasma is separated in a continuous manner, and the blood cells are returned to the patient. Automated equipment is most commonly used in therapeutic applications and is most useful in the processing of larger volumes of plasma. While centrifugal plasma exchange has been shown to be an effective treatment modality for various disease states, certain limitations exist in chronic applications. Equipment costs are high and the equipment is generally too bulky to make it portable. The equipment utilized is relatively complex, requiring the control of multiple paramaters on a continuous basis. Also, the separation between the plasma and blood cells is not complete, and the plasma contains significant concentrations of blood cells, particularly platelets (3). Blood cell losses can be quite high if multiple plasma exchanges are required, and may be a consideration in the course of therapy. This is particularly important when on-line processing of the plasma by sorption or filtration is considered. In such instances interferences by cellular elements can seriously hinder the treatment process.

Membrane technology, which has advanced rapidly in the past decade, has provided an alternative to centrifugal techniques. Within the past 5 years the application of microporous membranes to the separation of plasma from blood has received considerable attention as evidenced by the increased number of publications in this field. Both flat plate and hollow fiber designs are now available. Plasma separation occurs by application of a low hydraulic pressure. Equipment requirements are relatively minimal (only a blood and plasma pump and pressure monitors are required) and the system can be made portable. Sieving properties of macromolecular weight plasma solutes are generally greater than 90%, while passage of blood cellular elements or debris is nil in most instances. Plasma flow rates of 15–70 ml/min are achievable for blood flow rates of 50–200 ml/min (which are typically used clinically). Studies carried out to date with membrane systems indicate that they can potentially be made cost competitive with centrifugal methods, especially when used in conjunction with on-line plasma treatment schemes. Despite the lack of controlled studies of plasma exchange and plasma treatment techniques for most disease states being investigated, marketing analyses point toward a sharp rise in the use of this technology. In addition, these analyses recommend membrane technology for the on-line separation of plasma, particularly when treatment of the plasma and its reinfusion is to be employed.

DIALYSIS VERSUS MEMBRANE PLASMA SEPARATION

Because the appearance of the membrane plasma separators is so similar to hemodialyzers and hemofilters, first-time investigators operate them similarly. Dialyzers require higher operating transmembrane pressures and have lower filtrate fluxes than membrane plasma separators. While in operation, hemofilters yield filtrate fluxes similar to those from membrane plasma separators, but do not pass plasma proteins appreciably and require higher operating transmembrane pressures. Figures 1 and 2 compare the differences between the membrane filtration devices. Because of these differences a host of problems were subsequently associated with their use (4). Particular considerations of plasma separation for a given membrane system are that: (a) high plasma separation rates with high sieving are possible at low transmembrane pressures, generally below 50 mmHg (5); (b) increasing transmembrane pressure leads to deterioration of plasma flux, sieving, and hemolysis (6); and (c) the nature of the blood and its cellular and macromolecule concentrations will greatly dictate operational limits (7).

Thus membrane and module properties, blood properties, and operating conditions must be considered in the optimal selection and operation of membrane plasma separators. The evaluation of the individual parameters is best made through standardized testing using various solutions including bloods. Both *in vitro* and *ex vivo* studies are required for the full characterization of the modules for use in the various clinical situations being considered (8).

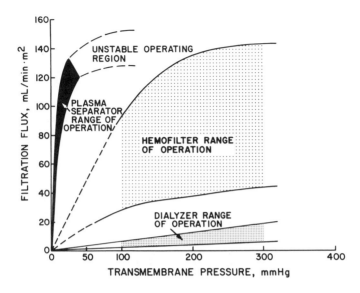

FIG. 1. Filtration flux as a function of transmembrane pressure for plasma separators, and ultrafiltration by hemofilters and dialyzers.

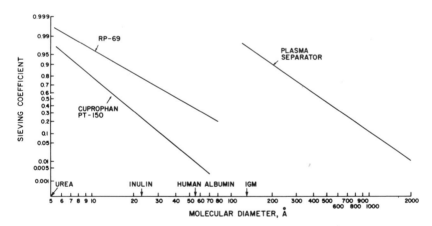

FIG. 2. Sieving as a function of molecular diameter for membranes used in plasma separation, hemofiltration (RP-69) and dialysis (Cuprophan PT-150). (Data for cuprophan PT-150 and RP-69 taken from Green et al., ASAIO, 22:627, 1976.)

MEMBRANE PLASMA SEPARATOR CONSIDERATIONS

Membrane Module Properties

Membrane properties for the various modules evaluated exhibit a wide range of differences with regards to polymer type, hydrophilicity, and microstructure (pore size and pore numbers). A given polymer type per se is not a unique requirement, and clinically acceptable plasma separators have been constructed with membranes of various composition including cellulose acetate, polyvinyl alcohol, polyolefins such as polyethylene and polypropylene, and polymethylmethacrylate. An individual polymer type may offer unique advantages in terms of operational features, cost, or biocompatibility. Candidate membranes must be hydrophilic or rendered hydrophilic, have a pore size adequate to allow the transfer of plasma solutes yet small enough to prevent the passage of blood cells, have adequate mechanical strength, exhibit low blood trauma and be free of pyrogens, and be sterilizable. Membrane structure for membranes of the same base polymer has been shown to be critically important to filtration and sieving properties (Table 1). Module properties of the various membrane plasma separators vary with regards to channel thickness, the number of parallel channels, channel length, and surface area.

In standardized *in vitro* (8) and *ex vivo* dog studies and in human studies, there are differences in filtration and sieving properties between the various modules and which are a function of the blood flow rate, channel dimensions, and the number of individual blood channels. But modules differ in the degree to which wall shear rate affects plasma flux (Fig. 3). Analysis of data obtained by Cleveland Clinic from the various plasma separators shows no correlation with concentration polarization theory as might be expected (Fig. 3) (9). Wall shear rate does not correlate to the one-third power and no correlation with length (from 14 to 29 cm) for a given membrane type has been seen. Comparison of the data with the deposition parameter theory (10) shows that wall shear rate to the three-halves power does not correlate even with membranes that produce hemolysis with the onset of deposition. At the point of maximal plasma flux where there is still high sieving and no hemolysis, the calculated deposition parameter is consistently higher by about an order of magnitude or more than that reported by Blackshear and Forstrom (Table 2). The inverse relationship of cell radius has been noted to correlate in comparing

TABLE 1. *Modules with membranes of same polymer type of varying porosity*

Property	Membrane type		
	F1	F2	F3
Module surface area, m²	1.1	0.77	0.63
Porosity (%)	41	64	67
Ultrafiltration coefficients at 25°C (ml/min-m²-mmHg)	1.0	18.5	20.4
Rejection (%) for particles:			
of 450 Å diameter	—	89	84
of 150 Å diameter	—	53	58
Maximum plasma flow rate (ml/min)	6	30	35
Sieving coefficient at Q_B = 100 ml/ min at maximum plasma flow rate			
Albumin	0.57	0.93	0.93
Total protein	0.51	0.90	0.89
Total cholesterol	0.22	0.73	0.76

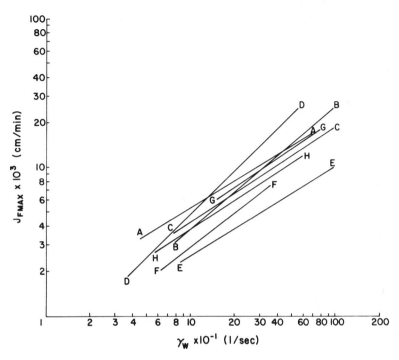

FIG. 3. Maximum plasma flux for various hollow fiber plasma separators as a function of average wall shear rate.

TABLE 2. *Results of in vitro studies with bovine blood at a blood flow of 100 ml/min (inlet hematocrit 30–40%)*

Module type	Maximum plasma flow rate (ml/min)	Sieving coefficient			D.P.[a] at inlet	Hematocrit at outlet	B parameter
		Total prot.	Albumin	Total cholesterol			
A	30–40	0.90–0.97	0.93–1.0	0.68–0.93	0.94–1.94	54–62	0.61
B	11–40	0.86–1.0	0.90–0.97	0.75–0.94	0.53–1.73	40–62	0.62–0.81
D	25–35	0.88–0.96	0.89–1.0	0.82–0.98	0.21–3.89	50–56	0.93
F	30–35	0.83–0.92	0.87–0.97	0.60–0.69	1.53	55–57	0.68–0.82
G	25–35	0.88–0.94	0.90–1.0	0.77–0.91	1.45–2.37	49–55	0.80–0.93
J	35–40	0.93–0.98	0.94–1.0	0.93–0.99	—	46–68	0.78

[a]D.P., deposition parameter.

bovine and dog blood; however, the correlation is not necessarily to the second power. The deposition parameter theory has been a useful guide to assess the axial changes in blood cell deposition (11) although the exact value of the parameter is variable and not reliable in design optimization.

Because of the importance of blood cell concentration on filtration flux and the effect of shear rate on blood cell dynamics, consideration of the effect of shear on blood cell distribution is important. Segre and Silberberg (12), working with dilute suspensions of rigid spheres, observed the phenomenon that rigid neutrally buoyant particles carried along in Poiseuille flow migrate to an equilibrium position from the axis. Thus two-way particle migration both away from the tube wall and the tube axis occurs, reaching equilibrium at an eccentric radial position. This phenomenon of particle migration is termed the "tubular pinch effect." Various investigators have studied this phenomenon and proposed theories to predict qualitatively the radial migration velocity. In general, the radial migration velocity is proportional to the wall shear rate squared and to the particle radius to the second to fourth powers, depending on particle size (13). Based upon the data available for particles the size of platelets and smaller, a power of 4 would be applicable, and for red and white cells a power of 3. Both values are higher than that given from the deposition parameter model.

Thus from consideration of the effect of wall shear rate alone, the data generated do not fit well with any of the above-mentioned theories with the shear rate dependency to the 0.6 to 0.9 power (Table 2). These theories, however, were not developed based upon the flow of a complex mixture such as blood or the filtration of a fluid such as plasma through membranes which would reject blood cellular elements while allowing all plasma components to pass.

In the evaluation of modules as candidates for plasma separation, distinct differences in their response to change in the plasma flow rate may be noted (8). In all modules there is a theoretical limit to the amount of plasma that can be extracted from the flowing blood. The unstability of plasma pumping is readily detected by an increase in the transmembrane pressure. With some modules the increased transmembrane pressure (a) is associated with the onset of hemolysis; (b) is not associated with hemolysis, and hemolysis occurs only at higher transmembrane pressures; and (c) may be associated with a decline in sieving for macromolecules in plasma. These differences appear to be closely related to membrane structure.

During extracorporeal circulation various hematologic changes can occur as changes in formed blood elements and activation of the coagulation and complement pathways. In the use of cellulose acetate hollow fiber modules and sorptive detoxification of the plasma with activated charcoal and an anionic resin for the treatment of hepatic insufficiency, leukopenia with complement activation was noted to occur (14). This occurrence was, however, less marked than that which occurs with standard hemodialysis using cellulosic membranes. In controlled *ex vivo* studies on dogs, decreases in total hemolytic complement (Fig. 4) and platelet count (with heparin as the anticoagulant) (Fig. 5) were noted for plasma separator modules containing varying polymer types (15). Changes in white blood cell counts (Fig. 6) were noted that appear related to the polymer type. While such changes occur and have been noted in the clinical studies of membrane plasma separators evaluated to date, they are not uniquely different from other extracorporeal devices with respect to biocompatibility. Due to the wide variance in patient populations poten-

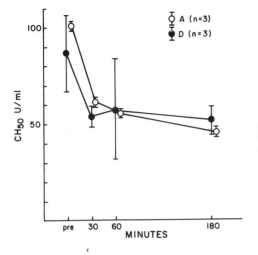

FIG. 4. Changes in total hemolytic complement (CH_{50}) as a function of perfusion time for two different polymer types of membrane plasma separators.

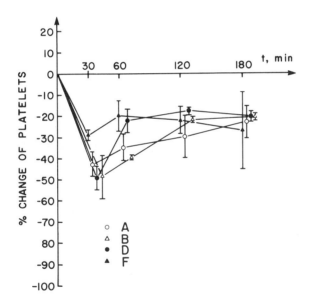

FIG. 5. Changes in platelet count in dogs as a function of perfusion time for different polymer types of membrane plasma separators.

tially treated with such devices, unique differences may be noted in the individual patient groups.

Blood Properties

For given membrane and module properties, the properties of blood and its concentrations of plasma solutes have been shown to affect the limits of the filtration

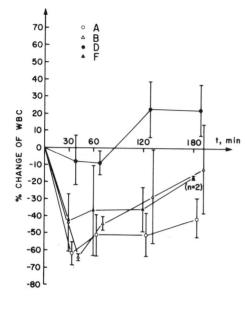

FIG. 6. Changes in white blood cell counts in dogs as a function of perfusion time for different polymer types of membrane plasma separators.

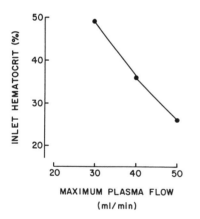

FIG. 7. Maximum plasma flow as a function of inlet hematocrit for one type of membrane plasma separator.

process. The maximal filtration rate is related to blood hematocrit (Fig. 7), and it is noted that for inlet hematocrits of 30–40%, outlet hematocrit approaches a maximum near 65% (Table 2). Support for the experimental evidence of a maximum in outlet hematocrit near 65% is given by the work of Tam (16) in which the drag on particles diverge as the particle concentration approached about 65%, by the calculations of Charm and Kurland (17) showing that the relative apparent viscosity sharply increased beyond an hematocrit of 60%, and by the work of Charm (18) showing that the marginal plasma layer decreases as the cell volume fraction decreases.

Devices meeting the clinical criteria of filtration and sieving have been shown to exhibit varying properties in pathologic states (Fig. 8) and with different com-

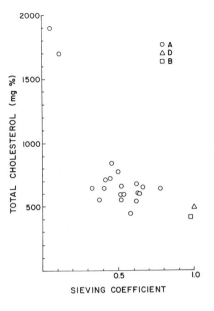

FIG. 8. Clinical sieving for total cholesterol as a function of total cholesterol content and for varying membrane module types in a patient with primary biliary cirrhosis.

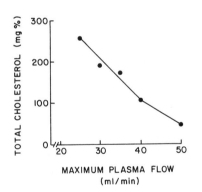

FIG. 9. Changes in the *in vitro* maximum plasma flow for a given membrane plasma separator with changes in total cholesterol concentration in bovine blood.

positions of blood (Fig. 9). Particularly noteworthy has been differences in total cholesterol sieving as related to membrane type, structure, and concentration.

Operating Conditions

For a given patient with set blood conditions and a given module type, the selection of operating conditions is of primary importance at the bedside in order to optimize the sieving of macromolecules and the plasma flux. Various considerations are the blood and plasma flow rates, maximum transmembrane pressure, position of module, and blood flow direction. *In vitro* evaluations coupled with clinical trials have been carried out to provide the guidelines for operation.

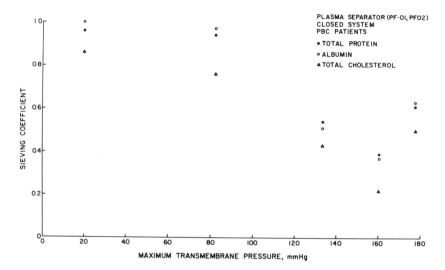

FIG. 10. Changes in sieving for total protein, albumin, and total cholesterol as a function of transmembrane pressure in patients with primary biliary cirrhosis.

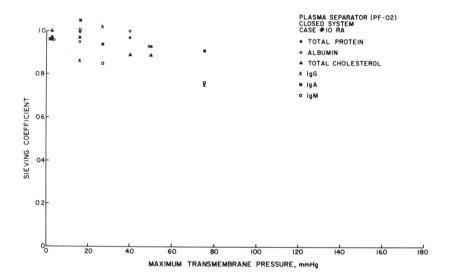

FIG. 11. Changes in sieving for total protein, albumin, total cholesterol, and the immunoglobulins G, A, and M as a function of transmembrane pressure in a patient with rheumatoid arthritis.

Unique differences exist among the available modules. The operational features of the Asahi plasma separators, which have been the modules predominantly used to date, are generally applicable (7,19). The filter is positioned vertically with blood flow downward. The plasma prime in the filtrate compartment should be kept to a minimum with plasma removal from the lower port. The plasma circuit should be closed with the plasma being pumped from the filtrate compartment, and the plasma flux should be selected to yield a blood outlet hematocrit of less than 65%. The maximum filtrate flow is best determined based upon empirical studies at a blood flow of clinical interest; however, operation should be at the lowest possible transmembrane pressure and generally less than 50 mmHg. Operation at low transmembrane pressures is also important to maintain high sieving (Figs. 10 and 11). In clinical operation, plasma flows may be lower than that achieved *in vitro* due to the specific disease state or to individual blood conditions. Stability of plasma pumping is best determined by monitoring the transmembrane pressure and regulation of the plasma flow rate (19).

CONCLUSIONS

Membrane plasma separation is a simple and efficient technique. It has been shown to be clinically acceptable and is the method of choice for the on-line treatment of plasma.

REFERENCES

1. Drees, T. C. (1979): Worldwide plasma supply and demand. *Plasma Forum*, edited by R. L. Crouch, p. 5. McNally & Loftin.
2. Malchesky, P. S., Asanuma, Y., Smith, J. W., Kayashima, K., Zawicki, I., Werynski, A., Blumstein, M., and Nosé, Y. (1981): Macromolecule removal from blood. *Trans. Am. Soc. Artif. Intern. Organs*, 27:439.
3. Chopek, M., and McCullough, J. (1980): Protein and biochemical changes during plasma exchange. *Therapeutic Hemapheresis*, edited by E. M. Berkman and J. Umlas, p. 13. American Association of Blood Banks, Washington, D.C.
4. Nosé, Y., and Malchesky, P. S. (1981): Technical aspects of membrane plasma treatment. *Artif. Organs*, 5(Suppl.):86.
5. Asanuma, Y., Smith, J. W., Suwa, S., Zawicki, I., Harasaki, H., Dixon, A. C., Malchesky, P. S., and Nosé, Y. (1979): Membrane plasmapheresis: Platelet and protein effects of filtration. *Proc. Eur. Soc. Artif. Organs*, 6:308.
6. Asanuma, Y., Malchesky, P. S., Zawicki, I., Smith, J. W., Carey, W. D., Ferguson, D. R., Hermann, R. E., and Nosé, Y. (1980): Clinical hepatic support by on-line plasma treatment with multiple sorbents. *Trans. Am. Soc. Artif. Intern. Organs*, 26:400.
7. Zawicki, I., Malchesky, P. S., Asanuma, Y., Smith, J. W., Kyo, A., Blumenstein, M., Shinagawa, S., Kayashima, K., and Nosé, Y. (1980): Quantitation of membrane plasma filtration. Presented at ISAO/IFAC Symp. on Automatic Control Aspects of Artificial Organs, Warsaw, Poland, Sept. 24–26, p. 87.
8. Werynski, A., Malchesky, P. S., Sueoka, A., Asanuma, Y., Smith, J. W., Kayashima, K., Herpy, E., Sato, H., and Nosé, Y. (1981): Membrane plasma separation: Toward improved clinical operation. *Trans. Am. Soc. Artif. Intern. Organs*, 27:539.
9. Blatt, W. F., Dravid, A., Michaels, A. S., and Nelson, L. (1970): Solute polarization and cake formation in membrane ultrafiltration: Cause, consequences and control techniques. In: *Membrane Science and Technology*, edited by J. E. Flynn, p. 47. Plenum Press, New York.
10. Forstrom, R. J., Bartelt, K., Blackshear, P. L., Jr., and Wood, T. (1975): Formed element deposition onto filtering walls. *Trans. Am. Soc. Artif. Intern. Organs*, 21:602.

11. Zawicki, I., Malchesky, P. S., Smith, J. W., Harasaki, H., Asanuma, Y., and Nosé, Y. (1981): Axial changes of blood and plasma flow, pressure, and cellular deposition in capillary plasma filters. *Artif. Organs*, 5:241.
12. Segre, G., and Silberberg, A. (1961): Radial particle displacements in Poiseuille flow of suspensions. *Nature*, 189:209.
13. Karnis, A., Goldsmith, H. L., and Mason, S. G. (1966): The flow of suspensions through tubes: V. Inertial effects. *Can. J. Chem. Eng.*, 44:181.
14. Malchesky, P. S., Asanuma, Y., Hammerschmidt, D. E., and Nosé, Y. (1980): Complement removal by sorbents in membrane plasmapheresis with on-line plasma treatment. *Trans. Am. Soc. Artif. Intern. Organs*, 26:541.
15. Matsubara, S., Malchesky, P. S., Shinagawa, S., and Nosé, Y. (1982): Preclinical evaluation of membrane plasma separation modules. *Abst. ASAIO*, 11:58.
16. Tam, K. W. (1969): The drag on a cloud of spherical particles in low Reynolds number flow. *Fluid Mech.*, 38:537.
17. Charm, S. E., and Kurland, G. S. (1972): Blood rheology. In: *Cardiovascular Fluid Dynamics*, edited by D. E. Bergel, p. 184. Academic Press, New York.
18. Charm, S. E., Kurland, G. S., and Brown, S. L. (1968): The influence of radial distribution and marginal plasma layer on the flow of red cell suspensions. *Biorheology*, 5:15.
19. Malchesky, P. S., Werynski, A., Asanuma, Y., Zawicki, I., Nosé, Y., Smith, J. W., Kayashima, K., and Gurland, H. (1981): Clinical operation of Asahi plasma separators. *Artif. Organs, 5 (Suppl.)*:113.

Plasmapheresis, edited by Y. Nosé, P. S. Malchesky, J. W. Smith, and R. S. Krakauer. Raven Press, New York © 1983.

An Evaluation of Polymethylmethacrylate Plasma Separator by Animal Experiment

Ichiro Iizuka, Zenya Yamazaki, Yoshizo Fujimori, Tatsuhiko Takahama, Fukuei Kanai, Tatsuo Wada, *Noboru Inoue, **Takeshi Sonoda, **Tachio Nogi, and **Mutsumi Kimura

*2nd Department of Surgery, University of Tokyo, Tokyo 113; *Department of Medicine, Oji National Hospital, Tokyo; **Toray Industry, Inc., Tokyo 103, Japan*

Membrane plasma separation is gaining increasing importance as a method of plasma exchange, which is one of the most promising therapies for hepatic failure (1–3), autoimmune diseases, and other disorders. Cellulose acetate membrane is already being used clinically, and new materials are being sought to obtain a membrane of higher blood compatibility and greater filtration efficiency.

Polymethylmethacrylate (PMMA) is a material of high blood compatibility which has less influence on the blood cells and platelets, and activates the complement system to a lesser extent than does cellulose membrane (4,5). It is now used clinically in hemodialysis for uremic patients. In this study, a newly developed plasma separator made of PMMA hollow fibers was evaluated for its efficiency to filtrate plasma and for blood compatibility.

MATERIALS AND METHODS

The plasma separator used was made of hollow fibers with a diameter of 370 μm, prepared from PMMA microporous membrane (maximum pore size 0.5 μm, thickness 85 μm). Three varieties of this device (Plasmax, Toray Industry, Inc., Tokyo, Japan) with total membrane areas of 0.5, 0.6, and 0.8 m^2 were employed. Extracorporeal circuits with V-V or A-V shunting were created on 20 adult mongrel dogs weighing 10–20 kg. The blood was introduced into the plasma separator, where it was separated into plasma and into blood rich in cellular components. The separated plasma was returned to the body without treatment after remixing. Heparin or sodium citrate was administered as anticoagulant.

Plasma separation was performed for 1–6 hr. The blood flow rate (Q_B) and the filtration pressure (transmembrane pressure, TMP) were in most cases kept at 100 ml/min and under 30 mmHg, respectively, and were changed on occasions to study the efficiency of plasma separation.

Serial blood and plasma samples were taken to compare the concentrations of protein components of the filtrated and the centrifuged plasma. Blood cell counts and several coagulation factors were also examined for blood compatibility.

In vitro studies of plasma separation using ACD blood were performed several times.

RESULTS

The change of plasma flux when the filtration pressure (TMP) was altered was studied by using a reservoir in the circuit, keeping the blood flow rate (Q_B) constant. The effect of TMP was small, plasma flux reached its maximum at the TMP of 25–30 mmHg and did not increase at higher TMP. Hemolysis was observed occasionally at a TMP greater than 50 mmHg.

Figure 1 shows the relationship of plasma flux and the blood flow rate (Q_B). Q_B had a great effect on the plasma flux, the increase of the latter being nearly proportional to the former under typical operating conditions. A smaller module with fewer fibers and smaller membrane area could produce nearly the same amount of plasma at the same Q_B.

Plasma flux was about 2 liters/hr under typical operating conditions; $Q_B = 6l/$ hr, TMP less than 30 mmHg, but usually around 10 mmHg. In other words, about 50% of the total plasma was extracted from the blood. Plasma flux decreased slightly with higher hematocrit levels. As long as Q_B was constant, there was no significant decrease in plasma flux during the experiments, which extended for up to 6 hr.

Table 1 presents the concentrations of various plasma proteins in plasma filtrated by the plasma separator and in plasma obtained from the whole blood by centrifugation at the same time. The concentrations are similar, regardless of the class of the proteins.

Figure 2 shows the sieving coefficients (concentration in filtered plasma/concentration in centrifuged plasma) and their change with the progress of plasma separation. Nearly 100% filtration is achieved for each protein investigated, and no signs of deterioration were observed.

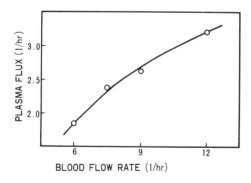

FIG. 1. Plasma flux versus blood flow rate for whole blood perfusion with 0.6-m² filter.

TABLE 1. *Composition of plasma proteins*

	Centrifuged plasma	Filtrated plasma
Total protein (g/dl)	5.7	5.5
β-Lipoprotein (mg/dl)	116	119
Fibrinogen (mg/dl)	356	350
A/G ratio	0.73	0.70

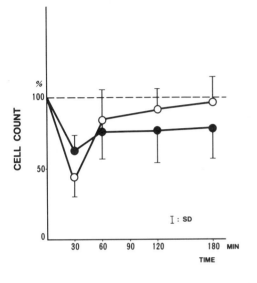

FIG. 2. Change of blood cells during plasma separation. *Open circles*, white blood cells; *filled circles*, platelets.

Hemolysis did not occur under the usual conditions of plasma separation with TMP under 30 mmHg, though it did occur occasionally when TMP was over 50 mmHg.

Figure 3 shows the change in the number of white blood cells and platelets during plasma separation. To rule out the effect of dilution by the priming fluid, the numbers were adjusted to the initial hematocrit values, which were taken as 100%. White blood cells rapidly declined by 50–60% (mean of 56% decrease at 30 min), returning to the initial level in about 1 hr. Platelets immediately decreased by 30–40% (mean of 38% decrease at 30 min) but were restored to about 80% of the initial value in 1 hr.

Fibrinogen decreased immediately after the beginning of plasma separation but the decline stopped after 15 min. In the experiments in which live animals were used, the decrease was about one-quarter of the initial level, but a much greater decrease was observed in the *in vitro* experiments. A certain amount of consumption was thought to take place and was estimated at about 130 mg per 0.1 m² of membrane surface. Prothrombin time was extended in the *in vitro* experiments, but there was no significant elongation in the animal experiments.

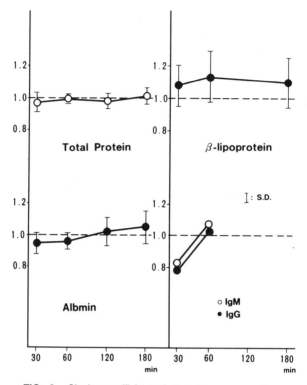

FIG. 3. Sieving coefficients during plasma separation.

Figure 4 gives the result of the assay of the 8th and 12th coagulation factors during plasma separation as measured by the method of Hardisty, with the average of several normal dogs taken as 100%. Both factors decreased to some extent in the *in vitro* experiments, but showed almost no change in the *ex vivo* studies.

The consumption of fibrinogen and coagulation factors occurred only at the beginning of plasma separation. There was a discrepancy in the extent of the decrease between the *in vitro* and the *ex vivo* experiments.

DISCUSSION

The clinical application of membrane plasma separators is plasma exchange for diseases such as hepatic failure and autoimmune disorders (1,2). In the future, it may be an important component of hepatic assist systems, extracting the plasma for treatments such as adsorption of harmful metabolites, and supplementing vital substances (3). For such purposes, the plasma separator must be capable of producing large amounts of plasma consistently for several hours. The filtrated plasma should have the same composition as the plasma in blood, that is, it should have

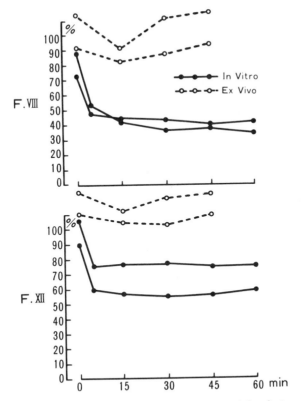

FIG. 4. Influence of plasma separation on coagulation factors.

sieving coefficient of 100%. Its influence on blood components should be as minimal as possible. Our investigation of the PMMA plasma separator focused on these points.

About 50% of total plasma was filtered out of the blood that went into the separator. Large amounts of plasma could be obtained by increasing the blood flow rate. This plasma-producing efficiency was nearly stable for up to 6 hr. Almost 100% of plasma proteins were filtered regardless of the nature or molecular size. This efficiency was also maintained throughout the experiments. Its fundamental efficiency in plasma separation thus proved to be excellent. The optimal filtration pressure was below 30 mmHg. Decreases in white blood cells, platelets, fibrinogen, and some coagulation factors were observed immediately after the beginning of plasma separation. This phenomenon has been reported frequently for white blood cells in hemodialysis (6,7). The degree of decrease of white blood cells was 50–60% in 30 min, and was restored almost completely to the initial level in about 1 hr. Though the restoration of platelets to the initial level was not complete, it was within the range in which no deterioration of coagulation would take place. Fibrinogen and the two coagulation factors examined in this study, Factors VIII and XII, seemed to be consumed on the membrane surface in the initial stage of plasma separation, but the decrease was not so great as to cause disorders in coagulation in normal animals. The large amount of blood in the animal's body and the animal's ability to compensate will explain the discrepancy in the degree of decrease between *in vitro* and *ex vivo* experiments.

These influences on blood cells and coagulation are probably not harmful to the normal subject because they are relatively slight, but one should be aware of such changes when employing this plasma separator on critically ill patients. Careful clinical evaluation is necessary.

CONCLUSION

PMMA membrane plasma separator has proved to have a high efficiency in plasma filtration. The large plasma flux and the membrane's near 100% sieving coefficient for various proteins were maintained throughout the experiments, which extended for up to 6 hr. Decreases in white blood cells, platelets, fibrinogen, and coagulation factors observed during the early stage of plasma separation appear to be within acceptable ranges for clinical use.

ACKNOWLEDGMENT

This study was supported by a grant for hepatic assist systems from the Industrial Technology Agency, Ministry of International Trade and Industry, Japan.

REFERENCES

1. Lepore, M. J., Stutman, L. J., Bonanno, C. A., Conclin, E. F., Robilotti, J. G., and McKenna, P. J. (1972): Plasmapheresis with plasma exchange in hepatic coma. *Arch. Intern. Med.*, 129:900.
2. Inoue, N., Yamazaki, Z., Fujimori, Y., and Sanjo, K. (1978): Clinical application of a new method for plasmapheresis using cellulose acetate hollow fiber as a plasma separator. (Japanese paper with English abstract.) *Jinko-zoki*, 7:1095.
3. Yamazaki, Z., Fujimori, Y., Sanjo, K., Kojima, Y., Sugiura, M., Wada, T., Inoue, N., Sakai, T., Oda, T., Kominami, N., Fujisaki, U., and Kataoka, K. (1978): New artificial liver support system (plasma perfusion detoxification) for hepatic coma. Proc. ISAO Vol. 1, 1977. *Artif. Organs*, 2:(suppl.) 273.
4. Hakim, R. M., and Lowrie, E. G. (1980): Effect of dialyzer reuse on leukopenia, hypoxemia and total hemolytic complement system. *Trans. Am. Soc. Artif. Intern. Organs*, 26:159.
5. Shibamoto, T., Matsui, N., Ozawa, K., Akiba, T., Yoshiyama, N., Nakagawa, S., Nomoto, T., and Kitaoka, T. (1981): Significance of serum β-thromboglobulin as a useful parameter of biocompatibility evaluation of dialyzer. (Japanese paper with English abstract.) *Jinko-zoki*, 10:98.
6. Kaplow, L. S., and Goffinet, J. A. (1968): Profound neutropenia during hemodialysis. *J.A.M.A.*, 203:1135.
7. Toren, M., Goffinet, J. A., and Kaplow, L. S. (1970): Pulmonary bed sequestration of neutrophils during hemodialysis. *Blood*, 36:337.

Plasmapheresis, edited by Y. Nosé, P. S.
Malchesky, J. W. Smith, and R. S. Krakauer.
Raven Press, New York © 1983.

Plasma Separation Using the Fenwal CPS-10™ Capillary Plasma Separator

D. H. Buchholz, J. Porten, M. Anderson, C. Helphingstine,
*A. Lin, *J. Smith, *M. Path, *J. McCullough, and **E. Snyder

*Fenwal Laboratories, Division of Travenol Laboratories, Inc.,
Round Lake, Illinois 60073; *Department of Laboratory Medicine, School of Medicine,
University of Minnesota, Minneapolis, Minnesota 55455; **Department of Laboratory
Medicine, Yale University School of Medicine, New Haven, Connecticut 06510*

Fenwal Laboratories, Division of Travenol Laboratories, Inc., has recently developed a disposable hollow fiber plasma filtration system, the CPS-10™ capillary plasma separator, which permits removal of cell-free plasma from donor/patient blood without the need of a centrifuge. The CPS-10™ device, shown schematically in Fig. 1, consists of approximately 800 hollow microporous polypropylene fibers enclosed in a rigid plastic casing. Each fiber has a 150-μ wall thickness, a 330-μ lumen, and contains numerous microscopic pores with a maximum diameter of ≅0.55 μ; total surface area is 0.17 m². When blood is pumped through the fibers at appropriate shear rates, plasma passes through the fiber pores and can be collected while the remaining blood elements are returned to the donor/patient. The present study was undertaken to establish the safety and efficacy of use of the CPS-10™ capillary plasma separator for both normal donor plasma collection and therapeutic plasma exchange. Since the "washout" associated with therapeutic plasma exchange may obscure subtle laboratory test findings, normal donors were extensively studied to detect the occurrence of coagulation, hematologic, or chemical changes consequent to exposure of donor blood to the device. After device safety was established, the CPS-10™ capillary plasma separator was also used to perform therapeutic plasma exchange transfusion.

MATERIALS AND METHODS

The studies described herein were performed as part of an experimental plan outlined in Investigational Device Exemption G810183 filed with the Bureau of Medical Devices, United States Food and Drug Administration. The study was approved by local institutional review boards at both Yale University and the University of Minnesota. Both normal volunteers as well as patients undergoing therapeutic plasma exchange were studied; informed consent was obtained from study participants in all instances.

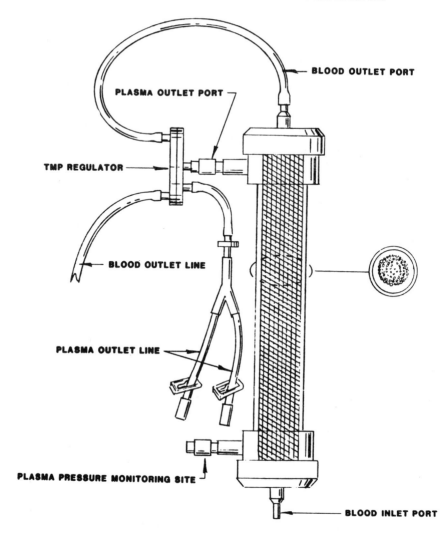

FIG. 1. CPS-10™ capillary plasma separator with TMP regulator.

The blood processing pathway and the CPS-10™ capillary plasma separator were primed with 0.9% sodium chloride injection prior to use. Each device and tubing set was used once and discarded. Following device priming, bilateral venipunctures were performed and blood was initially perfused through the collection system at 40 ml/min. After a period of approximately 5 min, blood withdrawal was increased to an arbitrarily selected rate of 70 ml/min and maintained at that rate throughout the remainder of the collection or exchange procedure. In most instances, blood was prevented from clotting using anticoagulant citrate dextrose (ACD) NIH formula

A, mixed with blood in a ratio of ≅1:13. In selected procedures sodium heparin USP (≅4,000 units) was used in place of ACD.

During plasma collection procedures (N = 43), sufficient blood was processed to harvest ≅550 ml of plasma; 10 normal donor sham plasma exchange procedures were also performed to study device performance over time, following which 12 therapeutic plasma exchange procedures were performed in patients with a variety of illnesses. Blood samples were obtained from the donor/patient before and after the procedure and from collected plasma at selected intervals for determining whether there were any hematologic, chemical, or coagulation test alterations resulting from exposure of the donor/patient blood to the CPS-10™ device and its associated blood pathway. Throughout these studies a prototype pump console containing two peristaltic pumps and a number of donor/patient safety monitors (hemolysis detector, air trap/bubble detector, occluded inlet vein sensor, system high pressure detector) was used. At the completion of each procedure, saline was pumped through the processing system to return red blood cells to the donor/patient.

NORMAL DONOR PLASMA COLLECTION

During plasma collection procedures donor blood was processed at 60–70 ml/min (mean, 69 ml/min), and the rate of plasma collection averaged 23 ml/min. An average of 536 ml of plasma was harvested in a total procedure time of 36 min (mean volume of blood processed, 1.9 liters). Additional operational parameters are shown in Table 1. Hematologic, blood chemical, and coagulation test results are shown in Table 2. There was no evidence of red blood cell hemolysis (plasma hemoglobin in collected plasma averaged 1 mg/dl and ranged from 0 to 5 mg/dl) and the collected plasma was virtually without cellular contamination (mean of 1, 3, and 6 red blood cells, platelets, and white blood cells per μl, respectively).

Taking into account the expected dilution of collected plasma and postprocedure donor blood samples due to ACD (≅130 ml) and saline (≅600 ml) administered to the donor during the procedure, there were no unexpected laboratory results noted in collected plasma or postdonation samples. In particular, coagulation Factors V, VII, VIII, and IX along with albumin and immunoglobulins G, A, and M appeared to pass the micropores of the hollow fiber device with ease.

NORMAL DONOR SHAM PLASMA EXCHANGE

In addition to the plasma collection studies, 10 2–3-liter sham plasma exchange procedures were performed in normal donors to establish device performance characteristics under conditions in which 4–7 liters of blood were processed. Separated plasma was collected, samples obtained, and the autologous plasma returned to the donor. Blood was processed at a mean rate of 69 ml/min and plasma was harvested

TABLE 1. *CPS-10™ capillary plasma separator operational parameters*

Parameters	Plasma collection (N = 43)		Sham exchange (N = 10)		Therapeutic exchange (N = 12)	
	Mean	Range	Mean	Range	Mean	Range
Whole blood flow rate (ml/min)	69	60–70	69	60–70	65	40–80
Blood volume processed (liters)	1.9	1.3–3.3	4.9	4.2–6.9	8.5	3.4–17.1
Plasma volume removed (liters)	0.54	0.37–0.60	1.7	1.5–2.0	3.4	1.3–6.7
Fluid volume replaced (liters)	0	—	1.7	1.5–2.0	3.7	2.0–6.5
Total procedure time (min)	36	25–60	81	69–96	142	67–261
Plasma separation rate (ml/min)	23	12–29	22	15–26	25	17–34
Plasma extraction efficiency (%)	52	29–71	65	40–74	60	45–70
Patient diseases	—	—	—	—	Myasthenia gravis Multiple sclerosis Pemphigus Polymyositis	

at 22 ml/min (range, 15–26 ml/min, Table 1). No unexpected or medically significant changes in laboratory values were seen (data not shown).

THERAPEUTIC PLASMA EXCHANGE

Device safety and efficacy was further documented by performing therapeutic plasma exchange in 12 patients with a variety of diseases (Table 1). A mean of 3.4 liters of plasma (range, 1.3–6.7) was exchanged during 142 min (average plasma separation rate, 25 ml/min). In most instances 5% albumin was used as replacement fluid and an average of 3.7 liters was administered. All procedures were tolerated without difficulty.

ADVERSE REACTIONS

No patient suffered any untoward response from therapeutic plasma exchange performed using the CPS-10™ capillary plasma separator. All donors and patients tolerated the blood processing procedure well. In 4 of 65 procedures the donor/patient experienced transient symptoms consistent with a vasovagal reaction, while mild or moderate symptoms attributable to "citrate toxicity" were seen in 4 persons. Three of these occurred during sham plasma exchange in which an average of 350 ml of ACD-A was administered and returned to the donor with separated autologous plasma. No donor or patient developed symptoms consistent with severe citrate toxicity.

TABLE 2. *Plasma collection using the CPS-10™ capillary plasma separator*

Test	N	Donor preprocedure (mean)	Donor postprocedure (mean)	N	Collected plasma (mean)
Hematocrit (%)	34	44	45	20	0.7 (RBC/μl)
Platelet (× 10³/μl)	34	245	239	19	3.0 (PLT/μl)
WBC (× 10³/μl)	34	5.9	6.1	20	6.0 (WBC/μl)
% PMN	34	58	61		
Plasma hemoglobin (mg/dl)	33	5	2	32	1
Glucose (mg/dl)	19	89	86	19	225
BUN (mg/dl)	19	15	15	19	13
Total bilirubin (mg/dl)	20	0.6	0.5	20	0.4
LDH (U/liter)					
Yale[a]	10	364	338	10	247
U of Minn[b]	10	224	217	10	188
GOT (U/liter)	20	21	20	20	17
Calcium (mg/dl)	20	9.7	9.0	20	8.0
Inorganic phosphate (mg/dl)	20	3.8	3.4	20	2.9
Uric acid (mg/dl)	20	5.8	5.5	20	4.9
Alk. phos. (U/liter)					
Yale[c]	10	29	25	10	24
U of Minn[d]	10	130	115	10	107
Cholesterol (mg/dl)	16	171	147	15	99
Triglyceride (mg/dl)	5	119	100	5	86
Sodium (mEq/liter)	19	141	141	19	151
Potassium (mEq/liter)	19	4.4	4.3	19	3.6
Creatinine (mg/dl)	19	1.0	1.0	19	0.9
Total protein (g/dl)	26	7.0	6.1	24	5.7
Albumin (g/dl)	26	4.3	3.7	24	3.5
Globulin (g/dl)	26	2.8	2.4	24	2.3
IgG (mg/dl)	20	976	847	20	757
IgA (mg/dl)	20	167	143	20	127
IgM (mg/dl)	20	141	115	20	103
PT (sec)	23	11.9	12.3	23	13.0
PTT (sec)	23	37.7	40.9	23	35.0
Fibrinogen (mg/dl)	19	208	177	19	214
FDP (μg/dl)	17	<10	<10	17	<10
Factor V (U/dl)	20	102	88	20	98
Factor VII (U/dl)	20	79	74	20	82
Factor VIII (U/dl)	20	86	78	20	86
Factor IX (U/dl)	20	104	99	20	118

[a]Normal value = 200–600 U/liter.
[b]Normal value = 136–309 U/liter.
[c]Normal value = 10–70 U/liter.
[d]Normal value = 61–220 U/liter.
WBC, white blood cells; PMN, polymorphonuclear neutrophil; BUN, blood urea nitrogen; LDH, lactic acid dehydrogenase; GOT, glutamic oxaloacetic transaminase; PT, prothrombin time; PTT, partial thromboplastin time; FDP, fibrin/fibrinogen degradation products.

COMPLEMENT ACTIVATION

Complement activation with associated marked donor/patient peripheral blood granulocytopenia presumably secondary to pulmonary leukosequestration has been reported to occur during hemodialysis and extracorporeal bypass procedures and during normal donor granulocyte collection procedures utilizing filtration leukapheresis. To evaluate the possibility that the polypropylene membrane material used in the CPS-10™ device activates complement, absolute circulating granulocyte counts were determined at periodic intervals during normal donor plasma collection procedures using both ACD and heparin anticoagulation; no granulocytopenia was seen. To further evaluate complement activation, total hemolytic complement activity (CH_{50}), alternative pathway hemolytic activity (AP_{50}), C3 conversion (assayed by immunoelectrophoresis), and C5a activity (assessed via *in vitro* leukocyte aggregating activity) were quantified in the laboratory of Augustine P. Dalmasso, M.D., Professor of Laboratory Medicine and Pathology, University of Minnesota Medical School. Complement studies are summarized in Table 3 and indicate that no complement activation was seen in either ACD or heparin anticoagulated donor blood before or after passage through the CPS-10™ device. Collected ACD plasma showed a similar lack of complement activation as assessed by each of the four assays. Some C3 conversion was seen in heparinized collected plasma, although none was detected in the donor. A number of the heparin plasma samples in which C3 conversion was demonstrated contained variable amounts of fibrin, suggesting inadequate sample anticoagulation. It is known that blood coagulation can induce

TABLE 3. *Changes in complement during blood processing with the CPS-10™ capillary plasma separator*

	ACD anticoagulation $(N = 5)$[a]		Heparin anticoagulation $(N = 4)$	
	CH_{50}	AP_{50}	CH_{50}	AP_{50}
Donor preprocedure	82 ($\pm$21)	18 ($\pm$3.1)	68 ($\pm$12)	18 ($\pm$2.9)
Donor postprocedure	77 ($\pm$20)	18 ($\pm$2.7)	68 ($\pm$16)	21 ($\pm$1.3)
Collected plasma	69 ($\pm$17)	17 ($\pm$2.6)	58 ($\pm$7)	16 ($\pm$1.3)
6 min				
Device inlet	69 ($\pm$14)	17 ($\pm$2.2)	59 ($\pm$18)	19 ($\pm$2.1)
Device outlet	73 ($\pm$25)	17 ($\pm$1.2)	67 ($\pm$10)	19 ($\pm$2.5)
16 min				
Device inlet	77 ($\pm$19)	18 ($\pm$2.8)	65 ($\pm$6)	19 ($\pm$1.7)
Device outlet	81 ($\pm$24)	18 ($\pm$3.1)	61 ($\pm$12)	18 ($\pm$1.5)
Collected plasma	64 ($\pm$15)	16 ($\pm$2.1)	54 ($\pm$5)	17 ($\pm$3.6)
21 min				
Device inlet	74 ($\pm$17)	18 ($\pm$2.7)	70 ($\pm$13)	19 ($\pm$1.6)
Device outlet	70 ($\pm$20)	18 ($\pm$2.2)	58 ($\pm$10)	18 ($\pm$0.5)
Collected plasma	74 ($\pm$24)	18 ($\pm$2.6)	60 ($\pm$3)	17 ($\pm$1.9)
26 min				
Device inlet	79 ($\pm$12)	19 ($\pm$1.9)	68 ($\pm$10)	18 ($\pm$2.5)
Device outlet	79 ($\pm$16)	19 ($\pm$3.1)	61 ($\pm$14)	19 ($\pm$1.3)
Collected plasma	78 ($\pm$15)	18 ($\pm$2.5)	60 ($\pm$4)	18 ($\pm$2.1)

Units expressed as mean and standard deviation.
[a]CH, classical pathway; AP, alternative pathway.

changes in the complement system, and studies are currently under way to understand the magnitude of coagulation-induced C3 conversion.

SIEVING COEFFICIENTS

In an effort to evaluate device performance over time, sieving coefficients for various blood parameters were determined. If a given molecular species freely passes the membrane pores, the amount seen in the collected plasma will be identical to that found in the blood entering the device, and the sieving coefficient will equal 1.00. Allowing for laboratory assay variability, sieving coefficients of 0.95–1.05 would be expected if there were no hindrance to passage of a given constituent, while lesser values would be seen for substances passing through membrane pores less easily.

TABLE 4. *CPS-10™ capillary plasma separator sieving coefficient (SC) values*

	Plasma collection: samples drawn after 200 ml plasma collected (N = 10)			
	SC			SC
Cholesterol	0.85	IgM		1.05
Total protein	0.97	IgA		0.97
Albumin	0.99	Factor V		0.88
IgG	0.99	Factor VII		1.00
		Factor VIII		0.97
		Factor IX		1.00

	Sham plasma exchange: samples drawn after 400–500 ml plasma collected (N = 10)			
	SC			SC
Cholesterol	0.95	IgM		1.01
Triglyceride	0.92	IgA		0.99
Total protein	0.99	Factor V		1.07
Albumin	1.03	Factor VII		0.97
Fibrinogen	1.06	Factor VIII		0.98
IgG	0.99	Factor IX		1.17

	Patient plasma exchange: samples drawn after 1,000 ml plasma collected			
	N	SC	N	SC
Cholesterol	9	0.99	IgM	11	1.00
Triglyceride	11	0.92	IgA	5	0.98
Total protein	5	0.96	Factor VIII	6	0.96
Albumin	5	0.94			
Fibrinogen	5	1.24[a]			
IgG	5	1.02			

[a]Suspected technical problem with assay.

TABLE 5. *Changes in sieving coefficients over time during therapeutic plasma exchange with the CPS-10™ capillary plasma separator*

	Plasma volume separated		
Plasma component	1,000 ml	3,000 ml	5,000 ml
Cholesterol	1.04 (4)	0.98 (4)	0.89 (3)
Triglyceride	0.94 (6)	0.89 (6)	0.86 (3)
IgM	1.03 (6)	1.00 (6)	0.91 (3)
Factor VIII	0.96 (6)	0.95 (1)	1.14 (1)

Number studied indicated in parentheses.

Sieving coefficients of various plasma components determined after 200, 400–500, 1,000, 3,000, and 5,000 ml of plasma had passed through the CPS-10™ device are summarized in Tables 4 and 5. As can be seen, most values are within ±0.10 of the theoretical value of 1.00, suggesting that even large molecular weight substances such as IgM and Factor VIII pass through the polypropylene fiber pores with ease. Even following separation of up to 5,000 ml of plasma during therapeutic plasma exchange, decline in device performance was minimal as reflected by sieving coefficient determination.

DISCUSSION

The above studies summarize and document the safety and efficacy of the CPS-10™ capillary plasma separator for use in the collection of normal donor plasma and for therapeutic plasma exchange. The constituent components present in separated plasma are nearly identical to those present in plasma before passage through the device, and as such, separation by membrane plasmapheresis techniques appears no different than that seen with centrifugal blood cell separators or Blood Pack units. No unexpected or medically significant changes in hematologic, blood chemistry, or coagulation test results were seen in donors or patients undergoing blood processing with the device. Collected plasma was virtually cell-free and did not differ significantly in the amount of albumin, globulin, IgG, IgA, IgM, Factor V, Factor VII, Factor VIII, and Factor IX when compared with predonation values after allowance for procedure-induced dilution with saline and ACD. Complement was not activated in pre- or postfilter donor blood using either heparin or ACD anticoagulation as assessed by changes in absolute granulocyte count, CH_{50}, AP_{50}, C3 conversion, and leukocyte aggregating (C5a) activity, nor was there evidence of complement activation in collected ACD plasma. All donors and patients tolerated exposure to the device without difficulty and no unexpected untoward donor/patient responses were seen. In summary, the CPS-10™ capillary plasma separator appears safe and efficacious for both normal donor plasma collection and therapeutic plasma exchange.

Plasmapheresis, edited by Y. Nosé, P. S. Malchesky, J. W. Smith, and R. S. Krakauer. Raven Press, New York © 1983.

Reuse of Membrane Plasma Filters

Horst Klinkmann, Eberhard Schmitt, Dieter Falkenhagen, Reinhard Schmidt, Bernd Osten, Peter Ahrenholtz, and Dieter Tessenow

University of Rostock, Klinik für Innere Medizin, DDR-25 Rostock 1, German Democratic Republic

Though still in the early stages of clinical application, the high cost of plasma exchange using plasma filters has imposed serious limitations on its availability and use in many countries.

These excessive costs are largely the result of the expensive homologous replacement solution and the recent high prices of membrane plasma filters.

In the literature there are a number of papers concerning the problem of the replacement solution. Studies, however, on the possibility of reusing plasma filters are very rare. It is our aim here to describe the reuse technique we have devised and to discuss the possibilities of reusing plasma filters.

METHODS AND RESULTS

To approach a possible technique for reuse, several basic properties of the plasma filters currently available for clinical use must be considered: (a) During treatment, the filtration rate decreases to varying degrees even when the transmembrane pressure (TMP) is kept constant. (b) Depending on the type of filter used, there can be a decrease over time in the sieving coefficient, even if the filtration rate is kept constant. (c) In order to maintain filtration rate, the TMP must often be increased, yet in all filters investigated, the TMP had to be limited to 100–150 mmHg because of the high risk for hemolysis.

The plasma filters used for this study were two filters with cellulose diacetate membrane (Plasmaflo, Asahi). One filter with a polypropylene membrane (Plasmaflux, Fresenius) and one experimental device with a polyethylene membrane (Cordis Dow Corp.).

We found that the main reasons for deterioration under clinical conditions were (a) obstruction of membrane pores by formed elements of the blood and protein absorption; and (b) formation of a secondary membrane on the inner membrane surface consisting of high concentrated gelled protein and a cell layer of blood constituents. Figure 1 shows a cell layer that formed after a 2-hr clinical application and a complete retransfusion of blood from the filter to a patient without anemia.

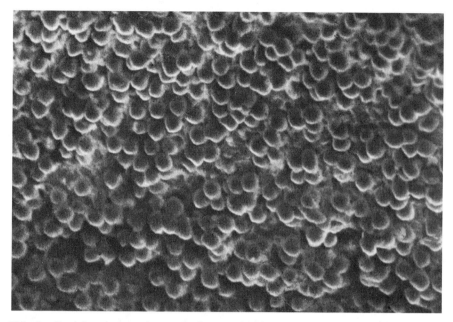

FIG. 1. Scanning electron microscope photograph of the "inner membrane" of a polypropylene membrane after 2 hr of clinical use and completed retransfusion to the patient.

To further investigate the obstruction of membrane pores and the formation of secondary membrane, two *in vivo* experiments were performed. In studying the efficiency of these plasma filters during prolonged clinical applications in acute hepatic coma in combination with an absorption device, we found that final capacity is not reached when the TMP in the filters is kept below 50 mmHg (Fig. 2). This figure demonstrates the mean values of four individual treatments with an overall mean filtration of 12.7 liters at a constant TMP of 40 mmHg. With respect to the seiving properties the decrease in efficiency is only about 10%.

Contrary to the results with our experimental device with the TMP increased to above 50 mmHg with 80 mmHg as an upper limit, the filtration rate could be kept constant as well, but the sieving coefficient dropped sharply (Fig. 3).

We concluded from these experiments that the possibility of reusing plasma filters differs with individual filters and depends largely on their first performance.

Our reuse technique is as follows: (a) After a complete reinfusion of the remaining blood from the filter to the patient, the filter is immediately rinsed with tap water for 10 mins. (b) For 30 min a reversed filtration from the filtrate compartment to the blood compartment is applied. (c) The filter is then primed with a 3% formaldehyde solution and stored. (d) Just before reuse another filtration procedure—this time in the direction from the blood compartment to the filtrate compartment—is carried out, using 4 liters of sterile 0.9% NaCl. The filtration procedure is interrupted several times by intermittent rinsing of the blood compartment with the same solution.

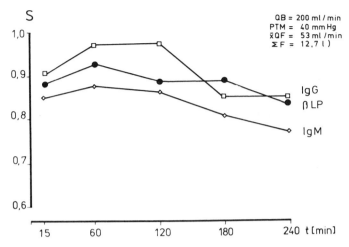

FIG. 2. Sieving coefficients during clinical application with constant TMP below 40 mmHg. Plasmasorption (Plasmaflux), $N = 4$.

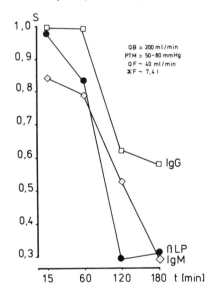

FIG. 3. Sieving coefficients during clinical applications with a TMP above 50 mmHg. Plasmasorption (CD-Plasmafilter), $N = 1$.

One important factor to be pointed out is that in filters with hydrophilic membranes which are originally hydrophobic, such as polypropylene and polyethylene, air contact with the membrane must be strictly avoided during the entire procedure. Before application such membranes have to be made hydrophilic by means of alcohol (e.g., ethanol, polyethyleneglycol). After the aqueous phase hydrophilicity will be lost when the membrane is in contact with air. If this happens, however, the hydrophilic property can be reestablished by incubating the membrane with 60% ethanol for 10 mins, followed by another rinsing procedure as described above.

Some preliminary clinical data on reused plasma filters are shown in Fig. 4. This figure demonstrates that there is only a slight difference between the four filters investigated in their efficiency during the first application. The differences in efficiency during clinical reuse can be clearly seen in Fig. 5. The device (no. 1) in which the TMP could be kept at approximately 30–40 mmHg during the first application as well as during the reuse, had sufficient efficiency. The other device (no. 2), which had a TMP above 50 mmHg in the first use and a TMP around 100 mmHg in the second use, had a distinct loss in efficiency during reuse for the parameters investigated. These results obviously do not depend on the different branches of filters used.

Figure 6 shows the result in reuse of three Asahi filters that require a high TMP during their first use. The loss in efficiency was as high as 30–70% during their clinical reuse.

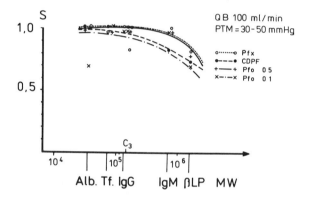

FIG. 4. Comparison of efficiency of four different plasma filters during clinical application. TMP is kept below 50 mmHg. Plasmafiltration, $N = 4$.

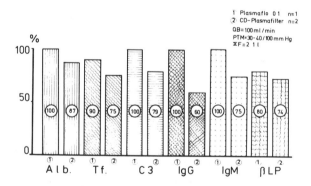

FIG. 5. Comparison of the loss of efficiency in reuse(s) in dependence from the TMP during first use. No. 1, TMP below 50 mmHg; no. 2, TMP above 50 mmHg.

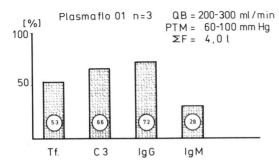

FIG. 6. Loss of efficiency during reuse in three plasma filters which needed a high TMP (60–100 mmHg) during first use.

CONCLUSIONS

During reuse no side effects in patients were observed. High TMP during the first use eliminates almost the possibility of reusing the same filter. A small decrease in efficiency can easily be compensated for by a prolonged treatment time. In hydrophobic membranes, air contact must be avoided in the preparation process for reuse.

We believe that reuse is generally possible but limited by several factors, and is at present certainly more cumbersome and complicated than the reuse of dialyzers. In our opinion, however, it is possible, and some general conclusions can be drawn from the experiences in reusing filtration devices, be they dialyzers, hemofilters, or plasma filters. If a device does not function properly in its first use, it is unlikely to be reusable. Therefore, the reuse possibility of a device depends upon a certain quality level as necessitated by its clinical application.

SUMMARY

Four plasma filters were investigated for reuse in clinical application. A special reuse technique is described. Filters requiring high TMP during the first use showed the highest loss of efficiency (up to 70%) during reuse and should be excluded. Filters in which the TMP could be kept below 50 mmHg during the first application showed only a very slight decrease in their efficiency during reuse. Despite the limitations described in this paper, plasma filters are reusable in clinical application.

BIBLIOGRAPHY

1. Jones, J. V. (1977): Plasmapheresis: Great economy in the use of horses. *N. Engl. J. Med.*, 297(21):1173.
2. Lockwood, C. M. (1979): Plasma exchange: an overview. *Plasma Ther.*, 1(1):1.
3. Frohlich, C. H., and Schneider, W. (1980): Plasmapherese: Therapeutische moglichkeiten. *Diagnostik und Intensivetherapie*, 5:89.
4. Ioue, N., Yamazaki, Z., Sakai, T., Kanai, K., Oda, T., Yoshiba, M., Fujiwara, K., Sanjo, K., Miake, A., Matsueda, K., Kominaga, N., and Kataoka, K. (1979): A new method for plasmapheresis using cellulose acetate hollow fibers as a plasma separator. *Artif. Organs*, 3:18 (abstr.).
5. Malchesky, P. S., Asanuma, Y., Zawicki, I., Blumenstein, M., Kyo, A., Calabrese, L., Krakauer,

R., and Nosé, Y. (1980): On line separation of macromolecules by membrane filtration with cryogelation. *Artif. Organs*, 4(3): 205.

6. Schmitt, E., Falkenhagen, D., Preussner, S., Tessenow, W., Holtz, M., and Klinkmann, H. (1980): Plasma separation (PS) and plasmapheresis (PP)—A comparative study. In: *Plasma Exchange*, edited by H. G. Sieberth, p. 99. Schattauer Verlag, Stuttgart, New York.

7. Sieberth, H. G. (1980): The elimination of defined substances from the blood and from separated plasma. In: *Plasma Exchange*, edited by H. G. Sieberth, p. 29. Schattauer Verlag, Stuttgart, New York.

8. Sieberth, H. G., Glockner, W., Hirsch, H. H., Borberg, H., Dotzauer, G., and Mathieu, P. (1980): Plasmaseparation mit hilfe von membranen-untersuchungen am menschen. *Klin. Wochenschr.*, 58:551–556.

9. Samtleben, W. (1981): Klinische aspekte zur membranplasmaphereses. In: *Plasma Exchange*, edited by H. J. Gurland, V. Heinze, and H. A. Lee, p. 23. Springer Verlag, Berlin, Heidelberg, New York.

Plasmapheresis, edited by Y. Nosé, P. S.
Malchesky, J. W. Smith, and R. S. Krakauer.
Raven Press, New York © 1983.

Factors Governing Mass Transport in Filters for Membrane Plasmapheresis

Michael J. Lysaght and *Matthias Schmidt

*Nephrology Division, Klinikum Grosshadern, University of Munich D-8000 Munich 70;
*Fachbereich Humanmedizin der Johann Wolfgang Goethe-Universität
D-6000 Frankfurt 70, Federal Republic of Germany*

The rapid evolution of membrane plasmapheresis over the past several years is in distinct contrast to the three preceding decades during which this technology lay dormant. The concept of membrane plasmapheresis is certainly old, and membranes with pores suitably sized to pass the plasma proteins and retain the formed elements have been available at least since the late 1940s. Progress was likely retarded by the almost universal consequences of casually filtering whole blood through such microporous membranes: hemolysis, plugging, and flux decay. Blatt et al. (1) appear to have been the first group to discover that such hemolysis and plugging could be avoided under special conditions of blood flow and channel geometry. In their 1972 patent (1), they disclosed a thin channel microporous membrane filter with tangential blood flow, and they specified the allowable ranges of velocities, transmembrane pressures, channel heights, and membrane pore sizes. Although strictly empirical and primarily intended for collection of plasma samples for subsequent analysis, their criteria apply to the larger devices currently employed for therapeutic and donor plasmapheresis.

In 1976 Castino et al. described the development of a microporous membrane device for blood detoxification at the Cleveland Clinic (2,3). The separated plasma was not collected as a discrete product but rather percolated through a layer of charcoal sandwiched between two microporous membrane sheets. Castino et al. based their design on the "deposition parameter" concept described by Forstrom and Blackshear 1 year earlier (4), and thus became the first to employ quantitative mass transfer theory to the problems of blood–plasma separation by microporous membranes. The year 1976 also saw the beginning of an NIH sponsored program conducted by the American Red Cross and Amicon corporation and aimed at evaluating the feasibility of large-scale donor plasmapheresis. Detailed transport studies were conducted, and the relationships between shear rate, filtration velocity, transmembrane pressure, and hemolysis were determined (5–8). Both the Cleveland Clinic's work and the Red Cross–Amicon project were based on the hypothesis that certain conditions of design and flow would lead to formation of a cell-free layer of plasma adjacent to the surface of the filtering membrane. Cells were thought to be excluded from this so-called skimming layer by radially directed forces whose magnitude increases with shear rate. Hemolysis-free filtration was possible only when these radial forces exceeded the oppositely directed Stokes law drag forces. The force balance was quantified in terms of the deposition parameter.

In 1978, the Asahi (Tokyo, Japan) hollow fiber plasma filters became available on a limited basis, and in 1980 Fresenius (Oberursel, FRG) introduced a hollow fiber plasma filter based on the Membrana (Wuppertal, FRG) polypropylene fibers. The design of these products does not appear to have been strongly influenced by previous work.

A number of additional studies on mass transfer in plasmapheresis have been undertaken. Chmiel has presented performance data at low wall shear rates (< 200 sec^{-1}) as well as studies on the radial distribution of erythrocyte density during capillary flow (9). Farrell et al. (10) and Schindhelm et al. (11) present kinetic data at medium shear rates (200–600 sec^{-1}) and also summarize time-dependent effects. Friedman et al. (12) have recently published the *in vitro* whole blood sieving coefficients and flux rates for a wide spectrum of commercially available microporous membranes. Randerson et al. (13) combine a comparison of *in vivo* and *in vitro* sieving coefficients for commercial plasma filters with a worthwhile discussion of methodological exactitude in the measurement of sieving coefficients. Asanuma et al. (14), Nosé et al. (15), and Werynski et al. (16) give the optimal operating conditions for available plasma filters compared with expectations from deposition parameter theory. They also provide a numerical integration of flow-dependent parameters to allow calculation of the deposition parameter at a point along the surface of a hollow fiber membrane (17). Solomon (18) recently analyzed polarization in plasmapheresis, especially the tendency of any rejected solute to form a secondary membrane which can reduce the sieving coefficients for smaller, normally unrejected cosolutes. Blackshear et al. (19) have provided an expanded treatment of his deposition parameter, and Drake and Eckstein (20) have recently published pertinent mechanistic studies of platelet and erythrocyte behaviour during blood filtration. In this chapter, we (a) summarize and correlate available data on filtration kinetics during plasmapheresis, (b) compare the performance of existing plasma filters with theoretical expectations, and (c) point out some of the problems with the skimming layer hypothesis and develop an alternative model.

FILTRATION KINETICS

Performance of Commercial Plasma Filters

To date (March 1982), three plasma filters are commercially available: The Plasmaflo I, the Plasmaflo II, and the Plasmaflux. Full design parameters and typical performance data for these filters are summarized in Table 1. All are hollow fiber designs; the Plasmaflo employ a cellulose-diacetate fiber, while the Plasmaflux is based on a polypropylene fiber. Area is about 0.5 m^2, fiber diameter is 320 μm.

TABLE 1. *Properties of commercial plasma filters*

Property	Plasmaflo I	Plasmaflo II	Plasmaflux
Area (m²)	0.75	0.5	0.5
No. of fibers	3,650	3,250	2,400
Inner diameter (μm)	360	320	320
Device length (cm)	28	26	25
Exposed fiber length (cm)	18	16	20
At inlet Q_B = 100 ml/min			
Filtration rate (ml/min)[a]	36	36	36
Filtration velocity (10^{-3} cm/min)[a]	5	7	7
Luminal velocity (cm/sec)[b]	0.4	0.5	0.7
Wall shear rate (sec⁻¹)[b]	80	130	180

[a]Maximum value.
[b]Average of inlet and outlet values.

TABLE 2. *Sieving coefficients in membrane plasmapheresis*

		Sieving coefficients	
Solute	MW	Nuclepore 0.4 μm	Membrana fiber in Plasmaflux
Albumin	69,000	1.0	1.0
IgG	150,000	0.99	0.98
α_2-Macroglobulin	725,000	—	0.97
IgM	950,000	0.92	0.99
β-Lipoprotein	2,400,000	1.0	1.0

Data are from Solomon et al., ref. 8 (Nuclepore), and Randerson et al., ref. 13 (Membrana fiber), *in vitro* with freshly drawn whole blood.

The luminal blood velocity (of about 0.4 cm/sec) is about a third, and the wall shear rates (80–160 sec⁻¹) are about a sixth of that normally found, for example, in hollow fiber dialyzers. Most strikingly, the filtration velocity (total filtration rate/ membrane surface area) is on the order of 0.5×10^{-2} cm/min, which is a full thousand times lower than the water flux of microporous membranes (6). This difference is too large to result from the increased viscosity of plasma relative to water and implies that a factor other than the membrane limits the rate of filtration. The overall filtration rate of 30–40 ml/min (at blood flows of about 100 ml/min which are typical for plasmapheresis access) is less than half of that easily achieved with hemofiltration cartridges of the same area (21). Direct comparison with hemo-filtration devices ignores many valid distinctions, but it is nevertheless disturbing that a protein-retentive filter operates at double the rate of a similarly sized protein-transmissive filter.

The sieving coefficients, defined as a solute's concentration ratio in the filtrate to the retentate, for the Plasmaflux are given in Table 2 along with comparable data for a 0.6 μm flat sheet membrane, which was used in several transport studies.

The data are from Randerson et al. (13) and Solomon et al. (8) based on *in vitro* experiments with freshly drawn whole blood. Both demonstrate complete passage of even the largest plasma proteins. Randerson gives equivalent results for the Plasmaflo II (the Plasmaflo I had lower sieving coefficients). Since the devices show no rejection of plasma proteins, not even β-lipoproteins, protein concentration polarization cannot possibly be responsible for the observed flux behavior. Randerson does report that the *in vivo* sieving coefficient is lower than the *in vitro* by about 15%, but since the *in vivo* filtration rate is the same as *in vitro*, the rejected plasma proteins are not influencing the flux.

Factors Controlling Filtration Flux

The filtration kinetics characteristics of plasmapheresis are illustrated in Fig. 1. Filtration rate per unit of membrane surface is plotted as a function of average transmembrane pressure. Filtration rate reaches a pressure-independent plateau where increases in pressure no longer result in increases in flux. The magnitude of the pressure-independent plateau increases with wall shear rate. For each plateau there is a transition pressure above which hemolysis will be observed. The transition pressure increases with wall shear rate. Figure 1 is plotted from the data of Solomon with 0.6 μm Nuclepore membranes (Pleasanton, CA) using freshly drawn whole blood (8). Similar curves with different systems have been presented by Castino et al. (7), Chmiel (9), and Farrell et al. (10). The latter two authors did not comment on the transition from regions of nonhemolysis to hemolysis, but the general form of this behavior can be assumed to be universal.

Of principal practical interest are the factors that affect the maximum permissible filtration rate. Data from available studies are given in Table 3 and summarized in Fig. 2. The ordinate of the graph is filtration rate divided by membrane surface

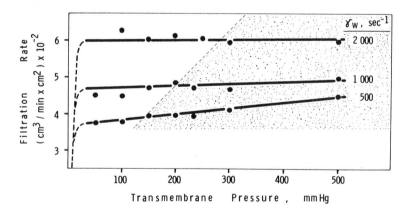

FIG. 1. Filtration behavior during plasmapheresis.

TABLE 3. *Summary of various studies on maximum filtration rate as a function of shear rate*

Study[c]	Membrane	Area (cm^2)	Length (cm)	γ_w (sec^{-1})	DP^{a}	FF (%)[b]	v_{uf} (10^{-2} ml/cm²min)
Chmiel (9)	"Plasmapheresis hollow fiber"	94	20	71	1.02	15.7	0.33
				142	0.43	9.3	0.39
				213	0.34	8.9	0.57
				284	0.26	7.9	0.67
Farrell et al. (10)	Cellulose-diacetate (Plasmaflo I)	≈40	8	320	0.18	<0.1	0.56
Solomon et al. (8)	Polycarbonate (Nuclepore 0.6 μm)	6	5	500	0.67	0.7	4.1
				1,000	0.34	0.5	5.8
				2,000	0.13	0.4	6.4
Friedman et al. (12)	Polycarbonate (Nuclepore 0.6 μm)	6	5	2,000	0.19	0.4	9.3
Castino et al. (7)	Polycarbonate (Nuclepore 0.6 μm)	6	5	1,400	0.29	0.5	8.4
				2,100	0.22	0.5	11.7
				2,800	0.20	0.5	15.8

[a]Blackshear's deposition parameter (calculated for $\nu = 0.015$ cm²/sec, $R = 3.5$ μm).
[b]Filtration fraction.
[c]All studies were at 37°C with whole blood at hematocrit of 35–40%, except Farrell's perfusate which was simulated plasma and Solomon's data which were collected at 21°C.

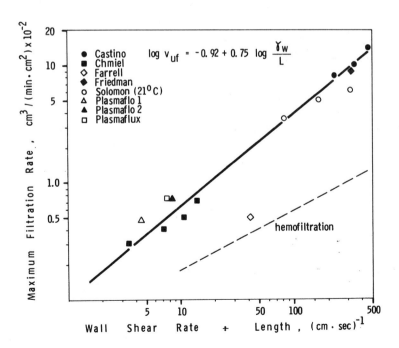

FIG. 2. Correlation of filtration rates reported for plasmapheresis.

area; the abscissa is wall shear rate divided by exposed fiber length. For hollow fibers, the latter term can be calculated as:

$$\frac{\gamma_w}{L} = \frac{4\bar{v}}{Lr} = \frac{4Q_B}{LN\pi r^3} \tag{1}$$

where:

γ_w = wall shear rate (sec^{-1})
L = effective length of the fibers (cm)
$\bar{v}$ = average velocity of the fluid along the x-axis (cm/sec)
Q_B = total flow rate through the filter (ml/min)
N = number of hollow fibers in the filter
r = inner radius of the hollow fiber (μm).

The expression for flat sheet modules (neglecting edge effects) is:

$$\frac{\gamma_w}{L} = \frac{3\bar{v}}{Lb} = \frac{3Q_B}{Lb^2w} \tag{2}$$

where:

b = channel half height (cm)
w = channel width (cm).

For the present, γ_w/L may be regarded as an expression which conveniently summarizes all parameters of design and flow; its theoretical significance is discussed later.

Data in Fig. 2 was collected in devices ranging in size from 40 to 7,500 cm^2, in both hollow fiber and flat sheet format. Flat sheet data is limited to Nuclepore 0.6 μm membrane, although data with other membrane types is quite consistent. Wall shear rates ranged from 120 to 2,600 sec^{-1}, filtration fraction varied from 0.5 to 30%. Solomon's points (open circles) are 21°C rather than at 37°C and were not included in the regression. Nor was Farrell's (open rhombus), because his data was not collected with whole blood. Friedman et al. (12) suggested that improper determination of membrane area may have given artificially high results in the Castino et al. (7) study, but the suspect results agree closely with his own and are thus included, although the time dependencies of the fluxes found by these two authors are surprisingly different.

The generally satisfactory fit of the data to the format of Fig. 2 is noteworthy, taking into account that even under identical test conditions, the filtration rate of blood from two different sources may vary as much as 30% (8).

Implications for Plasma Filter Design

The performance of commercially available (March 1982) plasma filters can be seen at the lower left portion of Fig. 2 (the data are from Table 1 and were included in the determination of the regression line). Because these devices have such low values of γ_w/L, their filtration flux is low and large areas are required to supply the filtration rates needed for plasmapheresis. The lengths of the plasma filters are unremarkable, but the wall shear rates are quite low. In hemodialysis device design, for example, γ_w is usually set at 500 sec^{-1} but the Plasmaflo and Plasmaflux devices have shear rates ranging from 80 to 160 sec^{-1}. Increases in shear rate and thus device efficiency are not difficult to achieve.

The most effective way to increase shear rate is to decrease fiber inside diameter for a hollow fiber or channel height for a parallel plate device. For hollow fibers, it can be seen from Eq. 1 that shear rate is inversely proportional to fiber diameter cubed, while membrane surface area is linear with diameter. Accordingly, decreases in diameter are highly leveraged and will yield the most significant improvement in overall filtration rate per unit area.

Shear rate may also be increased simply by putting fewer fibers or channels into the device and holding the blood flow constant. Again refer to Eqs. 1 and 2. Of course membrane surface area will also decrease, but according to Fig. 2 the increase in flow per unit area will substantially counterbalance this effect. Consider for example a hollow fiber device with a value for γ_w/L of 8 (cm·sec)$^{-1}$ and a flow per unit area of 0.6×10^{-2} ml/cm^{-2}min. If three-quarters of the fibers were removed from the device, the value of γ_w/L would increase to 32 (cm·sec)$^{-1}$ and the flux would increase to 1.6×10^{-2} ml/cm^{2}min. Since the area of the new device would be just 25% that of the old, its total filtration rate would be $\approx 70\%$ of its cohort with four times as many fibers.

Higher shear rate is necessarily linked to higher end-to-end pressure drops. Since relatively modest pressure differentials across the membrane can lead to hemolysis (see Fig. 1), more advanced designs may require methods of moderating or controlling transmembrane pressure. As in hemodialysis, these shear rates are not high enough to damage the blood cells.

In summary, this analysis predicts that future designs will pay substantially more attention to shear rate and will operate at much higher ratios of filtration rate to total membrane surface areas. It seems likely that tomorrow's plasma filters will bear no more relation to today's first generation models than does a contemporary hollow fiber dialyzer to a Kiil board.

MASS TRANSFER MODELS

The Skimming Layer Approach

Figure 3 (left) illustrates the time-honored model for mass transfer during plasmapheresis. It postulates a thin boundary layer adjacent to the membrane which is free of formed elements and from which filtration occurs. Consider a fluid whose lateral velocity is increasing in the radial direction. It is an established principle of fluid dynamics that a particle suspended in such a fluid will migrate in the direction of the increasing velocity and, moreover, the steeper the gradient in velocity, the greater will be the force for such migration. The magnitude of the radial forces can be calculated for a few limiting cases, for example, fully rigid or wholly deformable

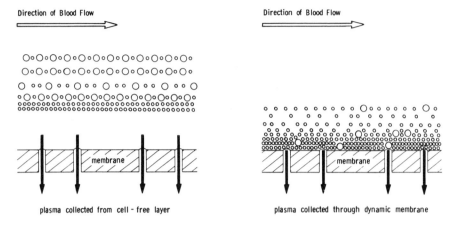

FIG. 3. Illustration of conventional skimming layer model **(left)** and proposed polarized secondary membrane model **(right)** for transport during plasmapheresis.

spheres, but none of the cases amenable to analytical solution represent blood. The subject is well reviewed by Brenner and Bungay (22). Incidentally, the density difference between the formed elements and plasma results in a small but real buoyant force which explains why device attitude plays some role in plasma filter performance.

From this simple qualitative picture and considering blood to be approximately described by Newtonian, laminar flow, in which fluid velocity increases parabolically from the wall to the midpoint, it follows that (a) red cells, white cells, and platelets will be subject to a repulsive (i.e., away from the wall-membrane surface) force when flowing through a capillary or a thin channel, (b) the magnitude of the force will decrease with distance from the wall because the velocity also decreases, and (c) the magnitude of the force will increase either if average fluid velocity increases or if the distance from the wall to the center decreases [both would increase velocity gradient and in turn $\gamma_w = (4\bar{v}/r)$]. If the wall is permeable, an oppositely directed force, called the Stokes law drag force, is superimposed on the particle. At some distance from the wall, these two forces will balance and that is where the particle will be found. The region between that point and the wall will be free of cells and represents the skimming layer. This is illustrated schematically in Fig. 4, where the formulae for the attractive and repulsive forces used for the derivation of the deposition parameter are drawn next to the vectors. The dependency of velocity, shear rate, and opposite forces on the distance from the wall are also shown.

For the case of plasmapheresis, the argument is carried one step further. For any given wall shear rate (i.e., repulsive force), there is a critical filtration rate above which the skimming layer disappears and particles deposit on the surface of the membrane. The allowable operating regions lie below this filtration velocity. This model successfully explains the shear dependency of filtration rate in plasmapheresis

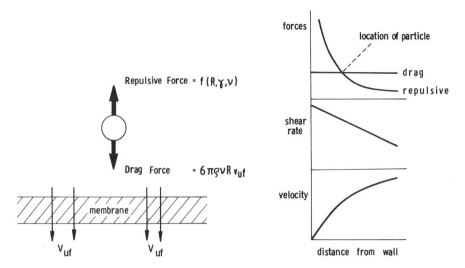

FIG. 4. Force balance on particle suspended in liquid. The full formula for the repulsive force is $6\rho\sqrt{\bar{\nu}}R^2\gamma^{3/2}y(1-f)$ (5). The graphs illustrate how velocity, shear rate, and forces vary with distance from the wall.

since the repulsive force—and hence the allowable Stokes law drag force—increases with shear rate. But the approach has several defects:

1. The rate of filtration from the skimming layer should be equivalent to that from particle-free plasma, which in turn should be only slightly smaller than water. As noted earlier, it is much lower. If proteins were rejected, a protein polarization phenomenon could limit flux from the skimming layer. No protein rejection is found except in the Plasmaflo I. Moreover, if proteins were being rejected, the flux would be expected to be quite similar to that during hemofiltration where protein polarization is indeed rate controlling. The observed relationship between γ_w/L and filtration rate in hemofiltration is in fact too low to fit the plasmapheresis model, as is illustrated by the dotted line in Fig. 2 which is drawn from the correlation of Isaacson (23).

2. The model does not explain the onset of a pressure-dependent, flux-independent onset of hemolysis nor why this onset should vary with shear rate.

3. Blackshear has derived and experimentally verified a correlation for predicting the conditions of shear rate and filtration velocity under which the cellular components of blood will deposit on the surface of a filtering membrane. They describe an "allowable" or hemolysis-free zone where the deposition parameter is less than 0.15. This deposition parameter was calculated for all the studies in Fig. 2 using averaged values for flow conditions. The results are summarized in Table 3. As Zawicki et al. (17) have pointed out, use of an integrated flow parameter will improve the estimation of the deposition parameter for devices with a high filtration

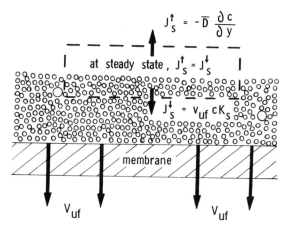

FIG. 5. Illustration of mass balance at some point x along the surface of the microporous membrane. Formed elements leave the secondary membrane by particle diffusion, i.e., Brownian motion, augmented by shear forces (20).

fraction. Nevertheless it is clear from Table 3 that the skimming layer approach is not quantitatively consistent with the deposition parameter approach.

Secondary Membrane Formation

We propose an alternative model, illustrated on the righthand side of Fig. 3, in which it is assumed that the microporous membrane is coated with a secondary membrane formed primarily of platelets but also containing some erythrocytes. The secondary membrane is described as dynamic since it continuously changes its thickness and hydrodynamic permeability in response to operating conditions; this feature distinguishes it from a fouling or plugging layer. Platelets and blood cells are brought to the secondary membrane by Stokes law forces and they are removed by shear augmented particle diffusion. At steady state, that is when flux is no longer changing with time, these two rates are necessarily equal. Stated alternatively, the secondary membrane will increase its hydraulic resistance (roughly thickness × compactness) until the forward filtration rate is low enough that the particles per unit time arriving by drag are equal to the number leaving by diffusion.

An approximate mathematical description of this model follows. Refer to Fig. 5, above, which depicts the boundaries of mass balance drawn at some point x along the full length L of a filtration membrane. The flux of formed elements $J_s(x)$ to and from the membrane is assumed to be

$$J_s(x) = v_{uf}(x)c(x)K_s - \overline{D}\,\frac{\partial c(x)}{\partial y} \qquad (3)$$

where:

$v_{uf}(x)$ = local filtration velocity (cm/sec)
$c(x)$ = concentration of the formed elements (particles/cm³)
x = distance from the entrance of the filter (cm)
y = distance from the membrane surface (cm)
K_s = proportionality constant assumed length-indendent
$\overline{D}$ = averaged particle diffusion coefficient (cm²/sec).

At steady state the boundary layer is by definition not changing. Therefore $J_s(x) = 0$ over the whole length, and the local filtration rate may be obtained by rearrangement of Eq. 3:

$$v_{uf}(x) = \frac{1}{c(x)} \frac{\overline{D}}{K_s} \frac{\partial c(x)}{\partial y} \tag{4}$$

Integration across the film yields:

$$v_{uf}(x) \int_0^\delta \partial y = \overline{D} \int_{c_p}^{c_w} c(x)^{-1} \partial c \tag{5}$$

so

$$v_{uf}(x) = \frac{\overline{D}}{\delta(x)K_s} \ln \frac{c_w(x)}{c_p(x)} \tag{6}$$

where:

$\delta(x)$ = thickness of the secondary membrane (in μm)
$c_w(x)$ = particle concentrations at the wall
$c_p(x)$ = particle concentrations in the bulk solution.

Finally, we replace $\{\overline{D}/\delta(x)K_s\}$ by $K_t(x)$, the local mass transfer coefficient. We represent $K_t(x)$ by an expression of the same general format employed for the description of the transport of large proteins from polarization layers during hemofiltration (24):

$$v_{uf}(x) = K_t(x) \ln \frac{c_w(x)}{c_p(x)} = \left(\frac{\gamma_w(x)K_b}{x} \right)^a \ln \frac{c_w(x)}{c_p(x)} \tag{7}$$

[This implicitly assumes that platelet transport from the boundary layer is physically similar to macromolecule transport (20).]

Predictions from this simple local transport model are consistent with observed behavior shown in Fig. 1. Equation 7 contains no pressure term, reflecting the independence of flux from pressure. Flux increases with shear rate. The secondary membrane is composed primarily of platelets, but we speculate that it contains a small fraction of red blood cells. Hemolysis then occurs when the applied pressure is high enough to extrude the cells into the membrane pores and rupture them. This is no doubt a statistical phenomenon. The fraction of the erythrocytes in the secondary membrane may be higher at higher shear rates. If so, this would account for the shear dependency of the transition from hemolysis-free to hemolytic regions.

A rigorous integration of Eq. 7 along the length of the membrane is not possible, since the exact profiles of $c_w(x)$, $c_p(x)$, and $\gamma(x)$ as a function of x are not known. In the absence of better information we assume that $\gamma_w(x)$ can be represented by the average of inlet and outlet conditions and that the ratio $c_w(x)/c_p(x)$ is independent of x. The integrated equation then takes the form:

$$\bar{v}_{uf} = (K_b)^a \left(\frac{\bar{\gamma}_w}{L}\right)^a \ln \frac{c_w}{c_p} \tag{8}$$

where:

$\bar{\gamma}_w$ = averages of inlet and outlet wall shear rate (sec^{-1})
c_w/c_p = the ratio of the wall concentration to the plasma concentration, assumed length-independent
K_b, a = constants.

The data in Fig. 2 does not allow the concentration term to be broken out and for the present we must be satisfied with an equation of the form

$$\bar{v}_{uf} = K \left(\frac{\bar{\gamma}_w}{L}\right)^a = 1.2 \times 10^{-3} \left(\frac{\bar{\gamma}_w}{L}\right)^{0.74} \tag{9}$$

where the numerical values of the constants are obtained from the regression line given in Fig. 2. The fit of the data to Eq. 9 provides some justification for the simplifying assumptions in the integration.

More data are required before this model can be considered fully developed. The effect of average particle concentration on filtration rate, representable either by hematocrit or platelet count, is a straightforward determination. The variation of γ_w and c_w along the length of the membrane can be approximated either analytically or numerically (17). But even in its present state of development, we believe this model provides an improved framework for the treatment of transport in plasmapheresis.

CONCLUSIONS

A wide range of available data on membrane plasmapheresis is well correlated by a log–log plot of filtration flux as a function of γ_w/L. Although existing commercial devices follow this correlation, they have low wall shear rates and consequently low filtration rates. Design of plasma filters with major improvements in efficiency is a realistic and practical goal. A transport model is proposed based upon a dynamic secondary membrane formed primarily of platelets. While relying upon the same basic radial forces, this analysis avoids many of the problems inherent in the skimming layer approach. It is hoped that further elaboration of this new model may lead to a better understanding of transport during plasmapheresis.

SYMBOLS

b = channel half-height (cm)

$c(x)$ = concentration of the formed elements at distance x (particles/cm^3)

$c_p(x)$ = particle concentration in the bulk solution at distance x (particles/cm^3)

$c_w(x)$ = particle concentration at the wall at distance x (particles/cm^3)

$\overline{D}$ = averaged particle diffusion coefficient (cm^2/sec)

$J_s(x)$ = net flux of formed elements to the membrane at distance x (particles/cm^{2}min)

$K_t(x)$ = local mass transfer coefficient (cm/sec)

L = length of the filter (cm)

N = number of fibers

Q_B = blood flow rate referring to the filter (cm^3/min)

R = radius of suspended particle (μm)

r = inner radius of the hollow fiber (μm)

$\overline{v}$ = blood velocity along the fiber, average of inlet and outlet value (cm/min)

$v_{uf}(x)$ = filtration velocity at distance x (cm/min)

$\overline{v}_{uf}$ = filtration velocity, device averaged (cm/min)

w = channel width (cm)

x = distance from the entrance of the filter (cm)

y = distance from the membrane surface (cm)

γ = shear rate (sec^{-1})

$\gamma_w(x)$ = wall shear rate at distance x (sec^{-1})

$\overline{\gamma}_w$ = wall shear rate, average of inlet and outlet value (sec^{-1})

$\delta(x)$ = thickness of the secondary membrane at distance x (μm)

ν = kinematic viscosity of the suspending fluid (cm^2/sec)

ρ = fluid density (g/cm^3)

a, K, K_s = dimensionless constants

K_b = constant (cm·sec)

ACKNOWLEDGMENTS

Fr. B. Schmidt, Klinikum Grosshadern, Munich, supplied some of the information for Table 1. The authors interest in this topic arose out of their investigations into mass transport in artificial organs at the Max Planck Institut für Biophysik, Frankfurt am Main, FRG.

REFERENCES

1. Blatt, W. F., Agranat, E. A., and Rigopulos, P. N. (1972): Blood fractionating process and apparatus for carrying out same. US Patent 3,705,100.
2. Castino, F., Scheucher, K., Malchesky, P. S., Koshino, I., and Nosé, Y. (1976): Microemboli-free blood detoxification utilizing plasma filtration. *Trans. Am. Soc. Artif. Intern. Organs*, 22:637.

3. Nosé, Y., Malchesky, P. S., Castino, F., Koshino, I., Scheucher, K., and Nokoff, R. (1976): Improved hemoperfusion systems for renal-hepatic support. *Kidney Int.*, 10:S244.
4. Forstrom, R. J., Bartelt, K., Blackshear, P. L., Jr., and Wood, T. (1975): Formed element deposition onto filtering walls. *Trans. Am. Soc. Artif. Intern. Organs*, 21:602.
5. Friedman, L. I., Castino, F., Lysaght, M. J., Solomon, B. A., Sanderson, J. E., and Wiltbank, T. B. (1979): A continuous flow plasmapheresis system. Final Report: Nat. Heart, Lung, and Blood Institute Contract No. 1-HB-6-2928, June 1976–April 1979.
6. Lysaght, M. J., Colton, C. K., Friedman, L. I., and Castino, F. (1977): Investigation of factors controlling the rate of plasma filtration with microporous membranes. *83rd National Meeting of the American Institute of Chemical Engineering*. Paper 69d, March 1977 (microfiche).
7. Castino, F., Friedman, L. I., Solomon, B. A., Colton, C. K., and Lysaght, M. J. (1978): The filtration of plasma from whole blood: A novel approach to clinical detoxification. In: *Artificial Kidney, Artificial Liver, and Artificial Cells*, edited by T. M. S. Chang, p. 259. Plenum, New York.
8. Solomon, B. A., Castino, F., Lysaght, M. J., Colton, C. K., and Friedman, L. I. (1978): Continuous flow membrane filtration of plasma from whole blood. *Trans. Am. Soc. Artif. Intern. Organs*, 24:21.
9. Chmiel, H. (1981): Technologische Aspekte zur Membranplasmapherese. In: *Therapeutic Plasma Exchange*, edited by H. J. Gurland, V. Heinze, and H. A. Lee, p. 15. Springer-Verlag, Berlin.
10. Farrell, P. C., Schindhelm, K., and Roberts, C. G. (1980): Membrane plasma separation. In: *Plasma Exchange*, edited by H. G. Sieberth, p. 37. Schattauer Verlag, Stuttgart.
11. Schindhelm, K., Roberts, C. G., and Farrell, P. C. (1981): Mass transfer characteristics of plasma filtration membranes. *Trans. Am. Soc. Artif. Intern. Organs*, 27:554.
12. Friedman, L. I., Hardwick, L. A., Daniels, J. R., Stromberg, R. R., and Ciarkowski, A. A. (1983): Evaluation of membranes for plasmapheresis. *Artif. Organs*, 7 *(in press)*.
13. Randerson, D. H., Blumenstein, M., Habersetzer, R., Samtleben, W., Schmidt, B., and Gurland, H. J. (1982): Mass transfer in membrane plasma exchange. *Artif. Organs*, 6:43.
14. Asanuma, Y., Smith, J. W., Suwa, S., Zawicki, I., Harasaki, H., Dixon, A. C., Malchesky, P. S., and Nosé, Y. (1979): Membrane plasmapheresis: Platelet and protein effects on filtration. *Proc. Soc. Artif. Organs*, 6:308.
15. Nosé, Y., Malchesky, P. S., Asanuma, Y., and Zawicki, I. (1981): Plasma filtration detoxification on hepatic patients: Its optimal operating conditions. In: *Therapeutic Plasma Exchange*, edited by H. J. Gurland, V. Heinze, and H. A. Lee, p. 125. Springer-Verlag, Berlin.
16. Werynski, A., Malchesky, P. S., Sueoka, A., Asanuma, Y., Smith, J. W., Kayashima, K., and Nosé, Y. (1981): Membrane plasma separation (MPS): Toward improved clinical operation. *Trans. Am. Soc. Artif. Intern. Organs*, 27:539.
17. Zawicki, I., Malchesky, P. S., Smith, J. W., Harasaki, H., Asanuma, Y., and Nosé, Y. (1981): Axial changes of blood and plasma flow, pressure and cellular deposition in capillary plasma filters. *Artif. Organs*, 5:241.
18. Solomon, B. A. (1981): Membrane separations: Technological principles and issues. *Trans. Am. Soc. Artif. Intern. Organs*, 27:345.
19. Blackshear, P. L., Bartelt, K. W., and Forstrom, R. J. (1979): Fluid dynamic factors affecting particle capture. *Ann. N.Y. Acad. Sci.*, 283:270.
20. Drake, K. L., and Eckstein, E. C. (1981): The effect of hemofiltration on fiber platelet concentration. *Artif. Organs*, 5:363.
21. Lysaght, M. J., Ford, C. A., Colton, C. K., Stone, R. W., and Henderson, L. W. (1978): Mass transfer in clinical blood ultrafiltration devices. In: *Technical Aspects of Renal Dialysis*, edited by T. H. Frost, p. 81. Pitman, United Kingdom.
22. Brenner, H., and Bungay, P. M. (1971): Rigid-particle and liquid-droplet models of red cell motion in capillary tubes. *Fed. Proc.*, 30:1565.
23. Isaacson, K. A., Ford, C. A., and Lysaght, M. J. (1980): Determination of Graetz solution constants for the ultrafiltration of albumin. In: *Ultrafiltration Membranes and Applications*, edited by A. R. Cooper, p. 507. Plenum, New York.
24. Colton, C. K., Henderson, L. W., Ford, C. A., and Lysaght, M. J. (1975): Kinetics of hemodi-

afiltration, I—*In-vitro* transport characteristics of a hollow fiber blood ultrafilter. *J. Lab. Clin. Med.*, 85:355.

25. Forstrom, R. J., Voss, G. O., and Blackshear, P. L. (1974): Fluid dynamics of particle (platelet) deposition for filtering walls: Relationship to artherosclerosis. *Trans. Am. Soc. Mech. Eng., J. Fluids Eng.*, 96 (Ser. 1):168.

Plasmapheresis, edited by Y. Nosé, P. S.
Malchesky, J. W. Smith, and R. S. Krakauer.
Raven Press, New York © 1983.

Plasma Water Removal by Membrane Filtration for the Treatment of Hemodilution

Roy L. Nelson, Yehuda Tamari, Anthony J. Tortolani,
Michael H. Hall, and Carmine G. Moccio

*Department of Surgery, Division of Cardiovascular Surgery, North Shore University
Hospital, Manhasset, New York 11030; and Department of Surgery, Cornell University
Medical College, New York, New York 14853*

Intentional hemodilution is employed during cardiopulmonary bypass for corrective cardiac surgery. The ability to control plasma volume during cardiopulmonary bypass would control the stability and degree of hemodilution. In addition, removal of plasma water at the conclusion of bypass could reverse the hemodilution, concentrate the blood, and restore to normal the levels of red blood cells and blood component. Currently available techniques of concentration employ a centrifuge device that is difficult to use during cardiopulmonary bypass, and discards all the blood components except the red blood cells.

It is our hypothesis that plasma water could be removed by ultrafiltration using a disposable dialyzer during and after cardiopulmonary bypass. In this manner, only the diluting fluid would be removed and all blood components could be concentrated.

MATERIALS AND METHODS

In 100 patients undergoing corrective cardiac surgery with hemodilution cardiopulmonary bypass (average hematocrit 18%), a disposable, hollow fiber dialyzer (TriEx-3, Extracorporeal Medical Specialties, King of Prussia, PA) was employed to control plasma volume during bypass and to concentrate the blood and plasma at the conclusion of the operation. The dialyzer was included in the bypass circuit in a parallel manner, and blood was taken from the coronary perfusion port (bottom) of the oxygenator and pumped through the dialyzer using a calibrated roller pump. Blood was returned to the oxygenator directly or via a cardiotomy reservoir. Provision was made for diversion of concentrated blood to transfusion bags for later infusion after the conclusion of the operation (Fig. 1). The dialysate inlet port of the dialyzer was occluded with a stopper and the dialysate outlet port was connected to a vacuum source that generated approximately 400 torr negative pressure. Inlet and outlet pressures were monitored with aneroid manometers (Tycos, Rochester, NY). Inlet pressures range between 40 and 60 torr and outlet pressures between 0

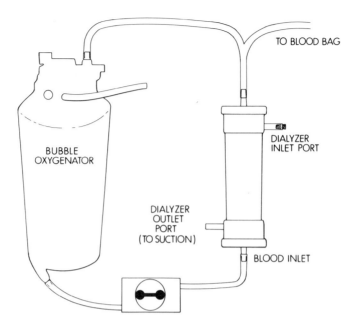

FIG. 1. Placement of dialyzer in bypass circuit. Blood is removed from the oxygenator and pumped through the dialyzer. Following concentration, the blood is either returned to the oxygenator or bagged for later reinfusion.

and 20 torr. The net transmembrane pressure was approximately 440 torr as calculated by the following formula:

$$P_m = \frac{(P_i + P_o)}{2} - P_u$$

P_m = mean transmembrane pressure (torr), P_i = pressure at blood inlet (torr), $\overline{P}_o$ = pressure at blood outlet (torr), and P_u = pressure in the ultrafiltration compartment (torr) (1). The filtration rate under these conditions was 33.3 ± 3.1 cc/min. Blood was circulated through the dialyzer at 350 cc/min.

For this study, data analysis was performed on the residual blood in the circuit at the conclusion of bypass in 20 patients. The dilute blood was circulated in a closed loop mode and measurements were performed before and after plasma water removal. The blood was maintained heparinized during the open heart procedure at 3 mg/kg of patient body weight with beef lung heparin, and no additional heparin was given. The ultrafiltration process took approximately 29 min. The initial volume was reduced by approximately one-half with the removal of 967 ± 81cc of plasma water.

Laboratory determinations performed pre- and postconcentration included a SMAC-20 (Technicon, Tarrytown, NY), a complete blood count and fibrinogen (2). Additional studies performed in 5 patients included platelet aggregation with ADP (2 μM), ristocetin and collagen (3) and, in another 5 patients osmotic fragility (4). Data obtained from pre- and postconcentration samples were anlayzed using the paired student's *t*-test.

RESULTS

The sodium, potassium, chloride, carbon dioxide, and glucose levels were unchanged by ultrafiltration (Table 1). Similarly, blood urea nitrogen, creatinine, uric acid, and phosphorous remained the same, while calcium increased by 50% from 9.3 ± 5.0 to 14.0 ± 4.0 mg/dl. Calculated osmolality was unchanged. Total protein increased 208% from 4.0 ± 0.4 to 12.3 ± 3.2 g/dl. Albumin rose 177% from 3.0 ± 0.3 to 8.3 ± 0.3 g/dl. In a similar manner, total bilirubin doubled from 0.5 ± 0.1 to 1.1 ± 0.5 mg/dl. However, lactic dehydrogenase (LDH) increased greater than threefold, 259 ± 71 versus 941 ± 218 U/liter.

Additional samples were subjected to hematologic evaluation (Table 2). Following ultrafiltration, the concentration of red blood cells doubled from 2.23 ± 0.45 to 4.52 ± 0.76 × 10^6. Similarly, hemoglobin increased from 7.4 ± 1.4 to 14.6 ± 2.0 g/dl. Red blood cell indices were within normal limits before hemoconcentration and were not significantly altered after concentration. There was no loss of white blood cells, indicating the absence of trapping by the membrane (5). Platelet counts rose from 156 ± 62 to 257 ± 113 × 10^3. Platelet aggregation was unchanged with ADP (2 μM), decreased with ristocytin and collagen, and increased with epinephrine. The changes in platelet aggregation were partially or totally reversible with the addition of platelet poor plasma. Osmotic fragility tests by the method of Dacie and Vaughn (4) showed no significant change before and after hemoconcentration by ultrafiltration.

TABLE 1. *Blood chemistry before and after ultrafiltration*

	Preconcentration	Postconcentration
Sodium (mEq/liter)	141 ± 3	142 ± 2
Potassium (mEq/liter)	4.5 ± 1.6	5.0 ± 0.8
Chloride (mEq/liter)	108 ± 5.0	93 ± 7.0
Carbon dioxide (mEq/liter)	20 ± 1.0	16.0 ± 2.0
Glucose (mg/dl)	178 ± 83	139 ± 69
BUN (mg/dl)	14 ± 2.0	14 ± 2.5
Creatinine (mg/dl)	1.2 ± 0.1	1.1 ± 0.1
Uric acid (mg/dl)	6.1 ± 1.1	5.4 ± 1.0
Calcium (mg/dl)	9.3 ± 5.0	14.0 ± 4.0
Phosphorus (mg/dl)	2.0 ± 0.5	1.8 ± 0.5
Osmolality (mOsm)	277 ± 7	277 ± 5
Total protein (gm/dl)	4.0 ± 0.4	12.3 ± 3.2[a]
Albumin (gm/dl)	3.0 ± 0.3	8.3 ± 0.3[a]
Total bilirubin (mg/dl)	0.5 ± 0.1	1.1 ± 0.5[a]
LDH (U/liter)	259 ± 71	941 ± 218[a]

[a] $p < 0.05$.
All values ± standard error of the mean.

TABLE 2. *Results of hematologic evaluation before and after ultrafiltration*

	Preconcentration	Postconcentration
White blood cells ($\times 10^3$)	11.4 ± 4.0	24.1 ± 8.4[a]
Red blood cells ($\times 10^6$)	2.23 ± 0.45	4.52 ± 0.76[a]
Hemoglobin (g/dl)	7.4 ± 1.4	14.6 ± 2.0[a]
Hematocrit (%)	20.7 ± 4.0	41.4 ± 5.8[a]
Mean corpuscular volume (μm^3)	92.7 ± 3.3	92.1 ± 3.2
Mean corpuscular hemoglobin ($\mu\mu g$)	33.1 ± 1.1	32.6 ± 1.2
Mean corpuscular hemoglobin concentration (g/dl)	35.7 ± 0.5	35.3 ± 0.4
Platelet count ($\times 10^3$)	155 ± 62	257 ± 113[a]
Fibrinogen (mg/dl)	120 ± 36	296 ± 55[a]

[a]$p < 0.05$.
All values ± standard error of the mean.

DISCUSSION

Commonly, cardiopulmonary bypass is performed using hemodilution. The hematocrit is lowered electively by priming the extracorporeal circuit with a crystalloid solution. In addition, during the course of the operation, there may be multiple infusions of additional quantities of crystalloid in the form of cardioplegia. The net effect is that during the course of the operation, the hematocrit may be reduced to unacceptably low levels (excessive hemodilution). In addition, at the conclusion of the operation, it is essential to remove the excess plasma water from the blood so that transfusion of dilute blood is avoided, thereby reducing the risk of circulatory overload.

It was our hypothesis that, by the application of modern ultrafiltration techniques, it would be possible to concentrate the blood by removing only the excess water (ultrafiltration) without loss of platelets or plasma proteins and without damaging the red blood cells. Hemoconcentration by ultrafiltration is not novel. Silverstein et al. (6), in one of the earliest reports, used an Amicon filter for the treatment of fluid overload by ultrafiltration. Ultrafiltration was used for hemoconcentration following hemodilution cardiopulmonary bypass by Romagnoli et al. in 1976 (7). This paralleled the introduction by Quellhorst et al. (8) of hemofiltration for the treatment of uremic patients. In 1977 Kramer et al. (9) introduced the concept of arteriovenous hemofiltration for the treatment of overhydrated patients resistant to diuretics. Similarly, in 1978 Lamar and associates (10) used an Amicon diafilter for fluid removal by ultrafiltration. Strife and McEnery (11) used the same diafilter successfully in small children. Application of ultrafiltration to the treatment of nonuremic hemodilution associated with cardiopulmonary bypass received no attention in the literature in the intervening years, presumably because of the unreliability of the equipment. With the advent of small, inexpensive, disposable, hollow fiber dialyzers that had a small priming volume, there was resurgence of interest, initially in Europe. In 1979 Darup et al. (12) published their experience with the successful use of an Amicon diafilter for ultrafiltration in association with cardiopulmonary bypass in 10 patients with reduced renal function.

Based on our studies, the application of currently available ultrafiltration techniques made it possible to concentrate the blood by removing only the excess water with minimal loss of platelets or plasma proteins and minimally damaging the red blood cells. While we employed the device both during and at the end of the operation, only the data derived at the conclusion of the operation, under stable conditions are reported here. Our studies using a hollow fiber dialyzer revealed no changes in the serum electrolyte determinations following ultrafiltration. Similarly, serum osmolality was unchanged. In addition, the normal pre- and postconcentration red blood cell indices indicate that there were no significant changes in the intracellular volume in the red blood cells subjected to ultrafiltration.

The disproportionate rise in the hematocrit compared with the albumin, along with the twofold increase in bilirubin and the threefold increase in plasma LDH, would indicate that there was some red blood cell destruction. While this destruction can be related in part to the flow rate through the dialyzer, which at 350 cc/minute may be excessive, it also may reflect distinction of the red blood cells that had been traumatized by the roller pumps and suction devices of the extracorporeal circuit. In addition, the value for plasma proteins may be artificially elevated because of interpretation of the spectrophotometric data using an automated analyzer. There may be some spillover in the color spectrum due to the presence of free plasma hemoglobin.

Platelet function was quite acceptable. In our laboratory, cardiopulmonary bypass alone has been associated with similar changes in platelet function as determined by aggregation.

The ability to return plasma proteins to the patient can provide long-term benefit in terms of hemodynamic stability as the oncotic pressure will be maintained. In addition, fibrinogen is active in the clotting process and, along with the platelets, has particular advantage in the postoperative open-heart patients. These patients have a bleeding tendency that is secondary to heparinization (even though it was reversed with protamine), as well as trauma due to the platelets, and also related to the dilution of the clotting factors. Consequently, the return of concentrated platelets and plasma proteins to the patient would be beneficial. The use of ultrafiltration for fluid removal in end-stage renal disease is limited by the patients' hemodynamic stability. Fluid removal by ultrafiltration in conjunction with cardiopulmonary bypass, where blood pressure is being maintained artificially by the extracorporeal circulation, is not limited as in the dialysis patient.

CONCLUSION

It is concluded that the use of a hollow fiber dialyzer can safely and effectively control plasma volume in connection with cardiopulmonary bypass. It can maintain a stable degree of hemodilution in the presence of infusions of additional volumes of diluting fluid. In addition, it can reverse hemodilution at the end of the procedure, returning to the patient concentrated levels of red blood cells and plasma proteins. The concentration process affects not only red blood cells but plasma proteins, fibrinogen, and platelets. These substances are beneficial in the postoperative open-heart patients for hemostasis.

The fluid removed does not change the electrolyte composition. There are no deleterious effects associated with transfusion of blood concentrated by ultrafiltration. The technique of plasma water removal by ultrafiltration in association with cardiopulmonary bypass is facile, safe, and effective. We would anticipate the widespread application of this device on an annual basis to the approximately 150,000 open-heart procedures performed annually in the United States and to another 150,000 procedures annually in Europe. In addition, any blood saved and returned to the patient reduces financial costs of blood, strain on blood banking facilities, and decreases the risk to the patient of hepatitis.

ACKNOWLEDGMENTS

This work was supported in part by NIH Grant S08-RR-09128-03 and by a grant-in-aid from the Suffolk County Chapter of the American Heart Association.

REFERENCES

1. Klein, E., Autian, J., Bower, J. D. et al. (1977): Evaluation of hemodialyzers and dialysis membranes. DHEW Publication No. (NIH) 77-1294. U.S. Government Printing Office, Washington, D.C.
2. Brown, B. A., editor (1976): *Principles and Procedures: Hematology.* Saunders, Philadelphia.
3. Day, H. G., and Holmson, H. (1972): Laboratory tests of platelet function. *Ann. Clin. Lab. Sci.*, 2:63.
4. Dacie, J. V., and Vaughn, J. M. (1938): The fragility of red blood cells: Its measurement and significance. *J. Pathol. Bact.*, 46:341.
5. Shin, J., Matuso, M., Shinka, S. et al. (1980): A study on hemodialysis leukopenia using various dialyzers. *Dialysis*, 4:51.
6. Silverstein, M. E., Ford, C. A., Lysaght, M. J. et al. (1974): Treatment of severe fluid overflow by ultrafiltration. *N. Engl. J. Med.*, 291:747.
7. Romagnoli, A., Hacker, J., Keats, A. S. et al. (1976): External hemoconcentration after deliberate hemodilation. *American Society of Anesthesiologist's Annual Meeting,* 269 (abstr.).
8. Quellhorst, E., Reiger, J., Dahr, B. et al. (1976): Treatment of chronic uremia by an ultrafiltration kidney. *Proceedings of the European Transplant Association: Vol. 13,* p. 314. Pitman, London.
9. Kramer, P., Wigger, W., Reiger, J., Matthaei, D., and Scheler, F. (1977): Arteriovenous haemofiltration: A new and simple method for treatment of over-hydrated patients resistant to diuretics. *Klin. Wochenschr.*, 55:1121.
10. Lamar, J., Briggs, W. A., and McDonald, F. D. (1978): Effective fluid removal with the Amicon diafilter. *Proc. Clin. Dialysis Transplant Forum,* 127–129.
11. Strife, C. F., and McEnery, P. T. (1977): Experience with low volume ultrafiltration cell in small children. *Clin. Nephrol.*, 8:410.
12. Darup, J., Bleese, N., Kalmar, P. et al. (1979): Hemofiltration during extracorporeal circulation. *Thorac. Cardiovasc. Surg.*, 27:227.

Plasmapheresis, edited by Y. Nosé, P.S.
Malchesky, J.W. Smith, and R.S. Krakauer.
Raven Press, New York © 1983.

The Shear Rate Filtration Rate Relationship of Membranes for Plasmapheresis

E. F. Leonard,

*Artificial Organs Research Laboratory, Columbia University,
New York, New York 10027*

Membrane plasmapheresis occurs when blood passes in shear flow over a porous surface, the membrane, whose pores are 0.1–1.0 μm in diameter. Up to a maximum value, the plasma flux increases more or less linearly, as the pressure difference across the membrane (TMP) increases. The maximum flux certainly increases with the strength of the shear flow, as characterized by the shear rate at the blood–membrane interface. Other factors in addition to shear rate, such as the microstructure of the membrane surface and possibly its chemistry as it affects cell–surface interaction, as well as properties of the blood (especially its hematocrit) may influence the maximum flux. At TMPs exceeding that producing the maximum flux, the observed flux may equal the maximum or be less.

Hemolysis may occur during membrane plasmapheresis when some or all of the pores in the membrane are inappropriately large, when the material of the membrane exerts a hemolytic effect, or when the shear rate exceeds a critical value for the blood being processed.

The phenomena described above have been qualitatively observed and confirmed. While quantitative data relating maximum flux to shear rate and hematocrit are available from a number of flow devices, and two correlations among these variables have been proposed (see below), the phenomena have not been well quantified. The configurations of devices currently in clinical trial appear to have been realized by essentially cut-and-dry methods. They are generally recognized as suboptimal in the sense that they do not make uniformly efficient use of the membrane they contain and do not minimize the area of membrane to which blood is exposed.

For a given combination of blood and membrane, imposition of a particular TMP and shear rate eventually results in a steady-state flux of plasma, at least for some values of these variables that constitute an operating range. It is uncertain how the flux varies with time as the steady state is approached. The rate of approach, the presence or absence of overshoot, and the dependence of these kinetics on blood and membrane properties all remain to be ascertained, although Malchesky et al. *(this volume)* report that the overall flux–pressure kinetics of clinical devices appear to vary with the nature of their membrane.

In addition to the phenomenological questions raised above, the underlying mechanism by which shear facilitates apheresis is in question. Cells may migrate away from the surface via a lift effect, the phenomenon on which Blackshear's (1) correlation is based, or the maximum rate may be due to a special realization of the classical concentration–polarization process in which shear–augmented diffusion of cells counterbalances convection, as Zydney and Colton (2) have suggested.

Study of the physics and surface chemistry of membrane plasmapheresis appears best undertaken in systems that expose all working parts of the membrane to the same conditions of pressure difference, hematocrit, and shear rate. This chapter describes one such device and preliminary observations made with it.

TEST SYSTEM PRINCIPLE

When a fluid is placed between a flat plate and a rotating cone whose included angle approaches pi radians (i.e., pi − 2 × theta), where theta is the gap angle shown in Fig. 1 (top), the shear rate in the gap is constant. This is so because both the tangential velocity of the cone surface and gap dimension are proportional to radius so that their quotient, which closely approximates the shear rate, is constant (Fig. 1, bottom). Under these conditions, fluid elements travel in concentric circles (Fig. 2, top). While one could thus envision a plasmapheresis test device in which the plate was a disc of membrane, and shear was provided on this surface by a rotating cone above it, such a design requires some augmentation. A means must be provided for removing blood whose hematocrit has been increased by filtration

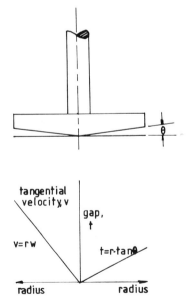

FIG. 1. Top: Basic cone plate configuration. Fluid is placed in the tapered, circular space between the plate (which is held stationary) and the cone (which is rotated about its axis). The design has been used primarily for studying the rheological behavior of fluids. **Bottom:** The graphs show that both gap and tangential velocity vary linearly with radius, both with zero value at the center. Thus their quotient, v/t, which is the shear rate, is a constant throughout the entire fluid space.

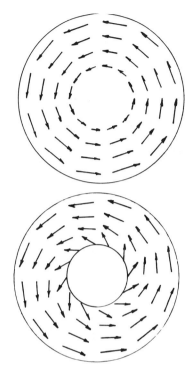

FIG. 2. Top: Velocity pattern of fluid in a classical cone-plate viscometer. Only the angular component is finite. **Bottom:** Velocity pattern of fluid in a modified cone-plate system in which a radial flow is purposely superimposed on the angular pattern. For a given radial flow, the velocity perturbation is greatest toward the center where the area for radial flow (circumference × gap) is smallest.

and replacing it with additional blood from a reservoir of substantial volume. This function can be provided by superimposing a shear-wise negligible radial flow so that fresh blood is provided at some small radius and removed at a larger one. Fluid elements then travel along spiral paths (Fig. 2, bottom).

TEST SYSTEM DESIGN

The actual test device, shown in Fig. 3, uses a hollow shaft, with ports for blood entry above the cone, to achieve the spiral flow pattern just described. The membrane is masked from its center to a radius corresponding to the inner radius of the shaft, 1.0 cm. A stepping motor coaxial with a photoelectric, digital tachometer is used to drive a cone with gap angle of 0.124 rads at speeds from 100 to 3000 rpm, the shear rate in reciprocal seconds being 0.845 × rpm. The working area of the membrane is an annulus of inner radius 2 cm and outer radius 4 cm, approximating 12 cm². The membrane is supported by a porous metal plate of negligible hydraulic resistance, on the lower side of which is a small reservoir maintained at reduced pressure. Flow rate is measured by injecting small air bubbles into the efflux from the reservoir which is passed through a 1-ml pipet, maintained in the horizontal position (Fig. 4).

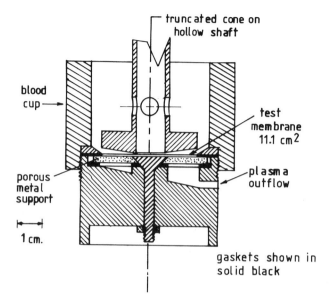

FIG. 3. Modified cone-plate system used in this study. Hollow shaft carries blood downward from side ports to the gap area to furnish the radial flow depicted in Fig. 2. The test membrane, an annulus of 15 mm inner diameter and 40.5 mm effective outer diameter, forms the plate. Vertical alignment is precise so that the virtual apex of the cone is coincident with the top center of the center pin of the plate.

PROCEDURE

Three sheet membranes were evaluated: Millipore (Bedford, MA) cellulose acetate type HA (catalog number HAWP 047 00, lot HIM66262 N) with a stated pore size of 0.45 μm; AMF (Stamford, CN) nylon 66 (sample no. S20881) stated to have a pore size of 0.45 μ and to be "uncharged"; and Membrana GmbH (Wuppertal, FRG) "Accural" polypropylene (type PS 508/2, run no. 236) with a stated pore size of 0.55 μm. None of these manufacturers offers the membrane for plasmapheresis, but each membrane has appropriate pore size and no characteristics that would indicate that it is biologically incompatible. The dry thickness of each membrane was measured with a "light wave" micrometer (van Keuren Co., NY). This device is a screw-type micrometer with a large, indexed wheel and vernier; its plunger simultaneously compresses the sample and a pair of cantilevered glass plates between which a reproducible pattern of Newton rings can be generated to accomplish a definite clamping pressure. Circles of approximately 4.7 cm in diameter were cut from the sheets of AMF and Membrana material. The Millipore material was precut. The Membrana material, which is hydrophobic, was prewetted by immersion in absolute ethanol. Each membrane was then placed in the test cell and the vertical elevation of the membrane's upper surface was adjusted relative to the lowest point on the cone surface, using a shim of 0.075 cm thickness. This

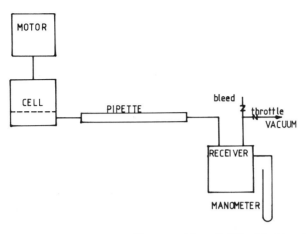

FIG. 4. Diagram of experimental system. The cone of the cell of Fig. 3 is driven by a concentric motor. Tubing connects the plasma outflow to a horizontal pipet used as a flowmeter (see text). Vacuum is applied to a receiver downstream of the pipet in order to create the desired pressure difference across the membrane. Pressures were measured with a manometer containing either water or carbon tetrachloride.

dimension corresponds to intersection of the virtual apex of the truncated cone with the membrane surface and provides a geometry consistent with constant shear rate over the membrane surface. Following this adjustment each membrane was rinsed with normal saline, drawn through it under vacuum. Thus the filtrate system was primed and it was possible to observe the pressure–flow relationship of saline through the membrane. Approximately 40 ml of outdated, banked blood were then added so that a sufficient level was achieved to cover the blood inlet ports in the shaft. Cone rotation was commenced and a blood sample was taken in a heparinized microhematocrit tube (Red-Tip, Fisher Scientific Co., cat. no. 02-668-66). After centrifuging in a "Readacrit" centrifuge (Clay-Adams Co., cat. no. 0591) at 8,000 rpm, 5,900 g for 5 min, and recording of the hematocrit, the tube was scored and broken to allow separation of 20 μl of plasma, which was then analyzed for hemoglobin using a method based on reaction with tetramethylbenzidene (see Appendix 1). Vacuum was then applied to the collection flask to achieve the desired TMP. Pressure relative to atmospheric was read on a single-leg manometer (Manostat Corp., NY) filled either with water or carbon tetrachloride (sp. gr. 1.594); all values were recorded as millimeters of mercury (torr). The reference leg of the manometer was kept level with the surface of the blood in the cell. Filtrate flowrate was measured, as noted above, by timing passage of a small bubble through a horizontal pipet using an observation volume that gave a passage time of at least 10 sec. Filtrate was sampled by syringe or micropipet for measurement of hemoglobin in a manner identical to that used on plasma from blood samples, as described above. These preliminary experiments were run at laboratory temperature, approximately 21°C.

RESULTS AND DISCUSSION

Table 1 gives values for the thickness and saline permeability of the three membranes studied.

Figure 5 (top) shows how flux through the Millipore membrane varies with shear rate at two different levels of shear. A clear effect of shear rate is shown at both TMP levels, although the curves suggest that a significant flux can occur at very low shear rates. The fluxes at the higher TMP (49 torr) are higher than at the lower TMP (30 torr), and appear to rise more rapidly with shear rate. However, the fluxes appear to rise with TMP at a less than proportionate rate. Figure 5 (middle and bottom) shows how flux through the AMF and Membrana membranes varies with TMP at two different levels of shear rate. Presuming that all fluxes are essentially zero at zero values of TMP, all curves exhibit a maximum at intermediate TMPs, then a region of decreasing flux, and at the highest TMPs studied, a flux that again increases.

It is possible to compare these results with Blackshear's (1) theory in two principal ways: (a) by a direct comparison of the flux levels seen here with those he predicts, and (b) by comparing the observed parametric sensitivities with those implied by the theory. Using a hematocrit of 0.4, a plasma viscosity of 2 cp, a cell radius of 4 μm, and a shear rate of 500 reciprocal seconds, the theory predicts a flux of about 175 ml/(min $\times$ m^2) in the middle range of values observed. Thus the quantitative agreement is remarkable.

The dependence on the square root of plasma viscosity and on the inverse square of cell diameter were not tested. Blackshear's theory suggests a 3/2 power dependency on shear rate which, as noted above, is considerably stronger than the data of this study suggest. His formula suggests a very strong hematocrit dependence. In numerous experimental runs during this study, hematocrit varied as much as 0.18 units (e.g., 0.34–0.52) with less than a factor of two drop in flux at a given TMP, while the theory would predict the flux to drop by a factor of 5.7.

The theory of Colton was not available when this chapter was written. If, as this author has been given to understand, it calls for a linear dependence on shear rate and a weaker hematocrit function, it would more nearly accord with the qualitative findings of this study.

TABLE 1. *Thickness and saline permeability of membranes*

Membrane type	Thickness (μm)	Saline permeability[a]
Millipore	135	493
Membrana	163	199
AMF	132	514

[a]ml/(m^2 $\times$ min $\times$ torr).

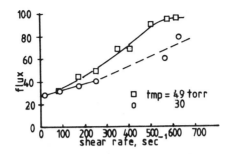

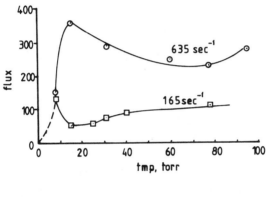

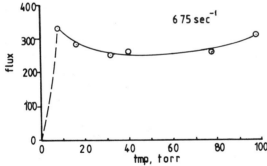

FIG. 5. **Top:** Flux [ml/(m × m²)] versus shear rate (reciprocal sec) for Millipore membrane at two different transmembrane pressures (TMP, torr). **Middle:** Flux versus TMP at two different shear rates, AMF membrane. **Bottom:** Flux versus TMP at 675 reciprocal sec, Enka membrane.

None of these membranes showed higher levels of plasma hemoglobin in the filtered plasma than in the plasma of the unfiltered blood. In many instances the hemoglobin level of the latter was, in fact, larger. It must be surmised that the pore size and surface chemistry of these membranes is such that flux is limited by cell accumulation and plugging, not by hemolysis, at least over the pressure range studied. The largest increment in plasma hemoglobin level observed was about 0.00015 g Hgb/ml.

APPENDIX 1: PLASMA HEMOGLOBIN DETERMINATION

Essentially the method of Standefer and Vanderjagt (3) was used, but with volumes adjusted to maximize sensitivity by reducing the volume of reacted solution to that required for the reading spectrophotometer. At present, the method is sensitive to 0.2% of the hemoglobin present in 1 ml of whole blood, that is, about 0.003 g Hgb/ml plasma. Limited stability of dilute hydrogen peroxide required three solutions to be used: 1 g of tetramethylbenzidine (TMB) (Sigma) dissolved in 100 ml 90% acetic acid; 1% hydrogen peroxide, prepared freshly by dilution of 1 ml of 30% solution with 29 ml of water; and 10% acetic acid in water as diluent. Lysate, consisting of 1 ml of whole blood in 19 ml of water, was prepared and used as a hemoglobin standard.

The assay is performed by combining 0.33 ml of TMB solution, 20 μl of plasma, and 0.33 ml of hydrogen peroxide solution, mixing, holding at room temperature for 20 min, adding 3.3 ml of 10% acetic acid solution, holding an additional 10 min at room temperature and reading optical absorbance in a Spectronic 20 spectrophotometer (Bausch & Lomb) at 600 mμ against a control containing 20 μl of water in place of plasma. The method was standardized by preparing dilutions of the 5% lysate. A straight line, passing through the origin, was obtained when absorbance was plotted versus the percentage lysis of the plasma sample over the range 0–5%. Hemoglobin content was reckoned from this calibration curve.

The principal difficulty with these measurements was the unexpectedly high level of plasma hemoglobin in the unfiltered plasma. The membrane was shown neither to be sieving nor adsorbing hemoglobin. Plasma hemoglobin levels decreased steadily with additional centrifugation of blood samples, suggesting that a few cells—insignificant for determining hematocrit—remained in the plasma layer of the blood samples and were responsible for the seemingly elevated levels of plasma hemoglobin.

ACKNOWLEDGMENTS

Specific data reported in this study were obtained at Columbia University by Mathew Dunleavy, Michael Giordano, Tova Stepner, and John Yin. Hemoglobin assays were adapted and tested by the latter (elaborations are presented in Appendix 1.) Research costs at Columbia University were borne in part by Grant GM 30205, from the National Institute of General Medical Sciences, National Institutes of Health. Initiation of the work was made possible by a grant from AMF, Inc. A suggestion of Lisa Moore led to the specific cone and plate geometry described here. Both she and John Munsch, who provided the motor drive, are employed by Travenol Laboratories, Round Lake, IL. Other parts of the system, most notably the plasmapheresis cell, were designed by Hermanus Bouwmann and constructed by him and Alfons Herremans who are employed by TERADEC, a Travenol subsidiary in Nivelles, Belgium. Valuable contributions were thus made from several parts of the Travenol organization and these are gratefully acknowledged.

REFERENCES

1. Forstrom, R. J., Bartelt, K., Blackshear, P. L., Jr., and Wood, T. (1975): Formed element deposition onto filtering walls. *Trans. ASAIO*, 21:602.
2. Zydney, A. L., and Colton, C. K. (1983): Continuous flow membrane plasmapheresis: Theoretical models for flux and hemolysis prediction. *Trans. ASAIO*, 28:408–412.
3. Standefer, J. C., and Vanderjagt, R. (1977): Use of tetramethylbenzidine in plasma hemoglobin assay. *Clin. Chem.*, 23:749.

Plasmapheresis, edited by Y. Nosé, P. S.
Malchesky, J. W. Smith, and R. S. Krakauer.
Raven Press, New York © 1983.

Membrane Plasmapheresis by Unipuncture Technique

Raymond VanHolder, Marc De Clippele, and Severin Ringoir

*Department of Internal Medicine, Renal Division, University Hospital,
B-9000 Gent, Belgium*

Plamapheresis has been described as a valuable technique in the treatment of several immunological disorders (1–4). Plasma exchange was originally performed using cell separators. However, due to the high complexity and cost of the equipment, this technique is only available in a limited number of hospitals. Membrane plasma exchange is a more simple technique, but is practiced almost exclusively in continuous flow on two needle systems.

Plasma exchange is performed in our unit using our conventional unipuncture dialysis equipment (5–8) and hollow fiber plasma separators. In the present chapter, this technique will be described. It is easily performed, well tolerated, and does not necessitate changes in the basic equipment if a unipuncture infrastructure of this type is already available.

METHODS

The basic technical equipment used in our unit for the performance of plasma exchange is illustrated in Fig. 1.

Blood access is obtained through a radioopaque Teflon catheter type Uldall SC-100 with an internal diameter of 1.8 mm and a length of 200 mm, introduced into the subclavian vein or through a 16-gauge single-lumen hemodialysis catheter (Deseret, Sandy, Utah), introduced into a peripheral brachial vein of sufficient internal diameter to allow the plasma exchange procedure.

In 3 patients (24 sessions) plasma exchange was carried out using a cellulose acetate hollow fiber plasma separator (Plasmaflo O1, Asahi Medical Co., Tokyo) with a surface area of 0.65 m^2 and a pore size less than 0.2 μm. In 2 other patients (9 sessions) exchanges were performed using a polypropylene CPS-10™ capillary plasma separator (Travenol Laboratories, S.A, Lessines, Belgium) (surface area: 0.17 m^2 and maximum pore size: 0.55 μm). The conventional unipuncture dialysis equipment of the double head pump type (Bellco BL 760, Mirandola, Italy) was used. The speed of the arterial and venous pumpheads was regulated in order to obtain a blood flow of about 150 ml/min. A positive pressure was allowed to build up in the blood compartment of the plasma filter to obtain a plasma filtration rate

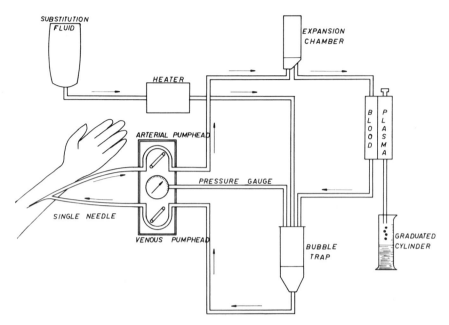

FIG. 1. Flow diagram of plasmapheresis unit, using conventional unipuncture dialysis equipment (BL 760).

of 20–40 ml/min, mean transmembrane pressures (TMP) ranging from 25 to 100 mmHg.

The ultrafiltration volume was substituted with 50% isotonic saline (+4 mEq KCl/liter) and 50% human plasma protein solution (SOPP) containing 4 g/100 ml of albumin. This substitution solution was infused at body temperature after passage through a fluid heater; the infusion rate was adjusted manually at regular 20-min intervals in order to keep a stable body weight. The patient was seated in a relaxing chair with continuous monitoring and instantaneous reading of body weight on a digital display (American Bed Scale Corp.).

At the start of each plasma exchange, 5,000 IU of heparin were administered intravenously. During the whole procedure, another 7,000–10,000 IU of heparin were given by continuous intravenous infusion in order to obtain blood clotting times between 10 and 25 min.

RESULTS

Table 1 summarizes some technical performance data. The filtered plasma volume per minute and the average TMP are slightly different for both plasma separators.

Some serum values before and after plasma exchange are reported for the Plasmaflo O1 separator in Table 2. Immunoglobulin, fibrinogen, and complement C3 levels decreased by at least 50% per plasma exchange session.

TABLE 1. *Technical performance (mean ± SEM)*

Plasma separator	Plasmaflo 01[a]	CPS-10™ capillary[b]
Total vol. of filtrate per session (ml)	3,224 ± 69	3,321 ± 72
Total duration per session (min)	119 ± 6	99 ± 8
Filtration vol. per min (ml/min)	28 ± 1	35 ± 2
Average TMP (mmHg)	61 ± 11	49 ± 7

[a]Asahi; 3 patients, 24 sessions.
[b]Travenol; 2 patients, 9 sessions.

TABLE 2. *Serum plasma exchange values (Plasmaflo 01; 3 patients)*

Components	Before	After	%
Total protein (g/100 ml)	6.42 ± 1.5	4.87 ± 0.10	− 24.14
IgA (g/liter)	2.24 ± 0.26	1.10 ± 0.15	− 55.28
IgG (g/liter)	7.16 ± 7.8	3.41 ± 0.38	− 52.37
IgM (g/liter)	1.00 ± 0.14	0.47 ± 0.06	− 53.42
Fibrinogen (mg/100 ml)	401 ± 31	171 ± 16	− 57.37
C3 (mg/100 ml)	105.62 ± 5.26	54.11 ± 2.17	− 48.77

Plasma exchange was well tolerated since no muscular cramps, headache, vomiting, or hypotensive episodes (systolic tension less than 100 mmHg) occurred. Continuous cardiac monitoring revealed no cardiac arrythmias.

CONCLUSION

Plasma exchange proved to be technically possible and well tolerated in 5 patients when performed by means of a hollow fiber plasma separator (Plasmaflo, Asahi, Tokyo, Japan or CPS-10™, Travenol, Lessines, Belgium) using conventional unipuncture dialysis equipment (double head pump Bellco, BL 760). Vascular access could be obtained by peripheral or subclavian vein catheterization. The heparin doses were adjusted to the clotting time values.

Appropriate blood compartment pressures were obtained and controlled using the double head pump TMP monitoring capacities. A plasma filtration rate of approximately 3 liters in 2 hr proved to be well tolerated without notable side effects.

Since the basic equipment is the same as that used in our hemodialysis unit (more than 100,000 conventional hemodialyses by unipuncture since 1973), no further costs or efforts were necessary for the introduction of plasma separation. The necessity of only a single vascular access site is in our opinion an advantage for the unipuncture approach.

ACKNOWLEDGMENT

We thank Mrs. I. Verslycken for secretarial assistance.

REFERENCES

1. Rossen, R., Hersh, E., Sharp, J., McCredie, K., Gyorkey, F., Suki, W., Eknoyan, G., and Reisberg, M. (1977): Effect of plasma exchanges on circulating immune complexes and antibody formation in patients treated with cyclophosphamide and prednisone. *Am. J. Med.*, 63:674.
2. Rizzo, G., Shires, D., Rifkin, S., De Quesada, A., and Pickering, J. (1981): Plasmapheresis treatment of rapidly progressive glomerulonephritis. *Dial. Transplant.*, 10:126.
3. Naik, R., Ashlin, R., Wilson, C., Smith, D., Lee, H., and Slapak, M. (1979): The role of plasmapheresis in renal transplantation. *Clin. Nephrol.*, 11:245.
4. Malchesky, P., Asanuma, Y., Hammersmidt, D., and Nosé, Y. (1980): Complement removal by sorbents in membrane plasmapheresis with on-line plasma treatment. *Trans. Am. Soc. Artif. Intern. Organs*, 26:541.
5. Ringoir, S., De Broe, M., Cardon, M., Van Waeleghem, J. P., and Boone, L. (1973): New pumpsystem for one needle dialysis. *Xth Congress of the European Dialysis and Transplant Association*, Vienna, p. 200 *(abstr.)*.
6. Hilderson, J., Ringoir, S., Van Waeleghem, J. P., van Egmond, J., Van Haelst, P., Schelstraete, K. (1975): Short dialysis with a polyacrylonitril membrane (RP6) without the use of a closed recirculating delivery system. *Clin. Nephrol.*, 4:18.
7. Ringoir, S., and Piron, M. (1979): An *in vitro* comparison of capillary flow dialyzer performances on a single needle system (double headpump). *Int. J. Artif. Organs*, 2:125.
8. Hoenich, N. A., Piron, M., De Cubber, A., Larno, L., and Ringoir, S. (1981): A study of the influence of single needle dialysis on the principal parameters of haemodialyser performance. *Int. J. Artif. Organs*, 4:168.

Plasmapheresis, edited by Y. Nosé, P. S. Malchesky, J. W. Smith, and R. S. Krakauer. Raven Press, New York © 1983.

Polyvinylalcohol Membranes for Plasma Separation

Akinori Sueoka, Jan Wojcicki, Paul S. Malchesky, and Yukihiko Nosé

Department of Artificial Organs, Cleveland Clinic Foundation, Cleveland, Ohio 44106

Membrane plasma separators are being used clinically for the removal of macromolecular weight solutes in autoimmune diseases (1). Until recently the major activity has centered about the use of cellulose acetate (2). Polyvinylalcohol (PVA) has been studied for use as a dialysis membrane and has been shown to have good permeability and biocompatibility (3–5). PVA is hydrophilic and easily modified structurally. Microporous PVA membranes of the hollow fiber type have been produced by Kuraray Co. (Osaka, Japan). These membranes have a high heat resistance and mechanical strength with high hydrophilicity. They are autoclavable and contain no additives.

MATERIALS AND METHODS

Membranes and Modules

Eight types of PVA plasma separators are listed in Table 1. They contain three types of membrane, S, M, and 400, with different membrane properties, membrane pore size, inner diameter, and wall thickness. The four module types, A, B, C, and N, have varying effective lengths, surface areas, and number of fibers. Scanning electron micrographs of the M and S type membrane are shown in Figs. 1 and 2.

In Vitro Experiments

In vitro evaluations were carried out (6) utilizing a closed plasma circuit as shown in Fig. 3. The sterile water prime was removed with 1 liter of normal saline. Prior to blood perfusion, the ultrafiltration rate for saline (UFR) was measured. The UFR value is corrected to 25°C based upon water viscosity data. Fresh bovine and human bloods of hematocrits of 33–39% were used. The blood was heparinized and kept at 37°C. Two types of test were carried out: (a) the determination of the maximum allowable plasma flux at a given blood flow rate, and (b) the determination of the stability of plasma flux as a function of time at a constant plasma flow selected to be below that of the maximum determined in step 1. The assessment of the maximum

TABLE 1. *Specifications of PVA plasma separators*

		Membrane				Module			
Filter type	Membrane type	Inner diam. (μm)	Outer diam. (μm)	Wall thickness (μm)	Pore size (μm)[a]	Module type	Effective length (cm)	No. of fibers	Surface area (m²)
SA	S	330	580	125	0.15	A	29	2100	0.63
SB	S	330	580	125	0.15	B	24	2100	0.52
SC	S	330	580	125	0.15	C	16	2100	0.35
MA	M	400	800	200	0.04	A	29	1100	0.40
MB	M	400	800	200	0.04	B	23	1100	0.32
MN	M	400	800	200	0.04	N	14.5	2400	0.43
400B	400	400	800	200	0.10	B	23	1100	0.32
400N	400	400	800	200	0.10	N	14.5	2400	0.43

Sterilization by steam autoclaving (121°C, 20 min) with sterile water.
[a]Determined by particle rejection studies.

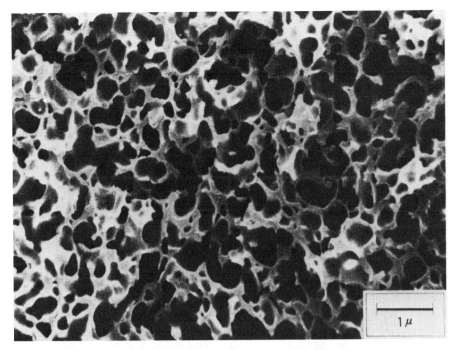

FIG. 1. Electron microscopic photograph showing a cross section of inner wall of M-type membrane.

plasma flux and its stability in time is made by following the course of the trans-membrane pressure (P_{TM}), plasma hemoglobin, and sieving coefficients for albumin, total protein, total cholesterol, fibrinogen, and immunoglobulins. The sieving coefficient is calculated as the concentration of the solute in the filtrate divided by its concentration in the incoming plasma. The different plasma flux tests were performed at varying constant blood flow rates (Q_B) of 50, 100, 200, and 500 ml/min, and in each test the plasma flow rate (Q_F) was increased at intervals of 30 min. The maximum Q_F ($Q_F$max) is defined as the maximum value of Q_F for which P_{TM} is constant and stable during the 30-min period with sieving of over 0.90 for albumin, and without hemolysis. The constant Q_F studies were carried out for 3 hr at constant Q_B, usually 100 ml/min, and constant Q_F equal to or below the $Q_F$max. The maximum plasma filtration rate ($J_F$max) normalized for $Q_F$max by surface area, and average wall shear rate ($\overline{\gamma}_w$) were discussed. $J_F$max (cm/min) was calculated as (7):

$$J_F\text{max} = \frac{Q_F\text{max}}{S}$$

where S is surface area (cm^2). $\overline{\gamma}_w$ (sec^{-1}) was calculated as:

$$\overline{\gamma}_w = \frac{2Q_{Bi} - Q_F\text{max}}{30\pi N r^3}$$

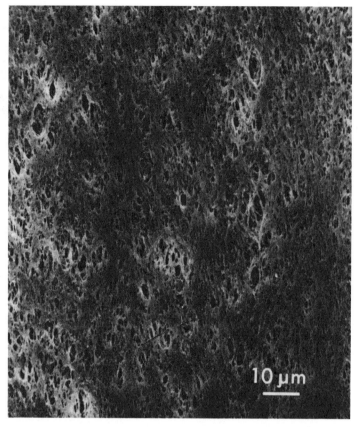

FIG. 2. Electron microscopic photograph showing inner surface of S-type membrane.

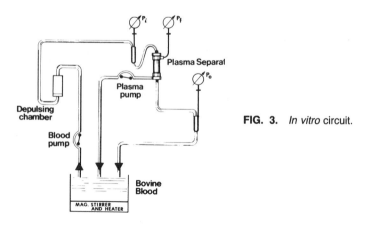

FIG. 3. *In vitro* circuit.

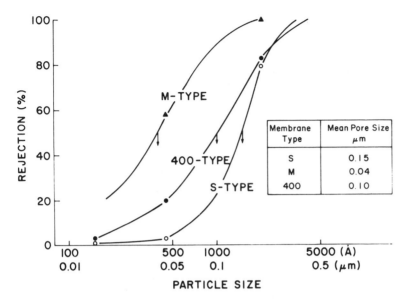

FIG. 4. Rejection curves of PVA membranes, S, M, and 400 type for particle of uniform size.

where Q_{Bi} is inlet blood flow rate (ml/min), N is number of fibers and r is inner radius of fiber (cm).

Ex Vivo Experiments

Ex vivo evaluations using male mongrel dogs were carried out to confirm *in vitro* results in the varying Q_F studies. The evaluations at constant Q_F were carried out to study blood cell damage and biocompatibility aspects of the module. Anesthesia was induced by sodium pentobarbital (10 mg/kg), and maintained by O_2 5 liters/min and halothene 0.2–0.4% throughout the perfusion. A femoral artery and vein or the A-V neck fistula was used for blood access. Heparin, 200 U/kg, was injected intravenously 5 min prior to the start of perfusion. The activated clotting time (ACT) was checked every 30–60 min, and 1,000 units of heparin were added when the ACT went below 200 sec.

Sampling was carried out for blood cell counts including red blood cells (RBC), white blood cells (WBC), and platelets (PLT), and for the marker macromolecular solutes such as albumin, total protein, total cholesterol, and fibrinogen. Samples were taken prior to the start of the perfusion, at 30, 60, 120, and 180 min during the perfusion.

Evaluation of Membrane Pore Size

Mean pore size of the membranes was evaluated by the filtration of 1% solution with particles of uniform size suspended in water. Studies were carried out at room

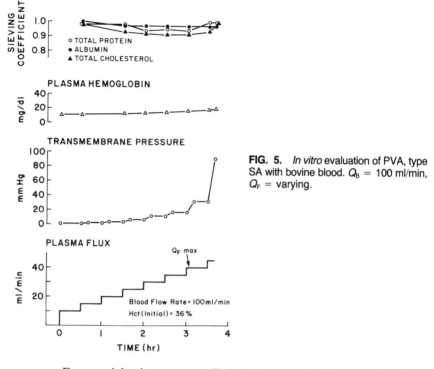

FIG. 5. *In vitro* evaluation of PVA, type SA with bovine blood. Q_B = 100 ml/min, Q_F = varying.

temperature. Four particle sizes were studied, 0.2 μm made of styrene-butadiene latex (Dow Chemical Co.) and 0.045, 0.015, and 0.008 μm made of colloidal silica (Nissan Chemical Co., Japan, and Dupont Co.). Particle solution flow rate was 100 ml/min and the filtrate rate was 5 ml/min. The circuit as outlined in Fig. 3 was utilized. Particle concentrations were measured through the weight determination of the solids following drying. The particle rejection was calculated as:

$$\text{Rejection (\%)} = \left(1 - \frac{\text{concentration of filtrate}}{\text{concentration of inlet solution}}\right) \times 100$$

The mean pore size of the membrane was defined as the value giving a 50% rejection as determined by the rejection curve (Fig. 4).

RESULTS

The particle rejection for three membrane types, S, M, and 400, are shown in Fig. 4. The evaluation of the pore size for tortuous membranes such as these and for those generally used for plasma separation is difficult due to their complicated pore structure. The method used in this study is preferred over the methods of the mercury penetration (8), bubble point (9), and air flow (10), since it is more relevant to the end use. From Fig. 4, the mean pore sizes obtained for the various membranes were 0.15 μm for S type, 0.04 μm for M type, and 0.10 μm for 400 type.

The ultrafiltration rates of saline (UFR) at 25°C were 46.2 ml/min·mmHg·m² for S type ($N = 29$), 40.7 for M type ($N = 13$), and 25.3 for 400 type ($N = 16$). The UFR relates to bulk membrane properties such as pore size, pore geometry, channel length, and pore density. Based upon UFR and pore size date, the S and M type are taken to have higher porosities than the 400-type membrane.

Examples of varying and constant plasma flow in *in vitro* studies using SA units are shown in Figs. 5 and 6. In the varying plasma flow study, P_{TM} gradually increased with increasing Q_F and remained stable and low at values of less than 40 mmHg. At Q_F 45 ml/min, the P_{TM} increased sharply. The plasma hemoglobin level showed no remarkable changes with time for 3.5 hr of pumping. Sieving coefficients were high, generally over 0.95 for total protein and albumin, and over 0.90 for total cholesterol. From these results, $Q_F$max was selected to be 40 ml/min at Q_B of 100 ml/min for the SA unit.

In the constant plasma flow study Q_F was 30 ml/min at Q_B of 100 ml/min with human blood. The P_{TM} and plasma hemoglobin were low and stable during the 3 hr. Sieving coefficients for albumin and immunoglobulin G (IgG) were over 0.95

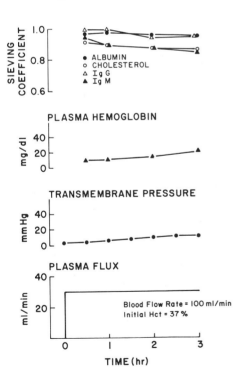

FIG. 6. *In vitro* evaluation of PVA, type SA with human blood. $Q_B = 100$ ml/min, $Q_F = 30$ ml/min.

TABLE 2. *Summary of* in vitro *tests with* Q_F *varying bovine blood*

Unit	Q_B (ml/min)	$Q_F$max (ml/min)	$J_F$max (cm/min $\times 10^{-2}$)	$\bar{\gamma}_w$ (sec^{-1})	Sieving coefficient Albumin	Total protein	Total cholesterol
SA	50	20	0.32	90	0.98	1.00	0.93
	100	40	0.63	188	0.97	0.96	0.93
	200	75	1.19	366	0.98	0.98	0.91
	500	170	2.70	934	0.94	0.93	0.89
SB	50	20	0.38	90	0.97	0.94	0.87
	100	35	0.67	186	0.98	0.94	0.86
	200	45	0.87	399	0.97	0.92	0.84
	500	110	2.12	1001	0.94	0.93	0.88
SC	50	10	0.29	101	0.97	0.93	0.88
	100	25	0.71	197	0.95	0.93	0.85
	200	40	1.14	405	0.97	0.95	0.88
	500	85	2.43	1029	0.94	0.92	0.87
MA	100	30	0.75	205	0.97	0.93	0.82
	200	45	1.13	428	0.96	0.96	0.84
	500	90	2.25	1170	0.92	0.89	0.70
MB	50	10	0.31	92	0.91	0.93	0.83
	100	25	0.78	213	0.95	0.95	0.84
	200	35	1.09	401	0.96	0.90	0.83
	500	55	1.72	1073	0.91	0.84	0.75
MN	100	15	0.35	102	0.97	0.94	0.85
	150	25	0.58	150	0.97	0.92	0.89
	200	25	0.58	193	0.97	0.93	0.83
400B	100	10	0.31	217	0.92	0.90	0.91
	200	20	0.63	458	0.93	0.91	0.86
	500	30	0.94	1145	0.94	0.92	0.85
400N	100	10	0.23	105	0.93	0.95	0.93
	200	15	0.35	204	0.95	0.94	0.91
	500	35	0.81	531	0.97	0.95	0.94

and for total cholesterol and IgM over 0.85 during this period. It must be noted that slight increases in plasma hemoglobin during *in vitro* tests are common due to trauma induced by the circuit and are quite distinguishable from increases due to trauma induced by the filtration process.

Figure 7 shows the results of *in vitro* tests of the three unit types, SA, MA, and 400N, operating under the same conditions of varying Q_F and constant Q_B, 100 ml/min, and using bovine blood. The $Q_F$max for each unit was 40 ml/min for SA, 30 ml/min for MN, and 15 ml/min for 400N. The sieving coefficient of albumin was generally over 0.95 for all units in the range of acceptable Q_F. The sieving coefficient of total cholesterol showed variability among the units; it was over 0.92 for S and 400, and between 0.80 and 0.85 for the M unit. For the M unit, the sieving coefficient decreased sharply for Q_F greater than $Q_F$max. It is noteworthy that the M-type membrane has the lowest mean pore size of the membranes evaluated.

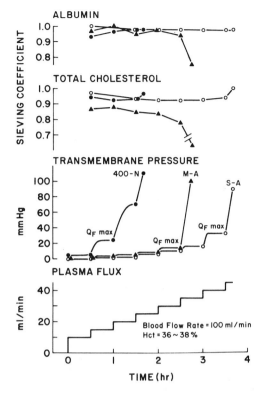

FIG. 7. *In vitro* evaluation of PVA, type SA, MA, and 400N with bovine blood. Q_B = 100 ml/min, Q_F = varying.

Results of *ex vivo* tests with the SA units at a constant Q_F of 30 ml/min and Q_B of 100 ml/min are shown in Fig. 8. No hemolysis was noted and P_{TM} was between 10 and 20 mmHg. Sieving coefficients were about 1.0 for albumin, total protein, and total cholesterol throughout the perfusion. The reduction ratios of WBC and PLT corrected for hemodilution by the RBC counts are shown in Fig. 8. The WBC and PLT counts decreased at 30 min into the perfusion, 30% for WBC and 50% for pre-perfusion, but gradually increased in time. The PLT counts post-perfusion were 80% and WBC were 65% of pre-perfusion values. These counts reached pre-perfusion values after 1 day.

DISCUSSION

The results of *in vitro* evaluations at constant Q_B of 50, 100, 200, and 500 ml/min and varying Q_F using bovine blood are summarized in Table 2 for the various units evaluated. The relationship between Q_B and $Q_F$max for the various units are shown in Fig. 9. Increasing Q_B and thus shear rate gave higher $Q_F$max for all units. The SA unit gave the highest $Q_F$max and the 400B unit the lowest throughout the

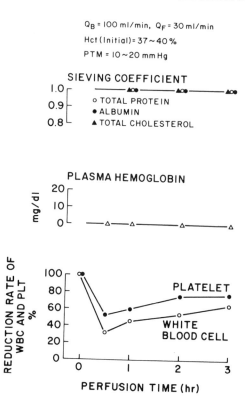

FIG. 8. *Ex vivo* evaluation of PVA, type SA with dog. Q_B = 100 ml/min, Q_F = 30 ml/min.

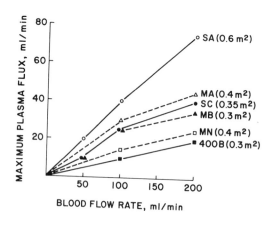

FIG. 9. Relationship of maximum plasma flux to blood flow rate for various PVA separators.

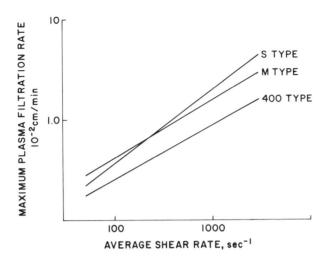

FIG. 10. Relationship of maximum plasma filtration rate to the average wall shear rate.

range of Q_B studied. The MN unit gave a lower $Q_F$max compared with the MA unit, even though both units contained the same surface area, 0.4 m². The major difference between these modules lies in the number of fibers. The MN unit has about two times the number of fibers, and therefore the shear rate is about one-half that for MA unit. The results of this study indicate that $Q_F$max is related to the membrane properties, in addition to module design and operating conditions.

The relationship of $J_F$max to $\bar{\gamma}_w$ for the various units are shown in Fig. 10. A good linear relationship between ln $J_F$max and ln $\bar{\gamma}_w$ was obtained for the S, M, and 400 type units with high correlation. The following relationships were obtained: S-type membrane: $J_F$max $= 8.7 \times 10^{-5} \bar{\gamma}_w^{0.81}$, correlation coefficient (c) $= 0.980$, $N = 12$. M-type membrane: $J_F$max $= 2.2 \times 10^{-4} \bar{\gamma}_w^{0.65}$, $c = 0.986$, $N = 11$. 400-type membrane: $J_F$max $= 1.3 \times 10^{-4}\bar{\gamma}_w^{0.62}$, $c = 0.950$, $N = 6$. These results show that $J_F$max directly relates to $\bar{\gamma}_w$ and that this relationship may be unique to the membrane properties. No correlation is noted with module length for a given membrane type. The highest $J_F$max is noted for the S-type units at high $\bar{\gamma}_w$ (>250 sec^{-1}) and for the M-type units at low $\bar{\gamma}_w$ (<250 sec $^{-1}$). The 400-type units had the lowest $J_F$max throughout the entire range of $\bar{\gamma}_w$. In general, the $J_F$max for the various membrane types parallels UFR, stressing the importance of overall membrane porosity, while the sieving data stresses the importance of pore size.

Sieving coefficients of total protein and albumin are generally over 0.90 for all units, as shown in Table 2. However, the sieving coefficient of total cholesterol was shown to be highly dependent on membrane type and its mean pore size. The large pore size membrane (>0.10 μm) are required to achieve high sieving of macromolecular weight solutes.

Reduction of WBC and PLT noted in *ex vivo* studies are typical in such extracorporeal perfusion and are not specific to the unit under investigation. These studies show the acceptability of PVA as a plasma separator membrane.

CONCLUSION

The SA unit, having the largest surface area, 0.63 m^2, a mean pore size of 0.15 μm, and a UFR of 46.2 ml/min·mmHg·m^2, has been selected for clinical use. Q_F is 20, 40, and 75 ml/min at Q_B 50, 100, and 200 ml/min, respectively, and sieving coefficients for total protein and albumin are over 0.95 and for total cholesterol over 0.90. PVA plasma separators exhibit no hemolysis when operated under the $Q_F$max and only minimal blood cell changes occur during perfusion. Plasma flux is directly related to wall shear rate, dependent upon the membrane type, and independent of module length. The properties of PVA make it a promising material for plasma separator construction.

REFERENCES

1. Malchesky, P. S., Asanuma, Y., Smith, J. W., Kayashima, K., Zawicki, I., Werynski, A., Blumenstein, M., and Nosé, Y. (1981): Macromolecule removal from blood. *Trans. Am. Soc. Artif. Intern. Organs*, 27:439.
2. Malchesky, P. S., Werynsky, A., Asanuma, Y., Zawicki, I., Nosé, Y., Smith, J. W., Kayashima, K., and Gurland, H. (1981): Clinical operation of Asahi plasma separators. *Artif. Organs*, 5(Suppl.):113.
3. Markle, R. A., Falb, R. D., and Leininger, R. I. (1964): Development of improved membranes for artificial kidney dialysis. *Trans. Am. Soc. Artif. Intern. Organs*, 10:22.
4. Odian, M., and Leonard, E. F. (1968): Synthesis and evaluation of graded polyvinylalcohol membranes. *Trans. Am. Soc. Artif. Intern. Organs*, 14:19.
5. Bernstein, B. S. (1968): *J. Polymer Sci, Part A*, 3:3405.
6. Asanuma, Y., Malchesky, P. S., Zawicki, I., Smith, J. W., Carey, W. D., Ferguson, D. R., Hermann, R. E., and Nosé, Y. (1980): Clinical hepatic support by on-line plasma treatment with multiple sorbents. *Trans. Am. Soc. Artif. Intern. Organs*, 26:400.
7. Werynski, A., Malcheski, P. S., Sueoka, A., Asanuma, Y., Smith, J. W., Kayashima, K., Herpy, E., Sato, H., and Nosé, Y. (1981): Membrane plasma separation: Toward improved clinical operation. *Trans. Am. Soc. Artif. Intern. Organs*, 27:539.
8. Washburn, E. W. (1966): *Proc. Natl. Acad. Sci., USA*, 7:115.
9. ASTM F316-70. Schweitzer, P. A. (1979): Handbook of Separation technique for chemical engineers. Section 2, pp. 89. McGraw-Hill Press, New York.
10. ASTM F301-70.

Plasmapheresis, edited by Y. Nosé, P. S.
Malchesky, J. W. Smith, and R. S. Krakauer.
Raven Press, New York © 1983.

Reuse of Membrane Plasma Separators

David H. Randerson, Matthias Blumenstein, Walter Samtleben,
Baerbel Schmidt, and Hans J. Gurland

*Medizinische Klinik I, Klinikum Grosshadern, University of Munich,
D-8000 Munich 70, Federal Republic of Germany*

Membrane plasma separation is routinely used for on-line plasmapheresis in a variety of immunologically mediated diseases. Polymeric membranes have been developed over the past 5 years that are capable of separating plasma with full protein complement and completely rejecting formed elements. However, the process remains costly because of the expense of reinfusion fluids and the disposable hollow fiber separators. Methods to reduce replacement solution requirement are being developed, such as cascade and cryoprecipitate filtration, and selective immunoadsorption systems. It is anticipated that the cost of the primary plasma separator will decrease over the next few years with greater production volume, particularly when Health Administration approval has been granted in the US, and with increased competition. Reuse, as commonly employed with hollow fiber hemodialyzers, will enable further reduction in plasmapheresis expenditure.

One published report on plasma separator reuse (1), in which the reduction in serum levels of proteins were compared following first and second uses, concluded that reuse was impractical because of increased solute rejection by the membrane, possibly the result of protein adsorption and cellular deposition. However, these findings have been contradicted by a more recent study (2) in which it was found that the reduction of serum immunoglobulin (IgG and IgA) levels was similar on first and third use of the filter, although IgM removal was reduced further. The latter study reports satisfactory experience up to six reuses. Both of these studies were performed using the prototype of plasma separators, the Plasmaflo 01. Two other devices have recently become available, the Plasmaflo 02, which has a thinner fiber wall and improved mass transfer characteristics, and the Plasmaflux, which features an increased maximum pore size. We have assessed these two newer devices for reuse, by measuring performance parameters both *in vitro* and *ex vivo* following first use in clinical plasmapheresis, and have attempted to define optimum operating conditions for reuse.

Present address of D. H. R.: School of Chemical Engineering, University of Queensland, St. Lucia, Qld. 4067, Australia.

MATERIALS AND METHODS

The Plasmaflo 02 (PF02) (Asahi Medical, Japan) is made with cellulose diacetate membrane, 0.5 m^2 surface area, wall thickness 75 μm, inner fiber diameter 330 μm, and maximum pore size 0.2 μm. The Plasmaflux (Px) (Fresenius MTS, FRG) is made with polypropylene membrane, 0.5 m^2 surface area, wall thickness 140 μm, inner fiber diameter 330 μm, and maximum pore size 0.5 μm.

Four parameters were used to characterize device performance: plasma flux rate, protein sieving coefficient, saline filtration rate, and maximum stable plasma filtration rate.

The plasma flux rate (ml/hr/m^2/mmHg) was determined at a fixed filtration rate (ml/min), normalized to transmembrane pressure (TMP) and surface area.

The sieving coefficient (SC) is the ratio of solute concentrations between blood and filtrate sides of the membrane. For a hollow fiber device, blood side concentration is generally taken as the mean inlet–outlet blood solute levels. SCs were measured simultaneously for a spectrum of endogenous proteins ranging in molecular weight (MW) from albumin (67,000 daltons) to β-lipoprotein (2.4 million daltons), using laser nephelometry (Behring Institute, Marburg, FRG) for protein determination.

Saline filtration rate was measured at 37 ± 0.5°C with isotonic (0.15 M) saline using a static technique. The plasma separator was deaerated and placed in a constant temperature bath, and a gravity-induced static pressure applied to the blood compartment. Filtration rate was measured by timed collection and TMP accurately measured by transducers (Bentley Trantec, Irvine, CA). Saline flux was measured at TMPs ranging from 1 to 20 mmHg and data expressed as filtration rate (ml/min) at 10 mmHg (Q_{10}) obtained by linear regression.

For any plasma separator design, there exists a maximum filtration rate (Q_{Fmax}): beyond which cellular matter is drawn into the membrane and operation at stable TMP is no longer possible (3). Q_{Fmax} was determined *in vitro* using fresh whole human blood from healthy volunteers with hematocrit adjusted to 40% employing a recirculation procedure at 37 ± 0.5°C. Plasma filtration was increased in steps of 4 ml/min from 16 ml/min, and TMP monitored for 15 min at each step. The procedure was continued until a filtration rate was obtained where TMP progressively increased, characterized by a rapidly falling filtrate chamber pressure. The highest filtration rate giving stable operation was taken as Q_{Fmax}.

Rinsing Procedures and Sterilization

Following clinical plasmapheresis *(ex vivo)* and *in vitro* assessment, 1 liter sterile saline was flushed through the blood side, arterial to venous, at 150–200 ml/min with filtrate chamber closed. Three liters were then run in the filtrate side and out the blood side under a gravity head of approximately 75 cm. The first liter was drained through the venous port, the second through the arterial, and the final liter through the venous port. During rinsing the module was tapped lightly to dislodge cells, and the filtrate chamber was free of air. Following rinsing, both blood and filtrate chambers were filled with 2% formaldehyde in sterile saline.

Before reuse, formaldehyde solution was drained from filtrate chamber of separators. One liter of sterile saline at 100 ml/min was passed through the blood side to purge fibers, with occasional filling and draining of filtrate chamber. An additional 3 liters were passed at 50 ml/min (for 1 hr) blood inlet to filtrate, to facilitate slow desorption of formaldehyde from the membrane.

In Vitro Evaluation

Three of each plasma separator were obtained following clinical usage, rinsed, and saline filtration rate measured. Following storage for 2–4 days, each device was evaluated for a second use *in vitro* using fresh whole human blood of the same ABO group as that of the patients. Flux rates and SCs were monitored over 2 hr at 37 $\pm$ 0.5°C using previously described recirculation procedures (4). Blood inlet rate was held constant at 100 ml/min and filtration rate adjusted to maintain constant TMP, but in any case never exceeded 30 ml/min. After the "second use" the plasma separators were again rinsed, Q_{10} determined, and stored for a further 2–4 days prior to a third *(in vitro)* evaluation. Q_{10} was determined following "third use," and finally the Q_{Fmax} measured. Q_{10} and Q_{Fmax} were also measured on new plasma separators for comparative purposes. These latter devices were not used clinically.

Ex Vivo Evaluation

Three of each PF02 and Px were reused a second time on patients. *Ex vivo* assessment comprised measurement of SCs and flux rates at 0.5-, 1.0-, 1.5-, and 2.0-liter exchange volumes. Patients received a bolus dose of 5,000 IU of heparin followed by a continuous infusion of 50 IU/min. Substitution fluid was albumin solution (Humalbin, Behring Institute, Marburg, FRG) diluted with electrolyte solution to 2.5% albumin.

Analysis of Data

Significance was assessed by analysis of variance for the *ex vivo*/*in vitro*/*in vitro* and the *ex vivo*/*ex vivo* studies. The influences of the following factors on SC variation were assessed: plasma separator (PF02, Px), use (1st, 2nd, 3rd), perfusion time (10, 30, 60, 90, and 120 min), and protein (albumin, IgG, IgA, IgM, α_2-macroglobulin and β-lipoprotein). The influences of device type, use, and time on flux rate were also assessed. All data are presented as mean $\pm$ SEM. SCs are expressed as a percentage.

RESULTS

Significant factors affecting SC of proteins obtained during the *in vitro* studies were the device ($p < 0.01$) and protein size ($p < 0.001$). The difference in SC values between uses was only significant at the 10% level, and the change in SC with perfusion time was not significant ($p < 0.1$). The interaction [plasma separator] $\times$ [use] was highly significant ($p < 0.001$). No other interactions were significant.

Mean SCs for the PF02 and Px are presented in Table 1, demonstrating the better performance of the Px. Table 2 presents mean SC data for the individual proteins showing the lower solute flux rate for the higher MW proteins. Mean SCs for the interaction [plasma separator] $\times$ [use] are presented in Table 3. Mean SCs decline substantially between the first and subsequent uses of the PF02, while the Px gave improved performance on the second and third uses compared with the initial use. Determination of Q_{Fmax} following the third use included determination of protein SCs (note there was a rinsing procedure and Q_{10} measurement prior to the Q_{Fmax} study). These data were not included in the statistical analysis because the test was not consistent with the study protocol; however, they provide a rough indication of suitability for a fourth use. Means SCs obtained at flow rates below Q_{Fmax} were 84.0 $\pm$ 1.2% and 90.3 $\pm$ 0.7% ($N = 54$) for the PF02 and Px, respectively.

Mean plasma flux rates for the three uses are presented in Table 4. There was no significant difference between uses because of the high variability of flux rate. Flux rates for the two plasma separators were also not significantly different.

Saline filtration results, expressed as Q_{10} values, obtained once on each of devices unused, and following each use, are presented in Table 5. The data suggest that the major loss of permeability occurred during the initial use, and that the drop was greater for the smaller pore PF02.

TABLE 1. *Mean sieving coefficients:*
comparison of plasma separators

Device	Plasmaflo 02	Plasmaflux
SC	88.1 $\pm$ 0.8	90.6 $\pm$ 0.7

Mean $\pm$ SEM, $N = 270$, $p < 0.01$.

TABLE 2. *Mean sieving coefficients: comparison of proteins*

Protein	Alb	IgG	IgA	IgM	α_2-macro	β-lipo
SC	95.0	92.1	90.4	86.9	85.9	85.9
	$\pm$0.8	$\pm$1.0	$\pm$0.9	$\pm$1.6	$\pm$1.5	$\pm$1.8

Mean $\pm$ SEM, $N = 90$, $p < 0.001$.

TABLE 3. *Mean sieving coefficients:*
[plasma separator] $\times$ [use] interaction

Device	Plasmaflo 02	Plasmaflux
1st use	95.1 $\pm$ 1.0	81.7 $\pm$ 1.3
2nd use	87.4 $\pm$ 1.7	95.1 $\pm$ 0.7
3rd use	81.9 $\pm$ 1.4	95.1 $\pm$ 0.6

Mean $\pm$ SEM, $N = 90$, $p < 0.001$.

TABLE 4. *Mean plasma flux rates: comparison of uses*

Use	1	2	3
Flux	290 ± 27	390 ± 44	290 ± 39
ml/hr/m²/mmHg			

Mean ± SEM, $N = 30$, differences not significant.

TABLE 5. *Saline filtration rate on new plasma separators and following each use*

Plasma separators	New ($N = 1$)	1st use ($N = 3$)	2nd use ($N = 3$)	3rd use ($N = 3$)
Plasmaflo 02	410	140 ± 26	140 ± 51	140 ± 13
Plasmaflux	310	160 ± 43	160 ± 65	150 ± 29

Q_{10}, ml/min at 10 mmHg, mean ± SEM.

TABLE 6. *Maximum plasma filtration rate on new plasma separators and following 3rd use*

Use		Plasmaflo 02	Plasmaflux
New ($N = 1$)	Q_{Fmax}(ml/min)	36	36
	Outlet hematocrit (%)	61	62
After 3rd use ($N = 3$)	Q_{Fmax}(ml/min)	32 ± 2.3	32 ± 2.3
	Outlet hematocrit (%)	56 ± 1.2	58 ± 2.7

Mean ± SEM, blood inlet flow rate 100 ml/min and inlet hematocrit 40%.

Results of the determination of maximum stable plasma filtration rate are presented in Table 6, and show that there was a similar drop for both plasma separators from 36 to 32 ± 2 ml/min ($N = 3$) over the three uses. The data include a Q_{Fmax} value of 28 ml/min obtained in one instance with both plasma separators. In both cases the initial use was on the same patient, who exhibited excessive loss of fiber bundle volume whenever undergoing membrane plasmapheresis. This may be related to elevated platelet counts (>400 × 10⁹/liter) and fibrinogen levels (5–8 g/liter).

A measure of the efficacy of the backrinse procedure can be obtained by comparison of SC and flux rate data taken at 10 min into each use. The data, presented in Table 7, show there was complete recovery of mass transfer properties following rinsing.

Comparison of the first and second use *ex vivo* data are presented in Table 8. Again, a significant decline in SC was observed for the PF02 ($p < 0.001$), while data for the Px remained unchanged between uses. Plasma flux rate for the PF02 dropped ($p < 0.001$), while the Px had a nonsignificant increase.

TABLE 7. *Comparison of sc and flux rate data obtained after 10 min of each use*

Parameter	1st use	2nd use	3rd use
SC (N = 36)	89.0 ± 1.5	88.4 ± 1.6	92.3 ± 1.6
Flux rate, ml/hr/m²/mmHg (N = 6)	350 ± 73	370 ± 83	310 ± 87

Mean ± SEM, differences between uses not significant.

TABLE 8. *Results of analysis involving two clinical plasmaphereses*

Parameter		Plasmaflo 02	Plasmaflux
SC (N = 60)	1st use	92.2 ± 1.3	95.5 ± 1.0
	2nd use	89.2 ± 1.2	96.8 ± 0.9
Flux rate, ml/hr/m²/mmHg (N = 12)	1st use	390 ± 46	320 ± 50
	2nd use	255 ± 13	360 ± 48

Mean ± SEM; SC, $p < 0.001$; Flux, $p < 0.001$.

DISCUSSION

Loss of sieving properties during membrane plasma exchange can result from protein adsorption by the membrane, occlusion of pores by macromolecules and formed elements, and clotting of fibers leading to loss of surface area. Although all three processes are essentially irreversible, it may be possible to dislodge formed elements deposited on the membrane surface, producing partial recovery of sieving properties, and to reuse in a manner compensating for loss of surface area, thus maintaining the filtering process at optimum efficiency.

The results demonstrate that membrane plasma separators can function efficiently for two or more treatments. Backrinsing is capable of removing most cellular debris such that the properties of the membrane are similar at the start of perfusion on second and third use as observed on initial use. Protein sorption probably occurs to the major extent in the first use, and is negligible thereafter, as exhibited by stable saline filtration characteristics.

The major factor causing loss of efficiency on reuse is fiber clotting, similar to that which restricts hemodialyzer efficiency. In two clinical treatments using the PF02 and one with the Px, considerable fiber clotting was visibly obvious. Backrinsing of these devices was ineffective in cleaning the clotted fibers, and Q_{Fmax} following final evaluation was reduced in all three devices. An attempt to reuse one device at a filtration rate of 30 ml/min resulted in rapid pore plugging with rising TMP and declining SCs. On the third use of this device, filtration rate was reduced to 24 ml/min and performance remained satisfactory with high SC values. The remaining two clotted devices were used at filtration rates reduced (20–26 ml/min) to maintain stable TMPs, and performance remained satisfactory. Therefore, if compensated for by reduced filtration rate, and thus longer treatment time, loss of fiber bundle volume need not represent a major restriction.

The slightly better performance of the Px on reuse relative to initial use may relate to incomplete hydrophilization during the manufacture of the device. First use of this device often required filtration rates considerably less than 30 ml/min to maintain stable operation. This is exemplified by measurement of Q_{Fmax} on two new devices giving values of 16 and 26 ml/min, and Q_{10} values of 57 and 160 ml/min. The data presented in Tables 5 and 6 for unused Px were obtained on a device hydrophilized in this laboratory. Usage and storage in aqueous media may partially improve hydrophilicity of the membrane. Fresenius has since advised us that hydrophilization problems have been overcome.

Although the rinse procedure was sufficient to avoid immediate symptoms such as burning sensation in fistula and hemolysis, the gradual appearance of anti-N-like antibodies remains a possibility that requires long-term investigation. However, as membrane plasmapheresis is not a long-term chronic treatment, as is hemodialysis, and that by definition plasmapheresis reduces antibody levels, it is unlikely that antibody formation is likely to be a serious complication of reuse.

ACKNOWLEDGMENTS

The authors are grateful to R. Gebhardt, H. Löbell, J. Nusser, and D. Woisetschläger for valuable technical assistance.

REFERENCES

1. Schmitt, E., Falkenhagen, D., Preussner, S., Tessenow, W., Holtz, M., and Klinkmann, H. (1980): Plasma separation and plasmapheresis — a comparative study. In: *Plasma Exchange. Plasmapheresis — Plasmaseparation*, edited by H. G. Sieberth, pp. 99. Schattauer, Stuttgart, New York.
2. Gajdos, Ph., Simon, N., Elkharrat, D., and Goulon, M. (1981): Essai d'une membrane de diacétate de cellulose pour les échanges plasmatiques. *Nouv. Presse Med.*, 10:3469.
3. Werynski, A., Malchesky, P. S., Sueoka, A., Asanuma, Y., Smith, J. W., Kayashima, K., and Nosé, Y. (1981): Membrane plasma separation: Toward improved clinical operation. *Trans. Am. Soc. Artif. Intern. Organs*, 27:539.
4. Randerson, D. H., Schmidt, B., Blumenstein, M., Samtleben, W., and Gurland, H. J. (1981): Comparison of membrane filtration properties with fresh and stored blood. *Artif. Organs*, 5(Suppl.):105.

Plasmapheresis, edited by Y. Nosé, P. S.
Malchesky, J. W. Smith, and R. S. Krakauer.
Raven Press, New York © 1983.

Automatic Control Apparatus for Membrane Plasmapheresis

T. Agishi, I. Kaneko, Y. Hasuo, K. Ota, H. Amemiya,
N. Sugino, *M. Abe

*Kidney Center, Tokyo Women's Medical College; *Kawasumi Laboratories, Inc.,
Tokyo, Japan*

Membrane plamapheresis is expected to become an increasingly significant therapeutic modality for the treatment of macromolecular disturbances such as immune diseases, hyperviscosity syndrome, and peripheral circulatory disorders. Possible major hazards in membrane plasmapheresis technology are hemolysis on the surface of the separation membrane and imbalance between the amount of the extracted and reinfused fluids. The former develops at improper transmembrane pressures (TMP) which are created in the process of filtration. The situation is further complicated in double filtration plasmapheresis (DFPP) (1–4), in which two membrane filters with different pore sizes are utilized to selectively remove pathogenic macromolecules in plasma. In this system, the four pumps, one for extracorporeal circulation, one for transferring the filtrate of the first filter to the second filter, one for discarding the macromolecular fraction, and one for infusing the replacement fluid, have to be strictly controlled.

Following is a report of an automatic control apparatus for membrane plasmapheresis which has been devised in an attempt to solve the problems mentioned above, and a discussion of the practical advantages observed in its clinical application.

MANUAL CONTROL

The principle and procedure of DFPP have been reported in detail elsewhere (1–4) and will thus be described only briefly here. Two filters with different pore sizes are installed in an extracorporeal circuit. Plasma is first separated from whole blood by a plasma separator with large pores. Plasma is then led to a second filter, the plasma filter, which has smaller pores and separates it into two components, one containing larger molecules and one containing smaller molecules. The filtrate of the second filter, which contains the smaller molecules, is mixed with the blood cell-rich component and returned to the patient. The component containing the larger molecules is discarded after selective concentration by the double-step filtration process. This rather complicated procedure was invented for the purpose of reducing the amount of replacement fluid—in other words, the amount of human blood product for substitution (3).

Figure 1 depicts the four pumps, one for extracorporeal circulation (A), one for transferring the filtrate of the first filter to the second (B), one for discarding the macromolecular component (C), and one for infusing the replacement fluid (D), which must be strictly controlled. TMP is created by the extracorporeal circulation pump (A) and the filtrate transferring pump (B). Improper control of either pump causes hemolysis. The balance between the amount of extracted plasma and that of the infusion fluid is maintained by two pumps—the one that discards the macromolecular component (C) and the one that infuses the replacment fluid (D). These fundamental concepts on hemolysis and fluid balance are, of course, applicable for simple standard membrane plasmapheresis.

FUNCTIONAL PRINCIPLES

The apparatus has three roller type pumps (Fig. 2 and 3). The extracorporeal circulation pump (I) delivers blood from the patient to the plasma separator at the maximum flow rate of 220 ml/min. Pump II transfers the filtrate of the first filter, the plasma separator, to the second filter, the plasma filter. Pump III works simultaneously both for removal of the macromolecular component and for infusion of the replacement fluid with two similar sized tubes. Pump I delivers blood at a steady blood flow rate, usually between 100 and 150 ml/min.

The pressure gradient at the blood inlet of the plasma separator and at the filtrate chamber of the plasma separator is continuously monitored. The desired upper and lower limit of the pressure gradient, representing the TMP, is set. Pumps II and III both function at the desired speed as long as the pressure gradient remains within the preset limit. Once the pressure gradient (TMP) exceeds the preset limit, both pumps stop instantaneously and automatically. Subsequently, the pressure gradient (TMP) returns to the preset level, and both pumps return to operation.

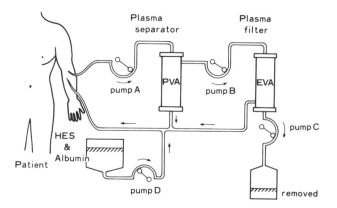

FIG. 1. Block diagram of manual DFPP.

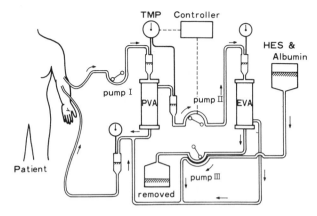

FIG. 2. Block diagram of automatic DFPP apparatus.

Balance between the amount of removal and replacement is theoretically made by the simultaneous squeezing movement of the similar sized bore tubes in the single rotating axis of pump III. The cumulative volume disposed by pumps II and III is recorded.

PLASMA SEPARATOR AND PLASMA FILTER

The plasma separator for the first step of filtration is composed of polyvinylalcohol hollow fibers, and the plasma filter for the secondary filtration process is made of ethylenevinylalcohol hollow fibers (Kuraray Co., and Kawasumi Laboratories, Tokyo, Japan).

RESULTS OF CLINICAL APPLICATION

TMP, which is represented as the gradient between the pressure at a blood inlet of the plasma separator and the filtrate chamber of the plasma separator, was set to be lower than 100 mmHg for this particular plasma separator. As a result, occurrence of hemolysis was markedly reduced. An average free hemoglobin concentration in the filtrate of the plasma separator was 1.9 mg/dl in the automatic control apparatus as compared with 24.9 mg/dl in the previous manual control system (Fig. 4).

There was a more steady flux of plasma in the plasma separator as compared with decreasing flux with time in the manual control system.

Evaluation of balancing function between removal and substitution was performed by direct comparison of the automatically removed and substituted amount. There was a good correlation between the amount removed and substituted (Fig. 5).

As mentioned previously, double filtration plasmapheresis was devised with the intention of selectively concentrating the pathogenic macromolecules. Concentration performance was expressed by the concentration coefficient (concentration coefficient = concentration of a particular solute in the removed plasma fraction to be

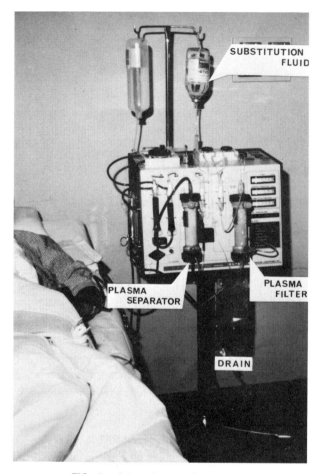

FIG. 3. Automatic control apparatus.

discarded/concentration of a particular solute in the separated plasma by a plasma separator). The concentration coefficient for electrolytes such as Na and K, and for small molecules such as urea, creatinine, and uric acid is approximately 1.0. No concentration of these substances occurred. The larger the molecular size of the solute, the larger was the concentration coefficient. The concentration coefficient was approximately 1.5 for albumin with a molecular weight of 68,000, 2.7 for IgG and IgA with a molecular weight of 160,000–170,000, and 3.5 for IgM with a molecular weight of 950,000 (Fig. 6).

DISCUSSION

An automatic control apparatus was built mainly for the purpose of making the double filtration plasmapheresis process easier. The apparatus is, of course, usable

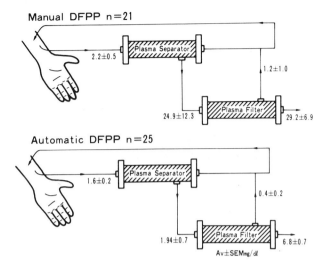

FIG. 4. Comparison of hemolysis between manual and automatic DFPP.

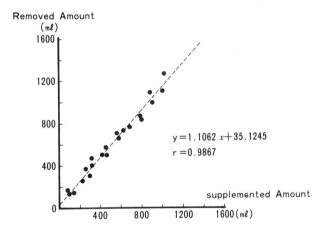

FIG. 5. Automatic removal versus supplementation.

for simple membrane plasmapheresis. Clinical application with this apparatus gave evidence that membrane plasmapheresis is performed not only in an easier way, but also in a safer and more effective manner. Hemolysis on the surface of the plasma separation membrane occurs much less frequently when the transmembrane pressure is strictly controlled so as not to exceed a preset limit. Automatic control of the transmembrane pressure also provides stable plasma filtration. Excessive application of transmembrane pressure is well known to cause an early fall in plasma flux due to plugging of the membrane pores with a protein cake. Regulation of transmembrane pressure will be of increasing concern as new membrane plasma

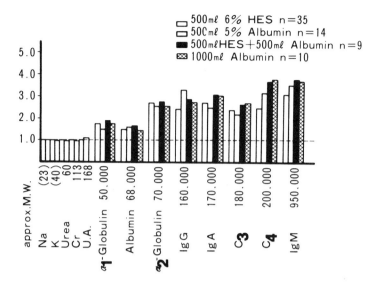

FIG. 6. Concentration performance of DFPP.

separators appear on the market that have various permeability properties requiring specific operating conditions.

Removal of the fractionated plasma and supplementation of the fluid is performed with balance. This is of major importance for safety in plasma exchange.

Concentration performance in double filtration plasmapheresis using a polyvinylalcohol plasma separator and an ethylenevinylalcohol plasma filter with the automatic control apparatus was acceptable. Selectivity in concentration of the solutes is more marked as the molecular size of the solutes increases. This is advantageous for removal of the large molecules. A solute with a concentration coefficient, for example, of 3.0 required only one-third the replacement fluid. Reduction of the amount of replacement fluid will save human blood products and lessen the chances of contracting transfusion hepatitis.

However, a considerable amount of albumin is leaked from this system. In order to decrease the leakage of albumin, alteration of the membrane properties of the second filter, the plasma filter, is necessary. It is , however, anticipated that a certain amount of macromolecules, which have a molecular size approximately similar to albumin, will be concomitantly returned to patients if retrieval of albumin is attempted using currently available membrane materials. Therefore, in order to avoid the situation in which the macromolecules that may contain pathogenic factors are again returned to the patient, the leakage of albumin must be tolerated as long as the membrane materials used in currently available plasma filters are utilized.

In conclusion, the newly devised control apparatus described herein has been found to be a simple, safe, and efficient system for membrane plasmapheresis.

REFERENCES

1. Agishi, T., Kaneko, I., Hasuo, Y., et al. (1979): Double filtration of selective removal or retrieval of plasma fraction. *Abstr. ASAIO*, 8:70.
2. Agishi, T., Kaneko, I., Hasuo, Y., et al. (1980): Double filtration plasmapheresis. *Trans. Am. Soc. Artif. Intern. Organs*, 26:406.
3. Agishi, T., Kaneko, I., Hasuo, Y., et al. (1980): Double filtration plasmapheresis with no or minimal amount of blood derivative for substitution. In: *Plasma Exchange*, edited by H. G. Sieberth, Schattauer-Verlag, Stuttgart, New York.
4. Agishi, T., Chikamori, M., Suzuki, T., Ota, K., Amemiya, H., and Sugino, N. (1981): Effect of double filtration plasmpheresis on peripheral circulation. In: *Therapuetic Plasmapheresis (I)*, edited by T. Oda, p. 119. Schattauer-Verlag, Stuttgart, New York.

Plasmapheresis, edited by Y. Nosé, P. S. Malchesky, J. W. Smith, and R. S. Krakauer. Raven Press, New York © 1983.

Clinical Evaluation of a Variable Geometry Membrane Plasma Exchange System

G. Delbert Antwiler, George W. Buffaloe, Ross R. Erickson, Frank Corbin, and Donn D. Lobdell

Cobe Laboratories, Inc., Lakewood, Colorado 80215

The Cobe Centry TPE System is a self-contained, integrated membrane plasma separation system intended for use in therapeutic plasma exchange (TPE). Plasma separation is accomplished by a variable geometry parallel plate membrane separator consisting of six blood channels. The total surface area of the separator is 0.13 m² with nominal pore size of 0.6 μm. Substantially improved operating characteristics over other previously described membrane separation devices has been accomplished because the system can control the geometry of the blood channels and transmembrane pressures in response to clinical conditions, for example, blood flow rate and hematocrit.

SYSTEM DESCRIPTION

It is well established that efficient membrane separation of plasma from whole blood without plugging of the membrane or hemolysis depends upon obtaining proper flow conditions in the blood channel. These conditions include the shear rate in the blood channel and the transmembrane pressure gradient down the channel. In general, the values of shear rate and transmembrane pressure, which provide the optimum filtration rate while keeping the hemolysis low, are a function of hematocrit. In conventional parallel plate membrane devices, including Cobe's, and in hollow fiber devices, the filtration from the blood to plasma compartments causes the shear rate to decrease, the transmembrane pressure to decrease, and the hematocrit to increase as the blood flows from the inlet to the outlet. Thus the setting of the optimum shear rate and transmembrane pressure for such devices must be based on average conditions in the channel.

One means of determining those average conditions is to ascertain the separator's efficiency and to have predetermined the blood flow rate and hematocrit which would flow into the separator. Then the separator could be designed with the proper geometry providing the optimum average shear rate and average transmembrane pressure. Because the range of blood flow rates obtainable from patients and the range of hematocrits is large, a single fixed geometry membrane separator cannot provide optimum separation.

Another approach would be to obtain a measure of the average condition and then change the geometry so that optimum separation can occur. One method to change the geometry in a parallel plate separator is to change the channel height (i.e., the blood film thickness). A measure of the average shear rate in the blood channel can be obtained from the pressure drop down the channel. The hematocrit of the blood is also important in that the greater the hematocrit the greater the viscosity, and thus the greater the pressure drop. The pressure in the filtrate channel can also be measured so that the transmembrane pressure can be determined. Thus, the pressures which can be measured external to the membrane separator can provide a measure (not independent of each other) of the hematocrit, shear rate, and trans-

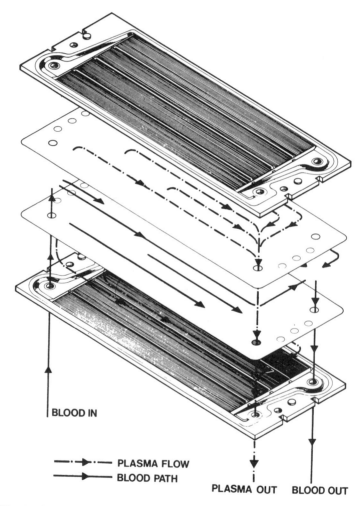

BLOOD IN

— · —▶— · — **PLASMA FLOW**
———————▶ **BLOOD PATH**

PLASMA OUT   BLOOD OUT

FIG. 1. Schematic of one channel of Cobe's parallel plate membrane separator.

membrane pressure gradient in the separator. The channel height could then be changed actively in response to the average condition seen from patient to patient or seen during a particular TPE procedure.

Through clinical experience, a set of external pressures have been found that describe a preferred relationship of shear rate and transmembrane pressure to blood flow rate and hematocrit. In the Cobe Centry TPE System, the pressure drop down the blood channel, along with the blood flow rate, is used to actively control the geometry of the blood channel by changing the channel height. The method for changing the channel height employs an hydraulic clamping system which responds according to the above relationship to either compress the separator, that is, decrease the blood channel height, or to release the separator, that is, increase the blood channel height. This actively controlled geometry combined with the controlling of transmembrane pressure employing the plasma pump, provides an efficient rate of filtration.

Figures 1 and 2 are a schematic representation of the membrane separator and a flow diagram of the control unit. The control unit consists of a blood pump, a plasma pump, and a replacement solution pump. In addition, there is a pump to deliver the prescribed amount of citrate anticoagulant. The control unit also consists of the proper pressure sensing transducers for automatic control of desired blood channel height and transmembrane pressure.

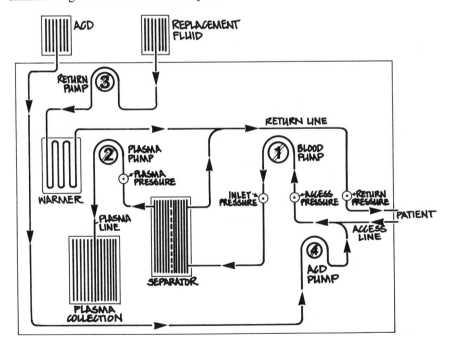

FIG. 2. Flow diagram of the control unit for the Cobe Centry TPE System.

CLINICAL STUDIES

Over 700 therapeutic plasma exchange procedures have been performed with the Cobe Centry TPE System. Table 1 lists the disease diagnoses from this clinical experience. Table 2 is a summary from 80 exchange procedures obtained from two trial centers. In Table 2 the maximum, minimum, and average values for the blood flow rate from the patient is given. The blood flow rate was also averaged for each TPE procedure, and the maximum, minimum, and average values for the average blood flow rate per procedure are also given. Table 2 also gives the data for the rate of filtration and for the ratio of filtration rate to blood flow rate. Values for

TABLE 1. *Disease diagnoses treated on the Cobe Centry TPE system*

Nephrologic	Rheumatologic
Rapidly progressive glomerulonephritis	Scleroderma
Goodpasture's syndrome	Rheumatoid arthritis (vasculitis)
Anti-GBM disease	Lupus vasculitis
Lupus nephritis	
	Neurologic
Hematologic	Guillain–Barré syndrome
Idiopathic thrombocytopenia purpura	Polymyositis
Waldenstrom's macroglobulinemia	Myasthenia gravis
Hemolytic anemia	Polyneuritis
Hyperviscosity syndrome	Eaton–Lambert's syndrome
Rh Incompatibility	Multiple sclerosis
Cryoglobulinemia	Dermatomyositis
Thrombotic thrombocytopenia purpura	

Other
Macrophage inhibitor disease
Hypercholesterolemia
Fibroblast inhibitor disease
Chronic liver disease
Multiple myeloma

TABLE 2. *Clinical experience with the Cobe Centry TPE system*

Parameters	Max.	Min.	Aver.
Blood flow rate (ml/min)	152	24	104
Aver. blood flow rate per procedure	135	58	106
Plasma flow rate (ml/min)	71	9	43
Aver. plasma flow rate per procedure	61	24	45
Plasma flow rate/blood flow rate	0.61	0.22	0.42
Aver. plasma/blood flow rate per procedure	0.54	0.30	0.43
Hematocrit (%)	45	20	35
Volume exchanged (liters)	6.08	2.58	3.83
Time for exchange (hr)	3.32	0.85	1.66

the patient's hematocrit, volume exchange, and time for exchange are also given. The time for exchange does not include set-up time or rinse back time.

The performance of the Cobe Centry TPE System is also illustrated in Fig. 3. In this figure the filtration flow rate is graphed as a function of blood flow rate for hematocrits ranging from 25 to 45%. The lines were obtained from a least squares curve fitting program which examined 3,011 clinical data points and had a correlation coefficient of 0.93.

Two-dimensional immunoelectrophoresis was performed on paired samples of inlet blood to the separator and plasma filtrate. Figure 4 shows two representative sets, one at the beginning and the other at the end of a procedure. These data strongly suggest that all the plasma components pass through the membrane unhindered, and that those plasma components that are not replaced have reduced concentrations at the end of the procedure. Quantitative techniques specific to individual plasma components were used to demonstrate that albumin, IgG, IgA, IgM, fibrinogen, cholesterol, triglycerides, and immune complexes (as measured by Clq binding) are not rejected by the membrane, that is, they all have sieving coefficients equal to 1.0.

Effects on the complement system were studied by measuring complement $C'3$ conversion by two-dimensional immunoelectrophoresis performed by Dr. Bruce McLeod, Rush–Presbyterian–St. Luke's Medical Center, Chicago, Illinois. Results were expressed as a percentage of the total $C'3$ present that is converted to $C'3b$. In 13 procedures, 38 patient blood samples were examined and no detectable $C'3$ conversion was found. In 25 plasma filtrate samples tested, 13 continued to show no detectable $C'3$ conversion and 12 samples showed slight $C'3$ conversion ranging from 2 to 10%, averaging 4%. These results suggest acceptable biocompatability with respect to the complement system.

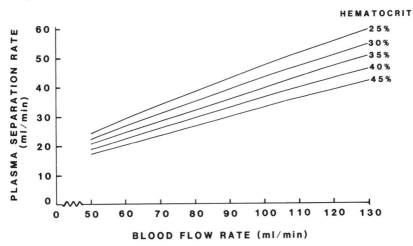

FIG. 3.   Plasma separation rate plotted as a function of blood flow rate at various inlet hematocrits for the Cobe Centry TPE System.

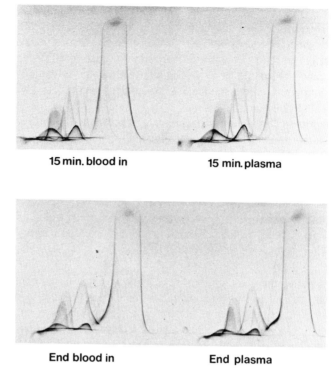

15 min. blood in   **15 min. plasma**

End blood in   **End plasma**

FIG. 4. Two-dimensional immunoelectropheresis of paired inlet blood and plasma samples taken at the beginning and end of a clinical procedure.

SUMMARY

   The overall clinical experience with the Cobe Centry TPE System has been very encouraging. The incidence of blood leaks in the membrane separator has been low with none occurring over the last 300 exchanges. Patient complications to the procedures have been rare and were mainly related to difficulties with vascular access.

Plasmapheresis, edited by Y. Nosé, P. S. Malchesky, J. W. Smith, and R. S. Krakauer. Raven Press, New York © 1983.

Effect of Repeated Plasma Exchange on Steady State Kinetics of Digoxin and Digitoxin

Frieder Keller, Andreas Hauff, Georg Schultze, Gerd Offermann, Sabine Reeck, Martin Molzahn, and *Gottfried Kreutz

*Departments of Medicine and *Clinical Pharmacology, Klinikum Steglitz, Free University, D-1000 Berlin 45, Federal Republic of Germany*

A single plasma exchange can eliminate a maximum of 1% of the amount of digoxin in the body, whereas the value for digitoxin is between 2 and 9% (1–3). These investigations are single-dose studies. In the present study, the effect of repeated plasma exchanges on the pharmacokinetics of digoxin and digitoxin after multiple dosing was investigated.

The effect of plasma exchange on digoxin is expected to be less distinct than on digitoxin due to the difference in pharmacokinetic parameters: plasma protein binding: 25% for digoxin, 97% for digitoxin; volume of distribution: 500 liters for digoxin, 40 liters for digitoxin; elimination half-life: 1.6 days for digoxin, 7 days for digitoxin; bioavailability: 0.8 for digoxin, 0.95 for digitoxin; therapeutic steady state plasma concentration: 1.0 ng/ml for digoxin, 15 ng/ml for digitoxin (4,5). The therapeutic amount in the body is the same in both drugs (500 μg).

METHODS

The kinetics of digoxin and digitoxin were investigated in 7 patients admitted to the hospital for plasma exchange treatment (Table 1). Six patients were already on digoxin or digitoxin before the first plasma exchange; one patient (U.D.) received a digoxin loading dose. Plasma exchange was performed by two central venous Shaldon catheters using a hollow fiber membrane (Asahi Plasmaflo 1). In each exchange, 4,000 ml plasma were filtered within 60–120 min and quantitatively replaced by an albumin (20 g/liter) containing physiological electrolyte solution (6).

At the start and end of each plasma exchange, 10 ml blood were withdrawn, centrifuged, and stored at −20°C. The filtered plasma was mixed, and an aliquot (10 ml) was stored with blood samples. Plasma protein binding of digitoxin was determined by ultracentrifuge.

Digoxin and digitoxin concentrations in blood plasma and filtered plasma were determined by radioimmunoassay (RIA NEN). Calculations were derived from the

TABLE 1. *Clinical data of 7 patients treated by repeated plasma exchange*

Pt.	Age (yr)	Diagnosis	Plasma exchange		Oral dose (μg/day)	Outcome
			N	days		
					Digoxin	
U. D.	37	Exophthalmus	11	24	250	Mild improvement
G. S.	56	Myasthenia gravis	5	10	213	Improvement
E. M.	77	Myasthenia gravis	9	15	400	Death
					Digitoxin	
A. B.	69	RPGN	12	29	75	Remission
U. K.	47	RPGN	12	29	100	Dialysis
M. M.	64	RPGN	13	27	75	Remission
S. W.	45	Goodpasture's syndrome	11	24	100	Remission

RPGN, rapidly progressing glomerulonephritis.

following considerations. Each plasma exchange leads to a fractional decrease in the plasma concentration ($-dC\%$).

$$-dC\% = \frac{C_{initial} - C_{final}}{C_{initial}} \tag{1}$$

The minute kinetics of intermittent plasma exchange only can be described with three independent rate constants, but the clinically relevant kinetics can be described by the effective elimination half-life ($T\frac{1}{2}^*$). The natural elimination half-life ($T\frac{1}{2}$) was calculated from the decrease of the plasma concentration after cessation of dosage (7).

$$C = C_o \exp\left(-\frac{\ln 2}{T\frac{1}{2}} t\right) \tag{2}$$

The volume of distribution (V_d) was calculated from the additional dose (D_a) and the difference between the extrapolated concentration (C_o) and the measured plasma concentration (C_{min}) before giving the additional dose.

$$V_d = \frac{D_a}{C_o - C_{min}} \tag{3}$$

The actual amount in the body is given by the calculated volume of distribution and the measured plasma concentration ($C \cdot V_d$). The amount eliminated by plasma exchange *(PE)* was calculated from the concentration (C_f) and volume (V_f) of the filtered plasma.

$$PE = C_f \cdot V_f \tag{4}$$

The fraction of the amount in the body eliminated by plasma exchange (*PE%*) was calculated from the volume of distribution and concentration at the start of each plasma exchange (C).

$$PE\% = 100 \frac{PE}{C \cdot V_d} \tag{5}$$

The theoretical amount in the body $(C_{min} \cdot V_d)$ can be derived from dose (D), bioavailability (F), dosing interval (Tau) and elimination half-life $(T\frac{1}{2})$ (7).

$$C_{min} \cdot V_d = \frac{F \cdot D}{\exp\left(\frac{\ln 2}{T\frac{1}{2}} \text{Tau}\right) - 1} \tag{6}$$

The amount in the body is decreased by the amount eliminated by plasma exchange resulting in the real amount in the body $(C_{min} \cdot V_d)^*$.

$$(C_{min} \cdot V_d)^* = C_{min} \cdot V_d - \frac{\Sigma PE}{t_{PE}} \tag{7}$$

From the real amount in the body the effect of repeated plasma exchanges during time (t_{PE}) was calculated resulting in the effective elimination half-life $(T\frac{1}{2}^*)$ (see Eq. 6).

The free fraction of drug in plasma (f_p) not bound to plasma proteins depends on the albumin concentration (C_{alb}), the molecular weight of albumin (MW = 69,000 g/mole), the number of binding sites (n), and the affinity constant (K_a) (8).

$$fp = \frac{1}{1 + \dfrac{n \cdot K_a \cdot C_{alb}}{MW}} \tag{8}$$

Binding sites and affinity constant were assumed to be constant despite of hypoalbuminemia.

The volume of distribution (V_d) increases if the free plasma fraction (fp) increases, depending on the plasma volume $(V_p = 2.5$ liters), the tissue water volume $(V_t = 39$ liters), and the free tissue fraction (ft) (8).

$$V_d = V_p + V_t \frac{fp}{ft} \tag{9}$$

The free tissue fraction (ft) is not changed by hypoalbuminemia. Thus, the increase in the free plasma fraction due to a decrease in plasma protein binding leads to a further decrease in elimination half-life $(T\frac{1}{2}^*)$ (9).

$$T\frac{1}{2}^* = T\frac{1}{2} \frac{fp}{fp^*} \frac{V_d^*}{V_d} \tag{10}$$

RESULTS

The effectiveness of plasma exchange was affirmed by the reference substances antithrombin III (65,000 daltons), antiplasmin (75,000 daltons), plasminogen (85,000 daltons), and IgM (900,000 daltons), which decreased by 63, 50, 31, and up to 70%, respectively, in the plasma.

Parameters given as medians were calculated from the measured concentrations of the 7 patients (Fig. 1). Median (range) of the minimal steady state plasma concentration (C_{min}*) of digoxin and digitoxin was 1.0 (0.62–2.03) ng/ml and 10 (8–20) ng/ml, respectively.

Median (range) of the fractional decrease ($-dC\%$) of plasma concentrations was 15% (2–35%) and 35% (0–75%) for digoxin and digitoxin, respectively. The median (range) amount eliminated by plasma exchange was 3 (0–5) μg and 16 (0–66) μg for digoxin and digitoxin, respectively, corresponding to 0.33% (0–1.8%) and 3.3% (0–6.4%) of the amount in the body. If the digitoxin dose was given within 2 hr before plasma exchange, the eliminated amount was 13–50% of the applied dose. Digoxin was eliminated by not more than 1.5% even immediately after dosing.

The plasma albumin concentration, which is 40 g/liter in normals, was decreased to 25 g/liters in the 7 patients. Accordingly, a decrease in plasma protein binding from 25 to 17% (digoxin) and from 97 to 95% (digitoxin) was calculated. Determination by ultracentrifuge revealed a median (range) plasma protein binding for digitoxin of 98.6% (100–93.6) before the first plasma exchange and the same value of 98.6% (99.7–97.9) after the last exchange. Because of the limitations of this method, the calculated values appear to be more reliable. The combined effects of repeated plasma exchange and decreased plasma protein binding on steady state kinetics was less pronounced on digoxin compared with digitoxin (Fig. 2).

DISCUSSION

In our study, two effects of repeated plasma exchange on pharmacokinetics of digoxin and digitoxin could be distinguished: first, the effect due to the amount eliminated by plasma exchange; secondly, the effect due to hypoalbuminemia. The former, the eliminative effect, can be confined to the plasma compartment. The median decrease of plasma concentrations was 15% for digoxin and 26% for digitoxin. However, after cessation of plasma exchange, a redistribution from tissue occurs (2). This redistribution corresponds to the rebound phenomenon after hemodialysis (10).

The amount actually eliminated by plasma exchange was only 0.5% (digoxin) and 3.3% (digitoxin) of the amount in the body, corresponding to the fraction of the body stores which is in the plasma compartment (0.5% for digoxin and 7% for digitoxin). Therefore, the eliminative effect of plasma exchange on the pharmacokinetics of digoxin and digitoxin was only marginal, as reflected by the small decrease in elimination half-life (Fig. 2). If plasma exchange was started, however, within 2 hr after dosage, during distribution phase, 13% to even 50% of the applied dose of digitoxin (not digoxin) was eliminated.

The second effect of plasma exchange, which is due to hypoalbuminemia and decreased plasma protein binding, leads to an increase in the volume of distribution and a shorter elimination half-life (Fig. 2). However, the increase in the volume

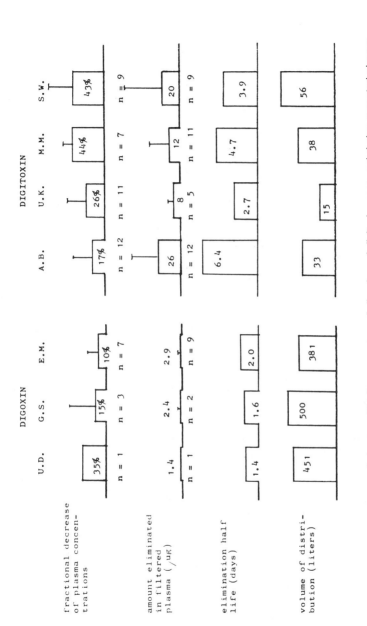

FIG. 1. Median and range of pharmacokinetic parameters of digoxin and digitoxin measured during repeated plasma exchanges and after cessation of treatment in 7 patients.

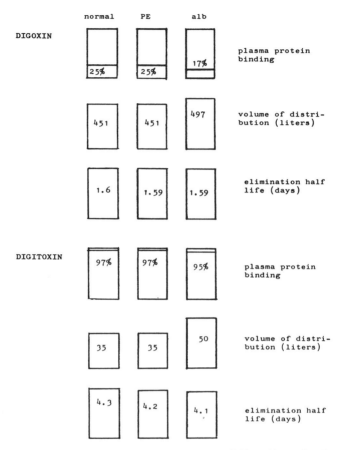

FIG. 2. Calculated effects of repeated plasma exchange (PE) and hypoalbuminemia (alb) on pharmacokinetics of digoxin and digitoxin.

of distribution is counteracted by a decrease in plasma concentrations. Thus, the amount bound to tissue remains unchanged (see Eq. 6).

Taking into consideration the eliminative effect as well as the decreased plasma protein binding, the calculated steady state concentrations completely agreed with the median of measured plasma concentrations (10 ng/ml) in the case of digitoxin. The calculated steady state plasma concentrations of digoxin (0.6 ng/ml) were lower than the median of measured concentrations (1.0 ng/ml).

CONCLUSIONS

Our conclusions on the effect of repeated plasma exchange on the pharmacokinetics of digoxin and digitoxin are as follows. The eliminative effect must be distinguished from the effects due to hypoalbuminemia. The eliminative effect on pharmacokinetics of digoxin and digitoxin is marginal and confined to the plasma

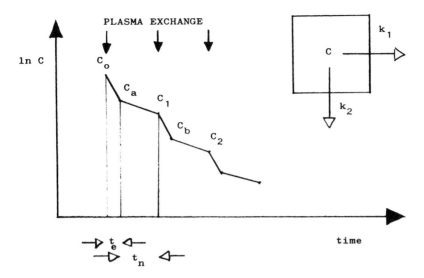

FIG. 3. Plasma exchange (k_2) intermittently added to natural elimination (k_1) leads to a sequential decrease of plasma concentrations. Duration of plasma exchange (t_e) is short compared with the time during which only natural elimination is at work (t_n).

compartment. Digitoxin (not digoxin) intoxication can be treated effectively if plasma exchange is established early. The decrease in plasma concentrations does not reflect the true amount eliminated, since a redistribution from tissue occurs. The decrease in plasma protein binding does not cause a significant change in the amount bound to tissue. Alteration of dosage is not recommended, but generally, drugs should be given after, not before, plasma exchange.

APPENDIX

To natural elimination (k_1) (Fig. 3)

$$-\frac{dC}{dt} = k_1C \tag{11}$$

$$C = C_o \exp(-k_1t) \tag{12}$$

plasma exchange (k_2) is intermittently added.

$$-\frac{dC}{dt} = k_1C + k_2C \tag{13}$$

$$C = C_o \exp(-k_1t - k_2t) \tag{14}$$

Intermittent plasma exchange leads to a sequential decrease of (C) (Fig. 1):

$C_a = C_o \exp(-k_1t_e - k_2t_e)$
$C_1 = C_a \exp(-k_1t_n)$

$$C_b = C_1 \exp(- k_1 t_e - k_2 t_e)$$
$$C_2 = C \exp(- k_1 t_n)$$

.
.
.

This sequential decrease can be simplified:

$$C = C_o \exp(-kt) \tag{15}$$

The constant *(k)* is defined by the duration of plasma exchange (t_e), the number of plasma exchanges (n_{PE}), the interval between plasma exchanges (t_n) and the duration of plasma exchange treatment (t_{PE}), which are also constants.

$$k = \frac{n_{PE}}{t_{PE}}(k_1 t_e + k_1 t_n + k_2 t_e) \tag{16}$$

Two intermittently combined first order linear processes $(k_1$ and $k_2)$ result in a single linear first order process from which the effective elimination half-life $(T^{1/2}*)$ was derived (where $\ln 2 = 0.693$).

$$T^1/_2* = \frac{\ln 2}{k} \tag{17}$$

ACKNOWLEDGMENT

Mss. Dalichow, Hess, and Grodzicki assisted in the laboratory. The manuscript was prepared by Mr. R. Condra.

REFERENCES

1. Peters, U., Risler, T., and Grabensee, B. (1980): Digitoxin elimination by plasma separation. In: *Plasma Exchange*, edited by H. G. Sieberth, p. 365. Schattauer-Verlag, Stuttgart.
2. Arsac, P., Credoz, D., Barret, L., and Faure, J. (1980): Intoxication digitalique traitée pa éxchange plasmatique. *Nouv. Presse Med.*, 9:3097.
3. Grabensee, B., Peters, U., and Risler, T. (1981): Digitalisglykoside und Niereninsuffizienz. *Internist*, 22:622.
4. Iisalo, E. (1977): Clinical pharmacokinetics of digoxin. *Clin. Pharmacokinet.*, 2:1.
5. Perrier, D., Mayersohn, M., and Marcus, F. (1977): Clinical pharmacokinetics of digitoxin. *Clin. Pharmacokinet.*, 2:292.
6. Sieberth, H. G., Glöckner, W., Hirsch, H. H., Borberg, H., Dotzauer, G., and Mathieu, P. (1980): Plasmaseparation mit hilfe von Membranen—Untersuchungen am Menschen. *Klin. Wochenschr.*, 58:551.
7. Gibaldi, M., and Perrier, D. (1975): *Pharmacokinetics*. Marcel Dekker, New York.
8. Gibaldi, M., and McNamara, P. J. (1978): Apparent volumes of distribution and drug binding to plasma proteins and tissues. *Eur. J. Clin. Pharmacol.*, 13:373.
9. Levy, G., and Yacobi, A. (1974): Effect of plasma protein binding on elimination of warfarin. *J. Pharm. Sci.*, 63:805.
10. Blair, A. D., Burgess, E. D., Maxwell, B. M., and Cutler, R. E. (1981): Sotalol kinetics in renal insufficiency. *Clin. Pharmacol. Ther.*, 29:457.

Plasmapheresis, edited by Y. Nosé, P. S. Malchesky, J. W. Smith, and R. S. Krakauer Raven Press, New York © 1983.

Cascade Filtration

H.-G. Sieberth, W. M. Glöckner, and H. Kierdorf

Department of Internal Medicine, II an der Rhein Westf. Techn. Hochschule Aachen, 5100 Aachen, Federal Republic of Germany

Plasma separation is currently being used in a range of diseases, but particularly in immunological diseases. Both cell centrifuge and membranes are used to unselectively separate all the proteins, which are then substituted by albumin or protein solutions. Current experimental work has as its goal the removal solely of pathogenic proteins from the body. Of the various methods available (1), the two most promising appear to be adsorption, especially immunoadsorption, and cascade filtration. In cascade filtration, the plasma is separated from the blood cells by using large pore membranes with high sieving; cell separators can also be used for this purpose. The plasma is then filtered through one more membrane filter of lower sieving. The filtrate from this contains the lower molecular plasma fractions and the residue the higher molecular fractions.

Filtration of the plasma has been carried out by various groups of workers with differing objectives in mind. Agishi et al. (2) used double filtration plasmapheresis primarily with the aim to reduce albumin loss. Malchesky et al. (3) removed aggregated cryoglobulins by a second filtration of the plasma through the same type of membrane; the aggregation of the cryoglobulins was by cooling the plasma. The function of cascade filtration is to eliminate the pathogenic proteins as selectively as possible and to reinfuse back all of the other proteins. Aside from the technical difficulties, which are discussed below, the problem is that the pathogenesis is only known for the antibody-induced immune diseases. The fact that plasmapheresis is effective in the immune complex diseases is probably due not only to the removal of circulating antigen–antibody–complement complexes but also to other mechanisms. This is supported by the fact that, in the majority of cases, plasma exchange treatment alone is not effective unless accompanied by immunosuppressive medication. It is also not clear why, in some cases, a long-lasting improvement or even a permanent cure can be produced by even short periods of combined plasma exchange and immunosuppressive treatment. This suggests that the immune system undergoes a long-lasting change of some sort. Therefore, further mechanisms for explaining the effectiveness of plasma exchange should be discussed.

Thus, in various immune diseases, plasma exchange causes normalization of the previously lowered activity of the reticuloendothelial system (RES). The lengthened half-life of heat-damaged, ^{51}chromium-tracer-marked erythrocytes becomes normal after a plasma exchange treatment, and the elimination through the spleen and the liver increases (4). The treatment also causes the Fc-receptor function on cell surfaces to normalize (5); it is assumed that this phenomenon is caused by the elimination of an RES blocking factor.

If the observed clinical improvement were solely attributable to the normalization of the phagocytosis of RES, then it would follow that a clinical improvement should be produced by plasmapheresis alone, without the accompanying immunosuppressive medication. This however seems not to be the case.

Both in animal experiments and in human beings, plasmapheresis induces rebound phenomenon of immunoglobulin production. It may thus be supposed that the B lymphocytes are stimulated, and possibly that certain T lymphocytes which activate the B lymphocytes are activated. The removal of circulating immune complexes can also stimulate the lymphocytes. Since plasma separation is usually only effective in combination with immunosuppressants, it is worth discussing whether the plasma separation does in fact stimulate the lymphocytic system and thus make it more responsive to immunosuppressive treatment (Fig. 1). From these considerations it is more difficult to decide which proteins or protein fractions should be removed.

On the other hand the selective elimination of proteins is also of considerable importance for explaining the pathological mechanism of immunological diseases and for explaining why plasma exchange treatment works.

TEST DESIGN AND MATERIALS

Work was carried out using cellulose diacetate hollow-fiber modules (Asahi Medical Co., Tokyo, Japan) of varying pore sizes. The membrane area was approximately 0.6 m^2 in each case. The various modules tested are designated XK 30, XK 30A, XK 30E, XK 60, and XK 100.

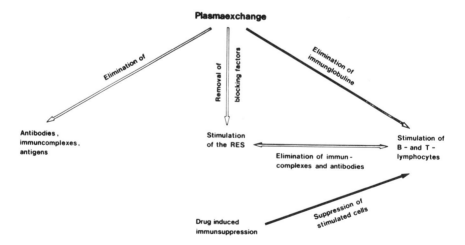

FIG. 1. Various routes of achieving effective plasma exchange.

The *in vitro* tests were made discontinuously using pooled human plasma which had been cooled. The plasma was rewarmed and then perfused through the plasma filter in a recirculation system (Fig. 2, top). In later tests, freshly separated plasma which was still warm was fed to the filter in a single pass; both filtrate and residue were then discarded.

In vivo tests, using the best filters available, were first carried out on dogs to test the toleration; here both filtrate and residue were reinfused to the conscious dog (Fig. 2, middle). Since there was no evidence of any reactions, plasma filtration was then carried out on humans; here the filtrate was reinfused together with an albumin solution of the same volume as the residue, controlled by a microprocessor-controlled balance (Fig. 2, bottom).

RESULTS

The Effect of Plasma Flow Rate, Transmembrane Pressure, and Colloidal Osmotic Pressure on the Quantity of Filtrate

With the outflow side of the module unrestricted, there is a close correlation between plasma flow rate and quantity of filtrate in the various modules we tested. As the plasma flow rate increases, the increase in filtrate lessens slightly and the curve drops off (Fig. 3).

If the pressure is increased at the output of the filter module by applying a throttle clamp, at constant flow rate, there is no effect on either the quantity or the composition of the filtrate (Table 1).

If the colloidal osmotic pressure in the plasma is raised by adding albumin, then the proportion of the various proteins contained in the filtrate drops (Fig. 4); it appears that this effect varies for different proteins. *In vitro* tests showed that cellulose diacetate membrane has a high permeability for pure albumin and pure IgG solutions, whereas if these two substances are mixed, the membrane is impermeable for both (Asahi Co., *personal communication*).

Permeability of the Various Membranes for Total Protein

Widely differing membranes were tested under unrestricted module outflow and at the same plasma flow rate. The lowest protein content, with only 30% protein, was given by the XK 30A module, and the highest, with 74% protein, by the XK 100 (Fig. 5). The explanation for this, for hydrophilic membranes, is probably that the proportion of pores available for passage of proteins varies. In between the sections of membrane that are open to the passage of proteins (the pores) there are sections of membrane that will only permit the convection of water and low molecular substances. Depending on the ratio of these two sections of membrane surface to one another, the plasma filtrate will be more or less diluted.

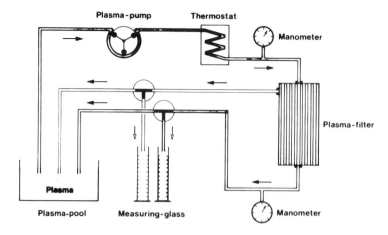

Plasma-pump   Thermostat   Manometer

Plasma-filter

Plasma

Plasma-pool   Measuring-glass   Manometer

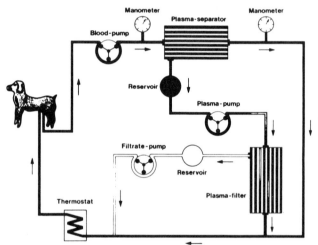

Manometer   Plasma-separator   Manometer

Blood-pump

Reservoir

Plasma-pump

Filtrate-pump

Reservoir

Thermostat   Plasma-filter

Cascade filtration in dogs

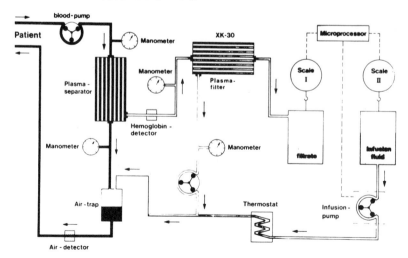

blood-pump

Patient

Manometer   XK-30   Microprocessor

Manometer   Scale I   Scale II

Plasma-separator   Plasma-filter

Hemoglobin-detector

Manometer   Manometer   filtrate   Infusion fluid

Air-trap   Thermostat   Infusion-pump

Air-detector

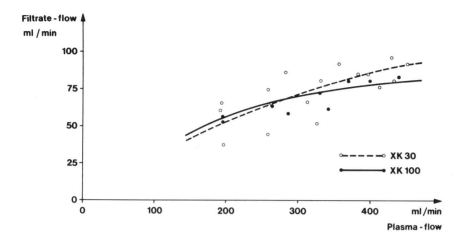

FIG. 3. Relationship between plasma flow and filtrate flow.

TABLE 1. *Percentage of protein concentration in plasma filtrate at different transmembrane pressures*

Component	N	TMP (mm Hg)		
		100	200	300
Total protein	3	$\overline{X}$ 0.36	$\overline{X}$ 0.33	$\overline{X}$ 0.37
Colloidal osmotic pressure	3	$\overline{X}$ 0.32	$\overline{X}$ 0.30	$\overline{X}$ 0.30
Albumin	2	$\overline{X}$ 0.35	$\overline{X}$ 0.35	$\overline{X}$ 0.36
IgG	2	$\underline{X}$ 0.30	$\overline{X}$ 0.30	$\overline{X}$ 0.29
IgA	2	X 0.31	X 0.28	X 0.29
IgM	2	—	—	—
Haptoglobin	2	$\overline{X}$ 0.31	$\overline{X}$ 0.2	$\overline{X}$ 0.37
Fibrinogen	2	—	—	—

TMP, transmembrane pressure. Protein concentration in pooled separated plasma = 100%, filter = XK 30. Plasma filtration at constant flow, 200 ml/min.

Sieving Properties of the Membrane

The sieving properties of a membrane are mainly dependent on the number of pores and their statistical size distribution. For cascade filtration we need membranes that are capable of separating proteins of different sizes well. On the basis of our

FIG. 2. Top: Plasma filtration *in vitro* with pooled human plasma. **Middle:** Plasma separation and filtration (cascade) in dogs. Both filtrate and retentate are reinfused. **Bottom:** Plasma separation and filtration in man. The filtrate is reinfused and the discarded retentate substituted by human albumin.

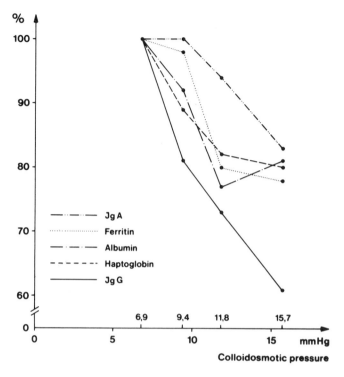

FIG. 4. Decrease of filtered protein with rising albumin concentration (colloidal osmotic pressure) in pooled human plasma.

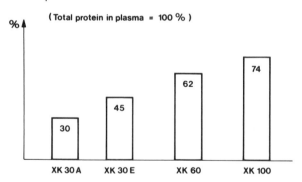

FIG. 5. Total protein concentration in plasma filtrate using different plasma filters (total protein in pooled plasma = 100%).

present ideas on the effectiveness of plasma separation, it would be desirable to have two different types of membrane available: membranes that could separate albumin of 69,000 daltons, from IgG of 160,000 daltons; and membranes that could separate the circulating immune complexes and IgM, having molecular weights over 700,000 and 900,000 daltons, respectively, from the lower molecular proteins

IgG and albumin. As has previously been shown (6), IgM and fibrinogen are fully rejected by the XK 30 membrane using pooled cooled plasma *in vitro*, while around 30% of the albumin appeared in the filtrate. Our explanation of this was that IgM could not pass through the membrane on account of this high molecular weight and that fibrinogen could not pass on account of its steric configuration. Later tests on freshly separated warm plasma showed, however, that the same membranes had a sieving coefficient of 0.2 for IgM, and a sieving coefficient of 0.7 for albumin and IgG. Comparative tests using the XK 30E and XK 60 membranes gave approximately comparable sieving coefficients. The highest quantitaties of filtrate were obtained by using the XK 60 filter which was then used for the subsequent work.

Thus our present test methods for new plasma filters are on line. The membrane properties are tested using freshly separated warm human plasma, and both filtrate and residue are discarded.

If, during the overall separation procedure, the plasma is also filtered, then the sieving coefficient for the substances under test rises and the total protein in the filtrate also increases (Table 2). This is opposite to the behavior of plasma separation filters, which show a drop in performance during the course of the treatment.

Possibly the rise in the sieving coefficients during longer periods of plasma filtration can be attributed to a loosening up of the membrane structure. It is also theoretically possible that the electric properties of the membrane are altered.

Pretreating the plasma exchange membranes with isotonic phosphate buffer solution of pH 7.4 led to an increase in the filtration performance and in the protein content of the separated plasma. This resulted in a considerable increase in the total protein separated per minute (Fig. 6). The lower line in the diagram shows the behavior with modules rinsed in 0.9 g/dl sodium solution, while the middle line refers to rinsing with additional heparin, and the upper line to rinsing with phosphate buffer solution. We think it possible that the phosphate buffer neutralizes fixed ions

TABLE 2. *Human protein content of filtered plasma at the beginning and at the end of four on-line plasma filtrations of approximately 120-min duration (N = 4; Plasma filter XK 60, plasma separator Plasmaflo Hi 05)*

	Start $\bar{X}$ %	N = 4	End $\bar{X}$ %
Colloidal osmotic pressure	67		86
Total protein	68		99
Albumin	100		100
IgG	52		86
IgA	59		97
IgM	18		41
α_2Macroglobuline	<20		55
Triglycerides	2		33
IgM/IgG	0.35		0.48

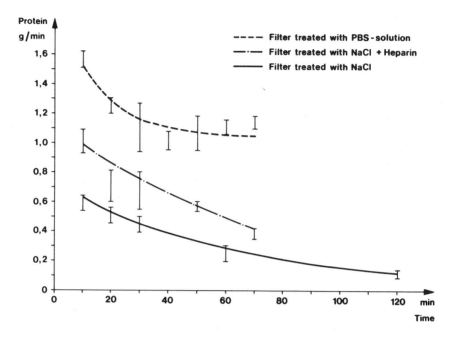

FIG. 6. Influence of a 3-hr prepriming with different solutions on plasma separation (Asahi Hi 02) under equal conditions: 0.9 g NaCl/100 ml, 0.9 g NaCl/100 ml + heparin, and isotonic phosphate buffer solution (PBS).

in the membrane which could otherwise bind the proteins; if fewer proteins are bound in the membrane, its permeability is larger. The possibility that the formation of secondary membranes is in part due to this effect should be discussed.

Where the plasma filtrate is reinfused into humans, the volume of the retransfused plasma filtrate was at least 50% and up to 75% of the volume of separated plasma. This enabled the amount of albumin required for substitution to be considerably reduced. The reduction of proteins in the plasma is, however, considerably lower than in conventional plasma exchange treatment (7).

Changes of Proteins on Passage Through the Membrane

There has been scarcely any work done on the change of the protein structure on passing through the membrane. In our own tests the proportion of immune globulins scarcely changed, and in acetate film electrophoresis the proportion of gamma globulins rose, directly after passing the membrane, to 170% of the value in the blood plasma. Tests carried out to date on immune complexes have also shown that the proportion of C4 complement increases on passage through the membrane (7).

When reinfusing plasma fractions that have been separated by means of membranes, the possibility that the proteins have been altered in the process should be borne in mind. Retransfusion of filtered plasma has been well tolerated by all patients. In 2 of 5 cases, a temporary rise in temperature to a maximum of 38.5°C was observed; complaints have not been reported at this time.

CONCLUSIONS

Discontinuous plasma filtration with cooled plasma is more selective than on-line filtration using only separated warm plasma. During plasma filtration with warm separated plasma, the sieving coefficients of the plasma filter membranes rise. These membranes become less selective. The sieving coefficient of membranes developed in the future should remain constant during use. Proteins may be altered by passing membranes.

REFERENCES

1. Sieberth, H. G. (1980): The elimination of defined substances from the blood and from separated plasma. In: *Plasma Exchange*, edited by H. G. Sieberth, p. 29. Schattauer-Verlag, Stuttgart, New York.
2. Agishi, T., Kaneko, I., Hasuo, Y., Hayasaka, Y., Sanaka, T., Ota, K., Amemiy, H., and Sugino, N. (1980): Double filtration plasmapheresis with no or minimal amount of blood derivate for substitution. In: *Plasma Exchange*, edited by H. G. Sieberth, p. 53. Schattauer-Verlag, Stuttgart, New York.
3. Malchesky, P. S., Asanuma, Y., Zawicke, I., Blumenstein, M., Calabrese, L., Kyo, A., Krakauer, R., and Nosé, Y. (1980): On-line separation of macromolecules by membrane filtration with cryogelation. In: *Plasma Exchange*, edited by H. G. Sieberth, p. 133. Schattauer-Verlag, Stuttgart, New York.
4. Lockwood, C. M., Worlledge, S., Path, F. R. C., Nicholas, A., Cotton, Ch., and Peters, K. (1979): Reversal of impaired splenic function in patients with nephritis or vasculitis (or both) by plasma exchange. *N. Engl. J. Med.*, 300:524.
5. Hoyoux, P., Malaise, M., Foidart, J. B., Rigo, P., Halleux, R., Hauwaert, C., Mahieu, P., and Franchimont, P. (1982): Effects of plasma separation by membranes on the Fc-receptor function in patients with severe rheumatoid arthritis. *Artif. Organs*, 5(S):144.
6. Sieberth, H. G., Kierdorf, H., and Glöckner, W. M. (1980): Cascade filtration for separating plasma proteins of different molecular weights. *Proc. EDTA: Vol. 17*, p. 347.
7. Sieberth, H. G., Glöckner, W. M., Dienst, C., Kierdorf, H., and Kindler, J. (1982): Cascade filtration in man. *Artif. Organs*, 5(S):122.

Plasmapheresis, edited by Y. Nosé, P. S.
Malchesky, J. W. Smith, and R. S. Krakauer.
Raven Press, New York © 1983.

On-Line Plasma Cryofiltration

J. W. Smith, K. Kayashima, T. Horiuchi, Y. Abe, C. Katsume,
M. Ueno, S. Shinagawa, S. Matsubara, J. Starre, P. S. Malchesky,
and Y. Nosé

Department of Artificial Organs, Cleveland Clinic Foundation, Cleveland, Ohio 44106

Plasma cryofiltration is an on-line plasma treatment system for the therapeutic removal of macromolecules from plasma. The system is a relatively recent development, introduced by Malchesky et al. in 1980 (1), and is undergoing clinical testing at this time. The system involves two stages of plasma filtration. The first stage, membrane plasma separation, involves the use of a hollow fiber plasma separator. Secondarily, the plasma is then cooled and filtered by a cryofilter in an on-line process to remove macromolecules. This represents a form of therapy directed at more specified removal of plasma components.

Plasma therapy may involve a number of methods for the removal of specified plasma components, but at present the method used predominantly is the general removal mode of plasma exchange. In this method all plasma solutes are separated from the blood cellular elements and the fluid portion of the blood is replaced by a variety of fluids including saline, albumin, or fresh frozen plasma. Other techniques for treatment of plasma would include sorptive processes such as charcoal (2) or ion exchange resins (3) or immunoadsorbents (4). Materials such as charcoal or protein A (5) have the capability to remove a variety of plasma components. Immunosorbents for specified removal of immunoglobulins or other plasma macromolecules are under evaluation (6). Various other techniques have been carried out using plasma filtration for specific component removal. Cascade filtration or double step filtration (7) has been used with successively more restrictive membranes to separate specified fractions from the plasma based upon molecular weight and steric properties. Other general techniques for plasma treatment include off-line processing; this could involve sorbent treatment or cold precipitation with subsequent reinfusion of the treated plasma into the patient.

The technique of cryofiltration involves an on-line, continuous process in which the plasma is cooled to 0–4°C in a short residence time circuit (15–20 min) and is filtered through a secondary filter also maintained in the cold. Figure 1 illustrates the process using a hollow fiber separator and hollow fiber cryofilter. The membrane plasma separator allows the separation of macromolecular plasma solutes such as immune complexes, rheumatoid factor, or cryoglobulins from the cellular elements of the blood. The platelet-free plasma obtained from this separator is then cooled

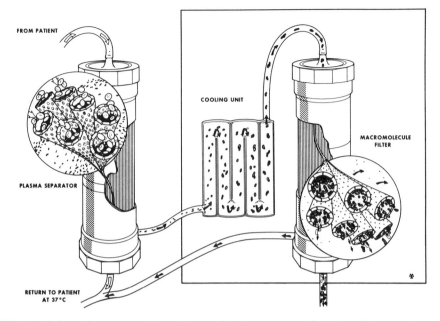

FIG. 1. Schematic representation of the cryofiltration process. The hollow fiber membrane separator produces cell-free plasma which is then cooled on-line to promote cryogelation. Macromolecule complexes are trapped in the cryofilter (macromolecule filter).

on-line and filtered through another hollow fiber membrane filter, or cryofilter. This device has more restricted sieving properties for macromolecular solutes and allows separation of large molecules from other plasma solutes such as albumin. The use of cold promotes on-line cryoaggregation of various materials from the plasma. This augments the removal of immune complexes and other macromolecular solutes in such a way that the cryofilter works more effectively.

METHODS

Both *in vitro* and clinical procedures have been carried out in evaluating the cryofiltration process. The system used clinically to perform cryofiltration is the Cryomax (Parker Hannifin Corp., Biomedical Div., Irvine, CA). The Asahi Plasmaflo Hi-05, 0.5-m² hollow fiber capillary module is used as the plasma separator, and the Plasmaflo 0.65-m² hollow fiber capillary filter module is used as the cryofilter. Both devices are manufactured by Asahi Medical Co., Tokyo, Japan. For *in vitro* experiments, plasma obtained by hollow fiber membrane plasma separation was maintained at 37°C and pumped through a cooling circuit and cryofilter to evaluate filtration under various conditions. The testing performed *in vitro* included the effects of temperature on the rate of transmembrane pressure increase versus the volume filtered, and the effect of patient disease on the transmembrane pressure versus volume filtered. In clinical trials, patients treated with the cryofiltration process included those with rheumatoid arthritis who demonstrated severe seropositive disease as indicated by elevated levels of rheumatoid factor, Clq-binding immune complexes, Westergren sedimentation rate, and cryoglobulins. The protocol used for evaluation of the cryofiltration system consisted of the treatment of patients twice per week for 5 weeks. Each procedure consisted of the processing of 3–5 liters of plasma in a procedure which took 3–4 hr. Biochemical and immunochemical evaluations were performed and included albumin, total protein, immunoglobulins, Clq-binding immune complexes, rheumatoid factor by nephelometry, quantitative cryoglobulins, Westergren sedimentation rate, and hematology profile. In addition, clinical evaluations were carried out on a schedule of once per week beginning with the first treatment and then every other treatment thereafter. Clinical evaluations include Ritchie index, grip strength, 50-foot walk time, and length of morning stiffness.

RESULTS

As the volume of plasma processed by cryofiltration increases, material accumulates on the cryofilter membrane and causes an increase in the transmembrane pressure with time. Figure 2 illustrates this process for *in vitro* cryofiltration carried out at various temperatures using normal human plasma. As is seen in this figure, procedures carried out at 4°C produce a rather dramatic increase in transmembrane pressure with filtration of approximately 1,000 cc plasma volume. Filtration at 25°C also produces an increase in transmembrane pressure, but requires a slightly larger fluid volume in order to effect the same change. Filtration at 37°C produces minimal change of transmembrane pressure even at 3 liters of volume filtered. Not only are

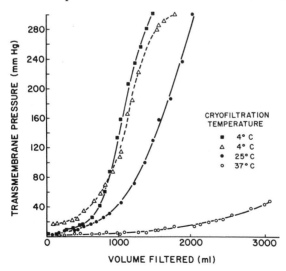

FIG. 2. *In vitro* cryofiltration using Asahi Plasmaflo—effect of temperature on filtration of normal human plasma. Cryofilter transmembrane pressure increases rapidly for plasma cooled to 4°C.

there effects produced by the temperature at which the process is carried out, but the cryofiltration process also varies depending upon the disease and patient.

Results of *in vitro* processing of plasma obtained by exchange from patients with a variety of diseases are shown in Fig. 3. These plasma samples were platelet-free, having been obtained by hollow fiber membrane plasma separation. One can see that plasma samples from patients with primary biliary cirrhosis and Sjogren's syndrome show very rapid increases in transmembrane pressure. The patient with rheumatoid arthritis had moderate elevations of rheumatoid factor and Clq-binding and showed a comparatively high transmembrane pressure increase versus volume filtered. The patient with diabetes and the "normal" patient showed a less rapid increase in transmembrane pressure versus the volume of filtration.

Regarding clinical results, the 6 patients summarized in this chapter comprise one portion of a multicenter study involving an evaluation of cryofiltration. Overall results have been quite favorable and indicate clinical usefulness of cryofiltration in the treatment of severe, seropositive rheumatoid arthritis. Figure 4 illustrates changes of transmembrane pressure, sieving coefficients, and the percentage of plasma solutes remaining in the plasma through the course of a typical cryofiltration procedure. The upper portion of the figure demonstrates sieving coefficients through the cryofilter as a function of the time of cryofiltration. A generally decreasing trend is noted for various materials; this indicates the increased amount of material deposited upon the cryofilter membrane which causes restricted sieving through the membrane. Average sieving coefficients for the cryofilter based upon a number of patients with various diseases, varying severity of disease, and varying concentrations of macromolecules are generally 0.7 for IgG, 0.7 for albumin, 0.4–0.5 for

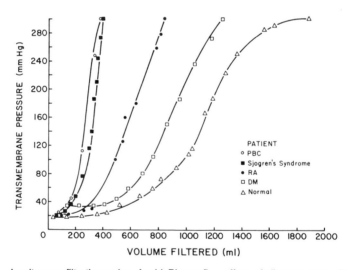

FIG. 3. *In vitro* cryofiltration using Asahi Plasmaflo—effect of disease state. Plasma from patients with various diseases exhibits cryofilter transmembrane pressure increases dependent upon volume of plasma processed and disease state. Elevated levels of plasma macromolecules cause more rapid increase of cryofilter transmembrane pressure.

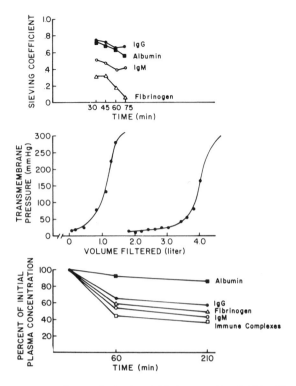

FIG. 4. Cryofiltration using Plasmaflo (patient MW, rheumatoid arthritis). **Top:** decreases of cryofilter sieving coefficients that occur during a clinical cryofiltration procedure. **Middle:** relation of cryofilter transmembrane pressure to volume of plasma filtered. **Bottom:** percentage of initial plasma concentration for various solutes remaining in the patient's circulating plasma through the course of a treatment.

IgM, and 0.1–0.3 for fibrinogen. The middle figure demonstrates the relationship of transmembrane pressure to the volume of plasma filtered. Transmembrane pressure is low initially and increases as the volume of filtration increases. Due to safety considerations, 300 mmHg transmembrane pressure is selected as the endpoint for processing using the present filter. If additional volume is to be treated, a second cryofilter may then be inserted into the circuit and the treatment continued. The lower figure demonstrates the percentage of initial plasma concentration remaining in the patient's blood during the course of treatment without correction for dilutional effects. Albumin can be seen to decrease 15%, IgG 40%, fibrinogen 50%, IgM 57%, and immune complexes 63% through a typical procedure.

Figure 5 demonstrates the changes that occurred in the course of treatment of 6 rheumatoid arthritis patients undergoing the 5-week protocol at the Cleveland Clinic. Tests shown here are Clq-binding immune complexes, Westergren sedimentation rate, and rheumatoid factor. Decreasing trends were noted for each of the immunochemical assessments, and the decrease of Westergren sedimentation rate achieved a level of significance at $p < 0.05$ using the paired t-test. Figure 6 illustrates further

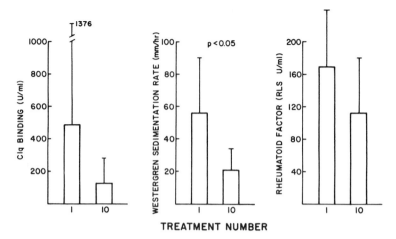

FIG. 5. Mean changes for 6 rheumatoid arthritis patients treated by cryofiltration. Values of Clq-binding immune complexes, Westergren sedimentation rate, and rheumatoid factor are plotted for the first and tenth cryofiltration procedures.

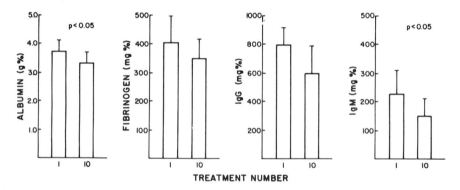

FIG. 6. Mean changes for plasma proteins of 6 rheumatoid arthritis patients during the cryofiltration protocol. First and tenth treatment values are given for albumin, fibrinogen, immunoglobulin G, and immunoglobulin M. A significant decrease ($p < 0.05$) is seen only for IgM.

immunologic and chemical parameters that were monitored routinely through the course of cryofiltration. Albumin and IgM showed significant decreases in levels through the course of 10 treatments. Fibrinogen and IgG also showed slightly decreasing trends; however, these were not significant. In general the decreases of these parameters were not clinically significant through the course of the 10 therapies. In relation to clinical parameters, Fig. 7 illustrates changes that occurred in the Ritchie index and the length of time of morning stiffness. A significant difference in the Ritchie index was found based upon values at the first and the tenth treatments using the paired t-test with a p value <0.05. Morning stiffness showed a dramatic decrease from the first through the tenth treatments; however, wide variations in initial values precluded statistical significance for the decrease that occurred. In

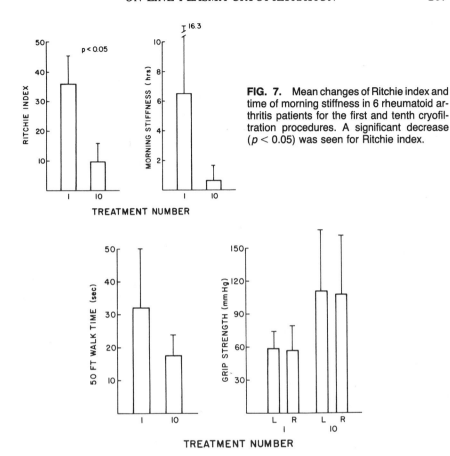

FIG. 7. Mean changes of Ritchie index and time of morning stiffness in 6 rheumatoid arthritis patients for the first and tenth cryofiltration procedures. A significant decrease ($p < 0.05$) was seen for Ritchie index.

FIG. 8. Mean decrease in time to walk 50 feet, and mean increase in grip strength for 6 rheumatoid arthritis patients at the first and tenth cryofiltration procedures.

Fig. 8 additional clinical parameters of 50-foot walk time and grip strength are summarized. There was an appreciable decrease in the length of time to walk 50 feet through the course of therapy. Grip strength showed a dramatic increase through the course of therapy.

DISCUSSION

The concept of cryofiltration evolved with the development of secondary filtration capability, the knowledge that many autoimmune diseases contain cryoprotein, and that cryogels are formed from plasma with cooling.

In many patients cryogel or cryoprotein contains immune complexes and other molecules believed to function in the pathogenesis of their diseases. It was found that rapid cooling of plasma promotes an on-line phenomenon of gelation of plasma macromolecules, and that these materials can then be easily trapped on a cryofilter membrane. The literature documents knowledge of the cold interaction of heparin with fibrin, fibrinogen, and fibronectin in plasma (8). It appears that the process of cryofiltration involves the formation of a cold-induced complex of these materials from heparinized plasma to form a basic cryogel matrix on the cryofilter membrane, after which further gel formation continues.

In vitro work supports the concept that cryofiltration occurs even with a moderate amount of cooling, for example, room temperature. With cooling to 0–4°C there is apparently optimum cryofiltration. Another factor noted from *in vitro* evaluations is that the phenomenon of cryogelation is not limited to occurrence in plasma from patients with various autoimmune diseases. Normal plasma also exhibits some cryogel formation, as evidenced by increasing cryofilter pressures through the course of the cryofiltration procedure. In the case of pathologic states, the cryofilter pressure rises more rapidly than in normal states. The increased cryogel formation occurring with disease states supports the fact that immune complexes and other molecules circulating in increased concentrations cause an increased amount of cryogel formation and aggregation on the membrane.

Regarding clinical use of the cryofiltration procedure, the multicenter trial involving 20 patients with rheumatoid arthritis has demonstrated favorable results. Overall the trends noted in these patients are similar to those seen with the 6 patients treated at the Cleveland Clinic. Immunochemical parameters are generally improved as evidenced by decreases of circulating immune complexes and quantitative cryoglobulins. Clq-binding immune complexes show reductions as great as 87% in single treatments, and cryoglobulins show up to 98% reductions in single treatments. Average reductions for these materials are 45% for immune complexes and 50% for cryoglobulins. Rheumatoid factor shows an average 40% reduction through a series of treatments. Immunoglobulins G, A, and M show average reductions of 35, 39, and 48%, respectively, and fibrinogen and albumin show 44 and 17% reductions, respectively. Clinical parameters of morning stiffness, 50-foot walk time, and Ritchie index have shown decreases of 50–75% in individual patients, while grip strength has increased as much as 400% for a given patient through the course of 10 treatments.

The process of cryofiltration is a clinically useful system which attempts to produce a more selected removal of plasma components from plasma. Increased selectivity in plasma therapy appears to be a new focus for additional research and will likely be involved in many new processes. Specified plasma therapy is of theoretical interest since it allows the manipulation of selected plasma components, thus providing another tool for investigating the pathogenesis of disease. It is also attractive from the standpoint that reductions of essential plasma solutes such as albumin are less, reducing the need for protein substitution fluids.

REFERENCES

1. Malchesky, P. S., Asanuma, Y., Zawicki, I., Blumenstein, M., Calabrese, L., Kyo, A., Krakauer, R., and Nosé, Y. (1980): On-line separation of macromolecules by membrane filtration with cryogelation. *Artif. Organs*, 400:205.

2. Asanuma, Y., Malchesky, P. S., Smith, J. W., Zawicki, I., Carey, W. D., Ferguson, D. R., Hermann, R. E., and Nosé, Y. (1980): Removal of protein-bound toxins from critical care patients. *Clin. Toxicol.*, 17:571.
3. Rosenbaum, J. L., Kramer, M. S., Raja, R., and Borejko, C. (1971): Resin hemoperfusion: A new treatment for acute drug intoxication. *N. Engl. J. Med.*, 284:874.
4. Terman, D. S., Buffaloe, G., Mattioli, C., Cook, G., Tillquist, R., Sullivan, M., and Angus, J. C. (1979): Extracorporeal immunoadsorption: Initial experience in human systemic lupus erythematosus. *Lancet*, 2:284.
5. Bansal, S. C., Bansal, B. R., Rhoads, J. E., Cooper, D. R., Boland, J. P., and Mark, R. (1978): *Ex-vivo* removal of mammalian immunoglobulin G: Method and immunological alterations. *Int. J. Artif. Organs*, 1:94.
6. Terman, D. S., and Buffaloe, G. (1978): Extracorporeal immunoadsorbents for specific extraction of circulating immune reactants. In: *Artificial Kidney, Artificial Liver, Artificial Cells*, edited by T. M. S. Chang, p. 99. Plenum Press, New York.
7. Agishi, T., Kaneko, I., Hasuo, Y., Hayasaka, Y., Sanaka, T., Ota, K., Amemiya, H., Sugino, N., Abe, M., Ono, T., Kawasai, S., and Yamame, T. (1980): Double filtration plasmapheresis. *Trans. Am. Soc. Artif. Intern. Organs*, 26:406.
8. Mosesson, M. W. (1978): Structure of human plasma cold-insoluble globulin and the mechanism of its precipitation in the cold with heparin or fibrin-fibrinogen complexes. *Ann. N.Y. Acad. Sci.*, 312:11.

Plasmapheresis, edited by Y. Nosé, P. S.
Malchesky, J. W. Smith, and R. S. Krakauer.
Raven Press, New York © 1983.

Selective Immunoadsorption

George W. Buffaloe

COBE Laboratories, Inc., Research and Development, Lakewood, Colorado 80215

As a result of the rapid growth of therapeutic plasma exchange (TPE), a need for improvements in the current practices has been recognized. These include: (a) more selective removal of pathogenic plasma components, and (b) reduction in treatment costs by the elimination of protein-containing replacement solutions. Selective immunoadsorption (SI) systems may address these needs. The development of practical therapy systems based on immunoadsorbent technology presents challenges to both researchers and engineers in the areas of safety, efficacy, and economics.

The rationale for the application of SI systems to TPE procedures is embodied in the knowledge of the specific circulating pathogenic species and the exploitation of the specific biological binding of immunologic reagents. The current debates associated with the rationale of TPE treatment in a number of diseases are pertinent to the design of SI systems. Indeed, one of the first contributions SI systems may make is in the elucidation of disease pathogenesis.

This chapter discusses the salient considerations for the development of SI systems from both theoretical and practical viewpoints and describes examples of current research that address such considerations.

DEFINITIONS AND CONCEPTS

SI systems can be defined as extracorporeal plasma treatment systems that employ immunologic reagents for the selective removal or modification of specific plasma components. Immunologic reagents in this discussion include not only antigens and antibodies, but also other molecules with similar binding properties, such as protein A from the Cowans I strain of *Staphylococcus aureus* that binds certain classes of mammalian immunoglobulin G (IgG), and bovine conglutinin that binds components of the complement system.

The use of SI techniques within therapy systems is generally viewed as the incorporation of SI "columns" into on-line, continuous-flow, extracorporeal plasma separation systems. This concept embraces a complex array of functions that suggests an integrated, systems design approach if such technology is to become more than a laboratory curiosity or research tool.

SI SYSTEM DESIGN

The SI system's contribution to disease treatment will be determined by its safety, efficacy, and economics. These three areas provide the framework for establishing system design approaches (Table 1).

Extracorporeal blood treatment systems must conform to general criteria of biological nonreactivity and physiological compatibility. The use of biological materials in SI systems presents a particular challenge in that this material may be immunogenic if released into the patient, and the process of binding of immune reactants may initiate undesirable biological reactions, such as complement activation. In addition, criteria of purity for biological "column" material presents interesting questions, particularly relating to original source materials. Additional challenges of rendering biological material sterile and pyrogen-free during the processing of SI systems is of particular note because of the fragile nature of many of these immunological reagents.

Efficacy considerations constitute, at present, the single most challenging area for the development of immunoadsorbent therapy systems. Identification of the specific pathogenic plasma components leads to delineation of their distribution and activity in the body and thus can indicate treatment regimens. Without such understanding, treatment efficacy is in serious question. In general, the more selective

TABLE 1. *SI system design*

Safety (biocompatibility)	
Biological nonreactivity	Physiological alignment
Sterility	Electrolytes
Pyrogen-free	Proteins
Nontoxicity	Temperature
Stability	pH
Thrombogenicity	Volume
Side reactions	
Purity	
Efficacy	
Disease	Treatment
Pathogenic plasma	Quantity
component identified	Frequency
Location	Duration
Quantity	
Generation rate	
Economics	
Cost	Value
Immunoadsorbant	Patient population
Immobilization	Reimbursement
technology	Cost/benefit
Complete therapy	Alternative treatments
system	

a system design may be, the more information is necessary concerning the disease pathogenesis. Maintenance of the desired biological activity of immune reactants during processing presents unique challenges. Technology developed from laboratory preparations of biological material may be helpful in this regard.

Economic criteria can be divided into cost and value considerations. At various points in the development of SI systems, economic factors dominate either the technical progress or the practical aspects of a project. The overall development costs of SI systems will likely be significant, thus the critical evaluation of economic factors may become a dominant consideration when compared with alternative approaches.

SI SYSTEM DEVELOPMENT

Table 2 is a general outline of experimental approaches to the development of SI systems. Appropriate overlap among laboratory, animal, and clinical studies at various stages of development can result in timely progress toward the realization of useful SI therapy systems.

Laboratory studies are helpful in a number of ways. The identification and quantitation of the particular circulating pathogenic species is a high priority for establishment of the basis of the SI system therapy protocols. Sizing experiments can yield valuable information concerning physical SI system design, cost, and compatibility with extracorporeal technology. Safety and biocompatibility testing will reflect the suitability of the system for animal and human exposure.

Animal models offer opportunities to study interrelationships between the SI system and living organisms that do not exist under laboratory conditions. Exper-

TABLE 2. *SI system development*

Studies	Advantages
Laboratory	Detection/quantitation of
Analytical methodology	pathogenic species
Immunoadsorbant isolation/	Sizing and cost projections
purification	
Safety testing	
Immobilization studies	
Animal	Removal specificity and
Normal	quantitation
Passive	Safety documentation
Active	Immune modulation
Induced disease	Projections to human disease
Spontaneous disease	states
	Treatment effectiveness
Clinical	Impact of treatment on disease
Normal subjects	process
Clinical diseases	Safety validation
	Contributions to disease
	pathogenesis understanding

iments using normal animals are useful in studying toxicity and biocompatibility, and, coupled with passive infusion of target material, the effectiveness of an experimental SI system may be examined. Models involving active immunization may be helpful in studying immune modulation and, in cases where disease or disease-like states are induced, studies might aid in projections of the effectiveness of the test SI system in the treatment of human disorders. Spontaneous animal disease models could be quite helpful in developing therapy strategies for clinical studies.

Experimental human studies involving SI systems present the same considerations as any new approach to disease treatment. Analysis of risk/benefit versus current therapy alternatives is the primary consideration. In many cases, TPE treatment regimens can serve as the "control" therapy for the evaluation of efficacy. The monitoring of long-term patient exposure to biological material, particularly immunologic parameters, should be a part of such studies.

RESEARCH ACTIVITIES

A number of creative research groups have contributed to the development of SI systems. This discussion will not attempt to review the current literature; however, a few examples will be extracted and used to demonstrate various approaches that have been taken toward the development of SI therapy systems.

Table 3 outlines SI system research from three groups of investigators that exemplifies different approaches to SI system development. Terman and Buffaloe (1) developed immunoadsorbent systems utilizing collodian-charcoal techniques for the immobilization of both antigens (deoxyribonucleic acid, DNA; bovine serum albumin, BSA; glomerular basement membrane, BSA) and antibodies. In laboratory

TABLE 3. *Examples of SI system research activities*

Authors	Animal studies	Clinical studies
Terman et al. (1–4) BSA–DNA collodian-charcoal columns	Passive canine Specific Ab removal Active canine Specific Ab rebound Rebound suppression	Lupus nephritis ssDNA Ab removal CIC removal Biochem/histologic improvement
Stoffel et al. (5,6) Anti-LDL agarose columns	Normal porcine Specific LDL removal Quantitative LDL removal	Hypercholesterolemia LDL/cholesterol removal Multiple treatments Column reuse
Bansal et al. (7,8) Staph A filters	Normal canine IgG removal	Colon carcinoma Tumor regression Side effects
Terman et al. (9–11) Staph A filters Protein A columns	Spontaneous canine carcinoma Tumoricidal effects Side effects	Breast adenocarcinoma Tumoricidal effects Side effects

and animal experiments they showed that these immunoadsorbent columns were capable of specifically removing the plasma proteins for which they were designed. Passively induced canine glomerulonephritis was attenuated by extracorporeal blood perfusion over GBM-columns, showing that these columns could effectively compete with the canine kidney for the binding of anti-GBM antibodies (2). In another group of canine experiments, actively immunized dogs (BSA and human serum albumin, HSA) were treated with BSA-columns and specific removal of anti-BSA antibody was observed. Furthermore, postperfusion anti-BSA antibody rebound was observed; this rebound could be suppressed by combination drug therapy (3). Animal studies revealed no significant toxicity or biocompatibility problems with the SI systems tested. The researchers then performed a single immunoadsorption procedure on a patient with lupus nephritis and demonstrated removal of anti-DNA antibody, immune complexes, and improvement in renal function, thus extending SI therapy to a clinical situation (4).

Stoffel and his colleagues have developed an SI system exploiting affinity chromatography to produce anti-low density lipoprotein (LDL) antibody columns for the treatment of familial hypercholesterolemia. After animal studies in normal pigs showed efficient removal of LDL and system safety (5), 3 patients were treated up to 12 times each and for up to 9 months (6). No untoward reactions were reported, and selective removal of cholesterol was demonstrated.

Bansal and co-workers developed an SI system for removal of mammalian IgG consisting of heat-filled, formalin-fixed *S. aureus* Cowan-I bacteria embedded in pleated membrane filters (7). After canine experiments with normal animals demonstrated effective IgG removal and low system toxicity, a patient with colon carcinoma was given a series of 20 treatments over a 5-month period, and showed improvement in general condition as well as decrease in tumor size among other positive results (8). A few undesirable side effects such as chills, hyperthermia, vasoconstriction followed by vasodilatation, and tachycardia were observed, and these symptoms were controlled with drugs and appropriate medical treatment. Terman et al., using this SI system and later collodian-charcoal immobilized protein A, treated spontaneous canine mammary carcinoma with similar results (9). In a preliminary report, 5 human patients with breast cancer were treated with both online and off-line systems. Tumoricidal effects were observed, as well as similar side effects (10). The results of these Staph/protein A studies suggest a role of such technology in the modulation of immune disorders, and also point out the risk of undesirable, sometimes severe, side reactions. In an editorial, Terman described adverse reactions and deaths in unreported animal studies, and discussed his approach to separating therapeutic effects from adverse reactions (11).

These three examples of the development and use of experimental SI systems have delineated different approaches toward exploitation of currently available technology for a more specific treatment of various diseases. These examples demonstrate the feasibility of SI system development; however, further work is needed in the demonstration of efficacy and safety.

CONCLUSIONS

The emerging technique of therapeutic plasma exchange suggests a role for selective immunoadsorption in the treatment of diseases mediated by humoral components. The challenges for successful development of new therapeutic SI systems lie in the definition of pathogenic species to be removed, creative exploitation of current and future technology, and well-designed clinical studies. Such efforts suggest the need for close working relationships among clinicians, scientists, and engineers in order to achieve the development of useful SI systems.

REFERENCES

1. Terman, D. S., and Buffaloe, G. (1978): Extracorporeal immunoadsorbants for specific extraction of circulating immune reactants. In: *Artificial Kidney, Artificial Liver, and Artificial Cells*, edited by T. M. S. Chang, p. 99. Plenum Press, New York.
2. Terman, D. S., Durante, D., Buffaloe, G., and McIntosh, R. (1977): Attenuation of canine nephrotoxic glomerulonephritis with an extracorporeal immunoadsorbent. *Scand. J. Immunol.*, 6:195.
3. Terman, D. S., Garcia-Rinaldi, R., Dannemann, B., Moore, D., Crumb, C., Tavel, A., and Poser, R. (1978): Specific suppression of antibody rebound after extracorporeal immunoadsorption. I. Comparison of single versus combination chemotherapeutic agents. *Clin. Exp. Immunol.*, 34:32.
4. Terman, D. S., Buffaloe, G., Mattioli, C., Cook, G., Tillquist, R., Sullivan, M., and Ayus, J. C. (1979): Extracorporeal immunoadsorption: Initial experience in systemic lupus erythematosus. *Lancet*, ii:824.
5. Stoffel, W., and Demant, T. (1981): Selective removal of apolipoprotein B-containing serum lipoproteins from blood plasma. *Proc. Natl. Acad. Sci. USA*, 78:611.
6. Stoffel, W., Borberg, H., and Greve, V. (1981): Application of specific extracorporeal removal of low density lipoprotein in familial hypercholesterolemia. *Lancet*, ii:1005.
7. Bansal, S. C., Bansal, B. R., Rhoads, J. E., Cooper, D. R., Boland, J. P., and Mark, R. (1978): *Ex-vivo* removal of mammalian immunoglobulin G: Method and immunological alterations. *Int. J. Artif. Organs*, 1:94.
8. Bansal, S. C., Bansal, B. R., Thomas, H. L., Siegel, P. D., Rhoads, J. E., Cooper, D. R., Terman, D. S., and Mark, R. (1978): *Ex-vivo* removal of serum IgG in a patient with colon carcinoma: Some biochemical, immunological, and histological observations. *Cancer*, 42:1.
9. Terman, D. S., Yamamoto, T., Tillquist, R. L., Henry, J. F., Cook, G. L., Silvers, A., and Shearer, W. T. (1980): Tumoricidal response induced by cytosine arabinoside after plasma perfusion over protein A. *Science*, 209:1257.
10. Terman, D. S., Young, J. B., Shearer, W. T., Ayus, C., Lehane, D., Mattioli, C., Espada, R., Howell, J. F., Yamamoto, T., Zeleski, H. I., Miller, L., Frommer, P., Feldman, L., Henry, J. F., Tillquist, R., Cook, G., and Daskal, Y. (1981): Preliminary observations of the effects on breast adenocarcinoma of plasma perfused over immobilized protein A. *N. Engl. J. Med.*, 305:1195.
11. Terman, D. S., Editorial (1982): Plasma perfusion over immobilized protein A from *Staphylococcus aureus* for treatment of cancer: Observations on the evolution of plasma perfusion systems. *Int. J. Artif. Organs*, 5:77.

Plasmapheresis, edited by Y. Nosé, P. S.
Malchesky, J. W. Smith, and R. S. Krakauer.
Raven Press, New York © 1983.

Plasmapheresis and Cryoglobulinemia: An Evaluation of Cold Precipitation as a Method for Removing Abnormal Protein

*†G. A. Rock, *V. A. Blanchette, **R. J. McKendry,
and *R. Kardish

*Canadian Red Cross Blood Transfusion Service, Ottawa Centre; **Department of
Medicine, Ottawa General Hospital; †Department of Medicine, University of Ottawa,
Ottawa, Ontario K1S 3E2, Canada

Plasmapheresis has been successfully used in the therapy of a wide variety of diseases, particularly in the management of autoimmune diseases. More recently, two modifications of the routine procedure for plasmapheresis of cryoglobulinemia patients have been proposed. One of these techniques recommends the on-line removal of the macromolecule from the plasma during the plasmapheresis procedure by cooling and membrane filtration. In the other, plasma removed by plasmapheresis is cold-incubated at 4°C for 48–72 hr, abnormal protein (cryoglobulin) is precipitated, and supernatant fluid is reinfused in a subsequent plasma exchange. It has been assumed that the supernatant fluid which is used as the replacement fluid represents physiological plasma minus the abnormal cryoprotein. However, our studies have indicated that the routine procedure for 4°C cryoprecipitation involving very short time periods is both inefficient in its removal of the cryoprotein and highly nonspecific, resulting in the coprecipitation of a number of other plasma proteins. This could result in a supernatant deficient in temperature labile coagulation factors and albumin. In addition, storage of plasma in an ice waterbath in the refrigerator can lead to problems of sterility.

RESULTS

The effectiveness of plasmapheresis in the management of cryoglobulinemia is illustrated in Fig. 1. The serum cryoglobulin in Patient 1 has been identified to be of type I classification—a monoclonal IgG with κ-light chains.

Cold-induced precipitation of the serum cryoglobulin is time dependent. A second cryoglobulinemia patient having an IgM cryoglobulin demonstrates similar time-dependent cryoprecipitation. Precipitation of the serum cryoglobulin is also dependent on the storage temperature. Decreasing temperatures from 4° to −80°C results in an increase in the quantity of the cold precipitable cryoglobulin. SDS-

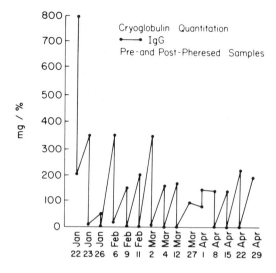

FIG. 1. Effectiveness of plasmapheresis in the treatment of cryoglobulinemia as monitored by immunoglobulin concentrations in the cold precipitable serum cryoglobulin in Patient 1.

polyacrylamide gel electrophoresis of the cold precipitated serum cryoglobulins demonstrates the presence of contaminating proteins coprecipitating with the serum cryoglobulin.

CONCLUSIONS

Plasmapheresis effectively reduced the cryoglobulins of a patient with κ-chain cryoglobulinemia.

Cryoprecipitation of the serum cryoglobulins is both a time- and temperature-dependent process. Cryoprecipitation is a non-specific process, resulting in the coprecipitation of a number of other serum proteins.

Proposed advances in plasmapheresis for the treatment of cryoglobulinemia patients, that is, cryofiltration and cryoglobulinpheresis involved procedures which are carried out at 4°C for very short periods of time. These procedures are therefore relatively inefficient in removing serum cryoglobulins, and the coprecipitation of other proteins could result in depletion of essential proteins. In conclusion, while these procedures would decrease the requirements for plasma or other replacement fluids it is unlikely that they would be as effective as more conventional plasma exchanges.

Plasmapheresis, edited by Y. Nosé, P. S.
Malchesky, J. W. Smith, and R. S. Krakauer.
Raven Press, New York © 1983.

Clinical Application of Newly Developed Immunoabsorbent Resin for Regeneration of Plasma from Autoimmune Disease Patients

K. Maeda, R. Sezaki, T. Shinzato, M. Usuda, A. Kawanishi,
T. Niwa, S. Kawaguchi, M. Shibata, *N. Yamawaki, *T. Furuta,
and *K. Inagaki

*Department of Internal Medicine, Nagoya University Branch Hospital, Nagoya 461;
*New Product Development Laboratory, Asahi Chemical Industry Co., Ltd.,
Tokyo, Japan*

In recent years, plasma exchange has been used for patients with various immunological abnormalities such as collagen disease (1,2) and nephritis (3). The use of replacement fluid is indispensable with plasma exchange, and fresh frozen plasma or human albumin solution is currently in widespread use for this purpose. However, the high cost and limits to the supply of fresh frozen plasma and human albumin have prevented further diffusion of plasma exchange. Certain medical problems also result from their use as a replacement fluid. For example, when fresh frozen plasma is employed for the replacement fluid, the risk of serum hepatitis is considerable. Moreover, when human albumin solution is used to avoid this, abnormalities may develop in the plasma composition; for example, abnormality in the coagulation system (4).

To resolve these problems, specific substances must be able to be selectively eliminated. With this as a background, the authors evaluated the adsorption capacity of a new resin for antinuclear antibodies and immune complex *in vitro*. The new resin was also clinically used for a patient with rheumatoid arthritis, and RA factor was removed.

METHOD

The new resin designated I-02 is a modified polyvinyl alcohol gel. As a control, a nonmodified polyvinyl alcohol gel was studied.

In Vitro Evaluation

Three milliliters of heparinized plasma obtained from 2 patients with mixed connective tissue disease and 6 systemic lupus erythematosus (SLE) patients was perfused through columns with 0.1 g of the modified polyvinyl alcohol gel (I-02) and with 0.1 g of the nonmodified polyvinyl alcohol gel (control) at the rate of 0.3 ml/min, respectively. In the pre- and postcolumn plasma, the respective concentrations of anti-DNA antibody, anti-RNP antibody, immune complex, complements (C3, C4), albumin, and electrolytes were measured, and the respective reduction rates were calculated, using the following formula:

$$\text{Reduction rate} = \frac{\text{precolumn concentration} - \text{postcolumn concentration}}{\text{precolumn concentration}}$$

Clinical Evaluation

The column with the modified polyvinyl alcohol gel (I-02) was used for four treatments of a 50-year-old male patient with an 8-year history of rheumatoid arthritis and suffering joint deformities. An internal arteriovenous fistula was used for blood access, and heparin was infused for anticoagulation at the initial dose of 5,000 U followed by the rate of 1,000 U/hr. Blood flow rate was 100 ml/min in the extracorporeal circulation. As shown in Fig. 1, a membrane plasma separator (Asahi Hi 05) was used to separate the plasma from the blood at the rate of 20 ml/min. The separated plasma was perfused through a column with 25 g of the modified polyvinyl alcohol gel (I-02). The plasma was then returned to the blood circuit on the venous side of the membrane plasma separator through a filter. The column was replaced with a new one 1 hr after the initiation of the treatment, and the treatment was then continued. Thus, approximately 2.4 liters of plasma was perfused through the columns during a 2-hr treatment.

Whole blood, immediately prior to being put into the plasma separator, and the separated plasma, immediately prior to and post perfusion through the adsorbing

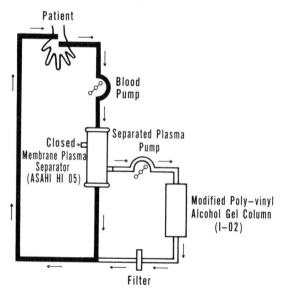

FIG. 1. Flow diagram of the extracorporeal circuit with modified polyvinyl alcohol gel column (I-02).

column (I-02), were sampled 15 min and 1.5 hr after every treatment. The RA factor was checked with the RA and RAHA tests.

Methods for Measuring Substances

Anti-DNA antibody was measured by the RIA method, anti-RNP antibody by indirect hemagglutination (RNase sensitivity), immune complex by the ACA method, complements (C3,C4) by laser immunoassay, albumin by HABCA method, and RA factor by RA test and RAHA test.

RESULTS

In Vitro Evaluation

As seen from Fig. 2, the mean reduction rate for anti-DNA antibody was 79% in the modified polyvinyl alcohol gel column (I-02) compared with 10% in the nonmodified polyvinyl alcohol gel column (control), and for the immune complex 75% in the modified polyvinyl alcohol gel column compared with 40% in the control in SLE patients. However, the level of anti-RNP antibody in patients with mixed connective tissue disease displayed no decrease after perfusion through the I-02 and control columns. The C4 concentration exhibited a slight decrease after perfusion through both columns, but C3, albumin, and electrolytes showed no variation thereafter.

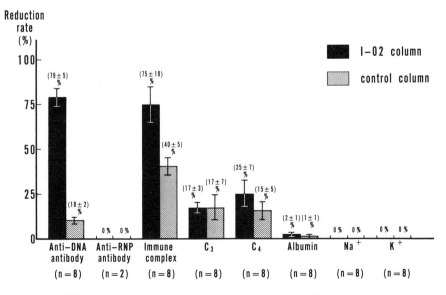

FIG. 2. Reduction rate of various substances according to column.

Clinical Evaluation

As seen in Table 1, RA test was positive and RAHA concentration was ×640–×320 before I-02 column perfusion, compared with a negative RA test and RAHA of ×40 or less after perfusion. Clearly, the modified polyvinyl alcohol gel adsorbed RA factor, but the patient showed only slight improvement of joint pain with these four treatments.

DISCUSSION

Recently, plasma exchange has been employed in the treatment of patients with antiglomerular basement membrane disease (5), renal transplant rejection episodes (6,7), SLE (3,8), polyarteritis nodosa (9), rheumatoid arthritis (1,2), circulating immune complex disease (10), and other diseases in which circulating mediators may be contributing factors. However, since fresh frozen plasma or albumin solution is used as the replacement fluid in plasma exchange, the cost and supply of the two are hindrances and the medical side effects are considerable.

To overcome these problems, a cascade filtration method (11) was developed in which the patient's plasma is returned to the body after a certain range of molecular weight substances is removed by filtering through two membranes, each with a different pore size. This system requires little replacement fluid.

The system presented here is another method to remove specific substances from the body and to eliminate the need for replacement fluid. Thus, RA factor, anti-DNA antibody, and immune complex can be selectively removed from the body of the patient without any great change in the plasma composition.

Also, in the treatment with the modified polyvinyl alcohol gel, by increasing the amount of the resin in the column, the plasma separation rate and operation time, it is possible to increase the total selective removal amount. However, it is not yet clear whether the RA factor, circulating immune complex, and antinuclear anti-

TABLE 1. *Plasma RA, RAHA elimination by column perfusion*

Treatment	Precolumn plasma	Postcolumn plasma
First treatment		
RA test	(+)	(−)
Plasma RAHA	×320	×40 ↓
Second treatment		
RA test	(+)	(−)
Plasma RAHA	×640	×40 ↓
Third treatment		
RA test	(+)	(−)
Plasma RAHA	×320	×40 ↓
Fourth treatment		
RA test	(+)	(−)
Plasma RAHA	×320	×40 ↓

bodies are disease-causing substances. Therefore, it is very important to determine if these substances are causes of disease by their selective removal and to investigate the subsequent clinical course.

The column with the modified polyvinyl alcohol gel (I-02) was used four times for the treatment of a single patient with rheumatoid arthritis, and only ambiguous signs of clinical improvement were noted. This was conceivably due to the fact that there were so few treatments with the modified polyvinyl alcohol gel column (I-02), or perhaps because the substances removed in these treatments were not important factors in causing the disease.

REFERENCES

1. Rothwell, R. S., Davis, P., Gordon, P. A., Dasgupta, M. K., Johny, K. V., Russell, A. S., and Percy, J. S. (1980): A controlled study of plasma exchange in the treatment of severe rheumatoid arthritis. *Arthritis Rheum.*, 23(7):785.
2. Kanamono, T., Iwata, H., Yamanaka, N., Ohta, K., Maeda, K., and Nakagawa, M. (1981): Plasma separation using various kinds of hemo-filters in rheumatoid arthritis. *Int. J. Artif. Organs (in press)*.
3. Clark, W. F., Lindsay, R. M., Ulan, R. A., Cordy, P. E., and Linton, A. L. (1981): Chronic plasma exchange therapy in SLE nephritis. *Clin. Nephrol.*, 16(1):20.
4. Sultan, Y., Bussel, A., Maisonneuve, P., Poupeney, M., Sitty, X., and Gajdos, P. (1979): Potential danger of thrombosis after plasma exchange in the treatment of patients with immune disease. *Transfusion*, 19(5):588.
5. Lockwood, C. M., Rees, A. J., Pearson, T. A., Evans, D. J., Peters, D. K., and Wilson, C. B. (1976): Immunosuppression and plasma-exchange in the treatment of Goodpasture's syndrome. *Lancet*, i:711.
6. Cardella, C. J., Sutton, D., Uldall, P. R., and DeVeber, G. A. (1977): Intensive plasma exchange and renal-transplant rejection. *Lancet*, i:264.
7. Graze, P. R., and Gale, R. P. (1979): Chronic graft versus host disease: A syndrome of disordered immunity. *Am. J. Med.*, 66:611.
8. Jones, J. V., Cumming, R. H., Bucknall, R. C., Asplin, C. M., Fraser, I. D., Bothamley, J., Davis, P., and Hamblin, T. J. (1976): Plasmapheresis in the management of acute systemic lupus erythematosus? *Lancet*, i:709.
9. Lockwood, C. M., Worlledge, S., Nicholas, A., Cotton, C., and Peters, D. K. (1979): Reversal of impaired splenic function in patients with nephritis or vasculitis (or both) by plasma exchange. *N. Engl. J. Med.*, 300:524.
10. Rossen, R. D., Hersh, E. M., Sharp, J. T., McCredie, K. B., Gyorkey, F., Suki, W. N., Eknoyan, G., and Reisberg, M. A. (1977): Effect of plasma exchange on circulating immune complexes and antibody formation in patients treated with cyclophosphamide and prednisone. *Am. J. Med.*, 63:674.
11. Nosé, Y., and Malchesky, P. S. (1981): *Therapeutic membrane plasmapheresis. Proceedings of the 1st Symposium on Therapeutic Plasmapheresis*, 1:3.

Plasmapheresis, edited by Y. Nosé, P. S.
Malchesky, J. W. Smith, and R. S. Krakauer.
Raven Press, New York © 1983.

Regeneration of Albumin During Plasmapheresis with a Selective Membrane Filtration System (Sedufark)

Thor M. Svartaas, Leif C. Smeby, and *Størker Jørstad

*Institute of Biophysics and *Department of Nephrology, University of Trondheim,
7034 Trondheim-NTH, Norway*

Plasma exchange has recently been used in the treatment of a wide variety of immunologically related diseases (1–3), but conventional techniques have severe limitations due to the requirement of plasma substitution fluid. The ideal method for treatment of these diseases would be selective removal of the harmful substances while all other plasma components are continuously returned to the patient. New membranes have led to systems in which on-line separation of essential plasma components from the disease-related substances is the main problem. Perfusion of plasma over affinity columns (2) or sorbents, chemical- (2) or cryoprecipitation combined with membrane separation (1), and double filtration systems (3,4) are examples of new techniques where the overall goal is removal of harmful substances without loss of other components from the patients' blood. Selective removal of "toxic" substances based on two or three membranes with different sieving characteristics was first used in treatment of uremic patients (5). The potential of this system in plasmapheresis is dependent on the availability of suitable membranes (4), and the possibility of separating albumin from "immunoactive" components with microporous membranes. Figure 1A shows a schematic outline of a *SE*lective *DU*al *F*iltration *AR*tificial *K*idney (SEDUFARK), and 1B gives the calculated (6) reduction of the concentration in a plasma pool of 5 liters when different membranes are used for 2 and 4 hr of treatment with SEDUFARK. This system has also been used for treatment of patients with different immune diseases *in vivo* (Svartaas et al., *unpublished results*) and the results have been promising. Due to the lack of a good second filter, we have used conventional hemofilters (as filter II) with nearly total rejection of albumin (>98%), hence infusion of about 100 g of albumin per 4 liters of filtrate has been necessary. As previously described (4), relatively high membrane rejection of albumin ($50\% < R_m < 80\%$) in the second filter in SEDUFARK can be preferable, and does not necessarily lead to loss of albumin due to the accumulative effect of the collecting container (CC). This is the main difference between SEDUFARK and other double filtration systems (3), where maximum regeneration is limited to about 30–50%.

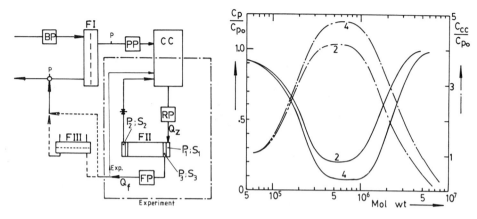

FIG. 1. **Left:** Outline of the main components in the SEDUFARK system. Blood is pumped through a filter (FI) with membranes permeable to substances with MW wt up to ~2 · 10⁶ daltons. Plasma filtrate is pumped into a collecting container (CC), and the fluid in CC recirculated through a second filter (FII) with cut-off at 80–100,000 daltons. Filtrate from this filter (FII) can then either be returned directly into the blood line, or the third filter in the original SEDUFARK design (5,6) (FIII with a cut-off at ~15,000 daltons) can be used as "albumin concentrator" where filtrate is returned to CC. The outlined parts (exp. —·—) represent the experimental configuration used for this chapter, with pressure ports P_1, P_2, and P_3 and sampling points S_1, S_2, and S_3. **Right:** Calculated (6) concentration (C_p) relative to beginning concentration (C_{po}) for different MW substances in a plasma pool of 5 liters after 2 and 4 hr of treatment with SEDUFARK using membranes with cut-off at 2 · 10⁶ (FI) and 100,000 daltons (FII), (FIII not connected). Broken lines (—·—) represent the relative concentration (C_{cc}/C_{po}) of different substances in the collecting container. All calculations were based on a fluid volume in CC of 0.5 liter.

The aim of the research described below was to explore the possibilities of predicting an optimal membrane for the second filter when the SEDUFARK system is used in plasmapheresis, and to examine how filter performance can be influenced by varying flow conditions and high protein concentrations.

MEMBRANE TRANSPORT

Solute (J_s) and volume (J_v) flux for nonelectrolytes in membranes can be described by (7):

$$J_s = P_m \Delta C + \overline{C}(1 - \sigma)J_v \; ; \; J_v = L_p \cdot (\Delta P - \sum_{i=1}^{n} \sigma_i \cdot \Delta \Pi_i) \tag{1}$$

where C is concentration and $\Delta \Pi$ the osmotic pressure difference. Spiegler and Kedem (8) showed that the mebrane rejection (R_m) of a given solute can be related to the Staverman reflection coefficient (σ) and the diffusive permeability (P_m) as:

$$R_m = \sigma \, (e^\alpha - 1)/(e^\alpha - \sigma)$$

where

$$\alpha = J_v(1 - \sigma)/P_m \; ; \; R_m = 1 - C_F/C_w = 1 - S_m \tag{2}$$

and S_m is the membrane sieving coefficient.

In order to reduce the number of experiments, and to enable prediction of P_m and σ for different substances on the basis of measurements on a single solute (i.e., albumin), one can use the "theory of equivalent pores" which relates σ, P_m, and hydraulic conductivity (L_p) to the mean pore dimensions of a membrane (9,10). According to these theories,

$$L_p = \left(A_p/A\Delta X\right) \cdot \left(r_p^2/8\mu\right) \tag{3}$$

$$P_m = \left(A_p/A\Delta X\right) \cdot \frac{D}{K_1} \cdot S_D \tag{4}$$

$$\sigma = 1 - \frac{K_2}{K_1} \cdot S_F - RT\overline{V}_s \left(\frac{P_m}{L_p}\right) \tag{5}$$

where

$$S_D = (1 - q)^2 \ ; \ S_F = (2 - S_D) \cdot S_D \ ; \ q = r_s/r_p$$

K_1 and K_2 are constants related to q, A_p/A is the relative pore area, D and μ are the fluid diffusivity and viscosity, ΔX is the effective diffusive length, r_p is the mean pore radius, and $\overline{V}_s$ is the molar volume.

For solutes where P_m is small compared with L_p, the last term in Eq. 5 can be neglected without significant errors in estimation of σ. The radius of the test solute (r_s) can be evaluated from the Stokes–Einstein relation with values of μ and D taken as reported (11) for albumin in dilute solutions $(C \to 0)$.

Assuming that globular molecules have similar densities, the radius of a different substance (r_x) with a given molecular weight (X) can be estimated from:

$$r_x = r_s \left[\frac{MW \ (x)}{MW \ (s)} \right]^{1/3} \tag{6}$$

CONCENTRATION POLARIZATION

Gill et al. (12) developed a boundary layer method which can be used to study concentration polarization with laminar flow in pipes and membranes with complete rejection $(R_m = 1.0)$ as:

$$[\theta_w] = 1 + 1.219\xi_t^{1/3} \ ; \ \xi_t < 0.04 \tag{7}$$

$$[\theta_w] = 0.5\xi_t + 6 - 5\exp[-\sqrt{\xi_t/6}] \ ; \ \xi_t \geq 0.04 \tag{8}$$

where

$$[\theta_w] = \frac{C_w}{C_b} \bigg|_{R_m = 1} \ ; \ \xi_t = P_t^2 E \ ; \ P_t = J_v R/2D \ ; \ E = 2J_v Z/(U_o R),$$

C_w is the concentration at the membrane wall, C_b is the bulk concentration, R is the pipe radius, Z is the axial distance, and U_o is the mean axial velocity at the inlet. These expressions are only valid when the diffusion boundary layer is thin compared with R, but with very high Schmidt numbers (as for protein solutions), these approximations are valid for considerable lengths downstream from the inlet as long as E is kept within reasonable limits. If the boundary layer extends over the full tube radius, the same authors (12) gave asymptotic expressions of $[\theta]_A$ for $R_m = 1$. It was also noted (12) that Eqs. 7 and 8 could be modified for $R_m < 1$ according to:

$$\theta_w = \frac{[\theta_w]}{R_m + (1 - R_m)\,[\theta_w]}. \tag{9}$$

It is not clear when to switch from Eqs. 7 or 8 to the asymptotic expressions, but Klein et al. (13) estimated a critical value of E (given value of P_t) at which $[\theta_w]_A = [\theta_w]$, and used this as a criterion for changing to asymptotic values. Albumin solutions with a concentration of 20 g/liter would then lead to asymptotic expressions for $E \geq 35\%$. With very high protein concentrations leading to $P_t \geq 3.3$ (see discussion on diffusivity below), extraction ratios (E) of more than 80% would be necessary to reach asymptotic values. By keeping $E \leq 30\%$, we based our calculations on Eqs. 7 and 8.

Diffusion of serum albumin in different solvents has been extensively examined. Keller et al. (14) gave the diffusivity of bovine serum albumin (BSA) in concentrations of 10–300 g/liter, pH 4.7 as:

$$D = D_o \tanh[15.89 \cdot 10^{-3} \cdot C]/[15.89 \cdot 10^{-3} \cdot C] \tag{10}$$

where

$$D_o = 7.1 \cdot 10^{-7} \text{ cm}^2/\text{sec}, \quad C \equiv \text{g/liter}.$$

Probstein et al. (15) referred to data at pH 7.1–7.7, where the diffusivity for BSA was more or less independent of concentration up to the solubility limit which they took as $C_g = 580$ g/liter. Trettin and Doshi (16) stated values $340 \leq C_g \leq 585$ g/liter, and stressed that buffer type and pH can have a strong influence on C_g.

Uncertainties about C_g, the effect of membrane surface charges, and possible chemical interactions between the membrane and proteins make it difficult to predict the influence of high protein concentrations, but our experimental results indicate that membrane gel formation can occur even for protein concentrations below 300 g/liter.

Nakao and Kimura (17) reported values for the reflection coefficient for vitamin B_{12} through ovalbumin gel layers as $\sigma_g = 99\%$, which indicate that gel formation will have a dramatic effect on albumin transport, and must be avoided.

Kozinski and Lightfoot (11) measured the effect of protein concentration on fluid viscosity and suggested the correlation

$$\frac{1}{\mu} = 1.11 - 5.42 \cdot 10^{-3} \cdot C + 6.71 \cdot 10^{-6} \cdot C^2, \tag{11}$$

which was used in our numerical computations.

Based on the foregoing discussion, we chose to analyze the transport and separation possibilities with hollow fiber filters using a computer program that could include the effects of varying diffusivity and viscosity. The main points in this program are that measured values for L_p and σ for a given test solute (such as albumin) were used to calculate mean pore radius, and then values of P_m and σ for other solutes were calculated from the pore theory. The true membrane rejection (R_m) was determined from Eq. 2. Numerical procedures allowing for adjustment of diffusivity and viscosity at each axial position combined with Eqs. 7–9, and mass balances to estimate bulk concentration, were then used to calculate polarization effects and the observed rejection (R_o) for different substances with a given filter.

EXPERIMENTAL PROCEDURES

Four Amicon H1p100-20 hollow fiber membrane cartridges (Amicon Corp., Lexington, MA), each unit containing approximately 240 capillaries (N) with a diameter of 0.5 mm and total membrane area of 0.07 m^2 were examined. Modified Amicon adapters, model DH4 with special pressure ports, were used with the filter units in our experiments.

BSA, fraction V (prod. no. A9647, Sigma Chemical Co., St. Louis, MO), was dissolved to concentrations of 0.5, 48, 92, and 134 g/liter in 0.9% NaCl solutions containing 0.02% NaN$_3$ to prevent bacterial growth. The pH of the solutions varied between 6.6 and 7.2, and the liquid temperature was kept at 37°C during all experiments. ^{14}C-labeled BSA (Code CFA 621, Amersham International Ltd., England) was added and isotope concentrations were measured with a scintillation counter, while concentrations of unlabeled BSA were determined with a spectrophotometer at 280 nm. The solutions were stored at 4°C between experiments, and no solution was reused if it was older than 14 days or if bacterial growth was discovered.

The Amicon filters were connected as FII in the SEDUFARK system (Fig. 1), and CC served as test solution pool. Filters I and III were disconnected and the filtrate (Q_F) was returned to CC. Test solution was recirculated through the filter by a peristaltic pump (RP) and the flow (Q_z) was monitored by a flow meter. Filtrate flow (Q_F) was controlled by a second pump (PF) and Q_F was calculated from measured volume versus time. Pressures were obtained at P_1, P_2, and P_3 (see Fig. 1), and concentration samples collected at $S_1(C_o)$ and S_2, while filtrate (C_F) was taken from the inside of the adapter close to the outlet from the cartridge (S_3).

Having connected a new filter in the system, it was first rinsed with 2–3 liters of distilled water and then with 1 liter 0.9% NaCl solution. After this rinse procedure, the filtrate side of the cartridge and the Q_F tubing were left fully primed (70 ml) while the rest of the system was drained. Test solution, 0.5 liters, was then poured into CC and the pump RP was started to prime the "blood side" of the filter before start of PF. Approximately 70 ml of filtrate was sent to drain before the Q_F was returned to CC.

The filters were tested with three different flow rates (Q_z) on each test solution, starting with 500 ml/min, reducing to 250 and then to 100 ml/min, giving shear rates ($\dot{\gamma}$) of about 2,870, 1,435, and 575 sec^{-1}. For each value of Q_z, Q_F was adjusted to 2 ml/min and then increased to 4, 7, and 10 ml/min. A total volume equal to twice the fluid volume outside the membranes (80 ml) was filtered for each Q_F before test samples were collected simultaneously at S_1, S_2, and S_3 (Fig. 1). After each sequence as described above, the filters were washed with an enzyme detergent (Biotex, Blumøller, Denmark) and rinsed with a large amount of distilled water. The filters were stored in 0.9% saline containing 0.1% NaN$_3$ between experiments and reused on protein solutions with increasing BSA concentrations from 0.5 g/liter to 48, 92, and 134 g/liter.

Observed membrane rejection was calculated from:

$$R_o = 1 - \frac{C_F}{C_o}. \tag{12}$$

No significant difference in C_F/C_o was detected when isotope concentrations were compared with total BSA concentrations; hence only isotope measurements were employed in Eq. 12.

Transmembrane pressure, ΔP, was calculated from

$$\Delta P = (P_1 + P_2)/2 - P_3 \tag{13}$$

where P_1, P_2, and P_3 refer to pressures as shown in Fig. 1.

Steady state conditions in plasmapheresis with SEDUFARK will give $Q_p \cdot S_1 \cdot C_p = Q_F \cdot S_2 \cdot C_{cc}$. When $Q_p = Q_F$, the steady state concentration of a given solute in CC will be:

$$C_{cc} = C_p \cdot S_1/S_2 \tag{14}$$

where C_p is the plasma concentration and S_1 and S_2 are the observed sieving coefficients $(1 - R_o)$ for FI and FII. It should be noted that the time to reach steady state in SEDUFARK depends on the volume (V_{cc}), flow (Q_F), in addition to S_1, S_2, and C_p.

RESULTS AND DISCUSSION

Figure 2 shows calculated rejection (R_o) for BSA and a 100,000 MW globular molecule (substance X) as a function of membrane pore radius ($R_p \cdot 10^{10}$ m) and the reflection coefficient for albumin (σ_A). Calculations were based on two different BSA concentrations (20 and 150 g/liter) in CC with $\dot{\gamma} = 2,866$ sec^{-1} and $J_v = 0.527 \cdot 10^{-4}$ cm/sec. Steady state ratio C_{cc}/C_p for these two molecules in SEDUFARK can now be predicted from Eq. 14 for filter II units with varying R_p and σ_A. At $\sigma_A = 0.9$, the ratios C_{cc}/C_p are 7 and 22 for BSA and substance X, respectively, while a reduction of σ_A to 0.75 gives the ratios 2.5 (BSA) and 4.4

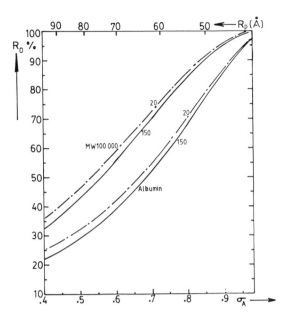

FIG. 2. Calculated rejection (R_o) of albumin and a substance with a MW of 100,000 when membranes with mean pore radius (R_p) of 40–95 · 10^{-10} m are used in FII and the albumin concentration in CC is 20 and 150 g/liter. Different values of the reflection coefficient for albumin (σ_A) and $L_p = 0.7 \cdot 10^{-5}$ cm/sec-mmHg were used to estimate R_p and membrane parameters for a substance with a MW of 100,000, and boundary layer analysis was used to calculate the filtrate concentration and the observed rejection with a shear rate $\dot{\gamma} = 2,866$ sec^{-1} and transmembrane velocity $J_v = 0.527 \cdot 10^{-4}$ cm/sec.

(X). The ratio between the observed sieving coefficients $S_{oA}S_{ox}$ is 3.1 at $\sigma_A = 0.9$, and 1.8 at $\sigma_A = 0.75$, hence the possibility of a good separation between these two molecules in SEDUFARK increases with increasing σ_A. An albumin rejection greater than 60% is necessary to obtain satisfactory retention of small ($>10^5$ daltons) immunoactive components, but too high rejection of proteins can lead to gel formation; hence a pore radius in the region of 45 · 10^{-10}–60 · 10^{-10} m should give the best result.

Experimental results for the Amicon H1P100-20 filter are shown in Figs. 3 and 4. Figure 3 shows mean R_o for albumin as a function of Q_F (or J_v) at two different concentrations (C_{Ao}) of BSA in CC. The shear rate varied between 575 and 2,870 sec^{-1} for each C_{Ao}. Observed rejection increased when Q_F and Q_z increased, and was highly dependent on BSA concentration. To prevent problems with gel formation at the membrane surface at high albumin concentrations, the shear rate should be high (i.e., high Q_z). The observed sieving coefficient (S_o) can be modified by adjusting Q_F, but J_v should be kept low to avoid protein–membrane interactions.

Figure 4 shows how R_o changes as a function of albumin concentration (C_o) in the container at constant shear rate ($\dot{\gamma} = 2,866$ sec^{-1}) and varying J_v corresponding to $Q_F = 2, 4, 7,$ and 10 ml/min. R_o decreases with increased C_o up to 92 g/liter, while R_o increases between 92 and 134 g/liter. When a filter which had been used with $C_o = 134$ g/liter was reused with $C_o = 0.5$ g/liter without the usual washing procedure between experiments, R_o was much higher than values obtained with "cleaned" filters. These results indicate increasing polarization for a given flow with increasing C_o and "gel" formation in experiments with $C_o > 92$ g/liter. With

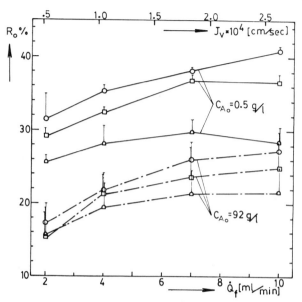

FIG. 3. Measured rejection (R_o) of BSA when Amicon H1P 100-20 filters were used as FII, and the concentration in CC (C_{Ao}) was 0.5 and 92 g/liter. The results are mean values + SEM from four filters used in experiments where $Q_z = 500$ ml/min (*circles*, $\dot\gamma \approx 2,866$ sec^{-1}), 250 ml/min (*square*, $\dot\gamma \approx 1,433$ sec^{-1}), and 100 ml/min (*domes*, $\dot\gamma \approx 573$ sec^{-1}), and Q_z varied from 2 to 10 ml/min, giving $0.527 \leqslant J_v \cdot 10^4 \leqslant 2,633$ cm/sec. With $\dot\gamma = 2,866$ sec^{-1} and $C_{Ao} = 92$ g/liter, a reduction of Q_F from 10 to 2 ml/min will give an increase in S_o from 72 to 83%.

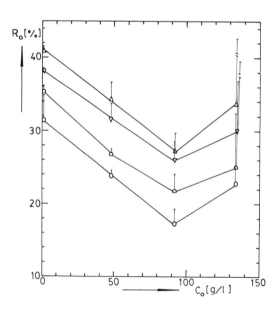

FIG. 4. Measured rejection of BSA (R_o) for Amicon H1P 100-20 filters as function of the albumin concentration in CC (C_o) with $Q_z = 500$ ml/min. The results are mean values + SEM for four filters in experiments with $J_v \cdot 10^4$ cm/sec equal to 0.527 (*circles*), 1.053 (*squares*), 1.843 *domes*, and 2.633 (*triangles*).

this filter used in SEDUFARK, C_o (in CC) will increase to a steady state value in the range 40–60 g/liter for $C_p = 35$ g/liter, and there will only be small variations in C_o for the different J_v's examined.

Multiple linear regression relating $\dot{\gamma}$, $\ln(J_v)$, and C_o to R_o for Amicon H1P100-20 filters when $1,433 \leqslant \dot{\gamma} \leqslant 2,866 \text{ sec}^{-1}$, $0.527 \cdot 10^{-4} \leqslant J_v \leqslant 2.633 \cdot 10^{-4}$ cm/sec, and $0.5 \leqslant C_o \leqslant 92$ g/liter, gives

$$R_o(\%) = 85.76 + 1.42 \cdot 10^{-3} \dot{\gamma} + 5.99 \ln(J_v) - 0.14 C_o$$

with a coefficient of determination (r^2) of 99%. With J_v instead of $\ln(J_v)$ in the correlation function, the coefficient of determination was 95%; that is, $\ln(J_v)$ gives a better correlation in the expression R_o.

It should be noted that experiments with $\dot{\gamma} = 573 \text{ sec}^{-1}$ ($Q_z = 100$ ml/min) showed a slightly different pattern, and that $C_o = 134$ g/liter resulted in problems with gel formation which should be avoided.

The Amicon filters used in these experiments had too large values for σ_A to obtain good retention of substances in the region 10^5 daltons, and results giving protein–membrane interaction even for concentrations below 200 g/liter could indicate charged membranes.

CONCLUSIONS

The second filter (FII) in SEDUFARK is the critical component when this system is used for plasmapheresis. Calculations and experiments indicate that this filter should have a mean pore radius in the region 45–60 Åm ($0.7 < \sigma_A < 0.9$) to obtain satisfactory regeneration of albumin and good removal of substances greater than 10^5 dalton. Axial flow rate (recirculation circuit) should be as high as possible, and transmembrane velocity (J_v) should be kept below 10^{-4} cm/sec to avoid a high degree of concentration polarization which can lead to gel formation and excessive osmotic pressures.

When such filters become available, and are used within specified limits, the SEDUFARK system should eliminate the need for additional fluid and (at least greatly reduce) albumin infusion during plasmapheresis treatment.

ACKNOWLEDGMENTS

This work was supported by The Royal Norwegian Council for Scientific and Industrial Research, and A/S Nor-Tron, Drammen, Norway.

REFERENCES

1. Malchesky, P. S., Asanuma, Y., Zawicki, I., Blumenstein, M., Calabrese, L., Kyo, A., Krakauer, R., and Nosé, Y. (1980): On-line separation of macromolecules by membrane filtration with cryogelation. In: *Plasma Exchange*, edited by H. G. Sieberth, p. 133. Schattauer-Verlag, Stuttgart, New York.
2. Pineda, A. A., and Taswell, H. F. (1980): Selective plasma component removal: Alternatives to plasma exchange. *Artif. Organs*, 5:3,234.
3. Agishi, T., Kaneko, I., Hauso, Y., Hayasaka, Y., Sanaka, T., Ota, K., Ameninja, H., and Sugino, N. (1980): Double filtration plasmapheresis with no or minimal amount of blood derivative for substitution. In: *Plasma Exchange*, edited by H. G. Sieberth, p. 53. Schattauer-Verlag, Stuttgart, New York.

4. Smeby, L. C., Jørstad, S., Svartås, T. M., and Widerøe, T.-E. (1981): Plasmapheresis with a selective filtration system. *Artif. Organs*, 5A:66.
5. Jørstad, S., Smeby, L. C., Widerøe, T.-E., and Berg, K. J. (1979): Removal of uraemic toxins by haemofiltration with different membranes. The benefit of regenerating haemofiltrate using a newly developed system. *Proc. EDTA*, 16:212.
6. Smeby, L. C., Jørstad, S., and Widerøe, T.-E. (1980): Design analysis of a new selective filtration system for removal of uremic toxins. *Clin. Nephrol.*, 13(3):125.
7. Katchalsky, A., and Curran, P. F. (1967): *Nonequilibrium Thermodynamics in Biophysics*. Harvard University Press, Cambridge, MA, p. 113.
8. Spiegler, K. S., and Kedem, O. (1966): Transport coefficients and salt rejection in uncharged hyperfiltration membranes. *Desalination*, 1:311.
9. Solomon, A. K. (1968): Characterization of biological membranes by equivalent pores. *J. Gen. Physiol.*, 51:335.
10. Verniory, A., DuBois, R., Decoodt, P., Gassee, J. P., and Lambert, P. P. (1973): Measurement of the permeability of biological membranes. *J. Gen. Physiol.*, 62:489.
11. Kozinski, A. A., and Lightfoot, E. N. (1972): Protein ultrafiltration: A general example of boundary layer filtration. *AICHE J.*, 18(5):1030.
12. Gill, W. N., Derzansky, L. J., and Doshi, M. R. (1971): Convective diffusion in laminar and turbulent hyperfiltration (reverse osmosis) systems. In: *Surface and Colloid Science, Vol. 4*, edited by M. Matijević, p. 262. Wiley-Interscience, New York.
13. Klein, E., Holland, F. F., and Eberle, K. (1981): Ultrafiltration rates and rejection of solutes by cellulosic hollow fibers. In: *Synthetic Membranes, Vol. II*, edited by A. F. Turbac, p. 75. American Chemical Society, Washington, D.C.
14. Keller, K. H., Canales, E. R., and Yum, S. I. (1971): Tracer and mutual diffusion coefficients of proteins. *J. Phys. Chem.*, 75(3):379.
15. Probstein, R. F., Shen, J. S., and Leung, W. F. (1978): Ultrafiltration of macromolecular solutions at high polarization in laminar channel flow. *Desalination*, 24:1.
16. Trettin, D. R., and Doshi, M. R. (1981): Pressure-independent ultrafiltration—Is it gel limited or osmotic pressure limited? In: *Synthetic Membranes, Vol. II*, edited by A. F. Turbak, p. 373. American Chemical Society, Washington, D.C.
17. Nakao, S.-I., and Kimura, S. (1981): Effect of gel layer on rejection and fractionation of different-molecular-weight solutes by ultrafiltration. In: *Synthetic Membranes, Vol. II*, edited by A. F. Turbak, p. 119. American Chemical Society, Washington D.C.

Plasmapheresis, edited by Y. Nosé, P. S.
Malchesky, J. W. Smith, and R. S. Krakauer.
Raven Press, New York © 1983.

Basic Studies on a New Immunosorbent (I-02)

Z. Yamazaki, Y. Fujimori, T. Wada, *M. Kazama, *M. Morioka,
*T. Abe, **N. Inoue, †N. Yamawaki, and †K. Inagaki

*2nd Department of Surgery, University of Tokyo, Tokyo 113; *Teikyo University,
Tokyo 173; **Internal Medicine, Oji National Hospital, Tokyo; †Asahi Chemical
Industry Co., Ltd., Tokyo, Japan*

Plasma exchange therapy, using cell separators (centrifuge) or plasma separators (membrane filter), has been applied to the treatment of intractable diseases, such as hepatic (1), renal (2), and immune (3) diseases with increasing frequency. The disadvantages of this therapy are well known, namely the loss of essential plasma components and the demand for a plasma substitute. The elimination of specific high molecular weight toxins, that is, pathogenic immune reactant, would be most desirable. To this end, cascade filtration (4), double filtration plasmapheresis (5), continuous cryogel filtration or cryogelpheresis (6), and immunosorption (7) have been developed and investigated. Our research team has recently developed a new immunosorbent, I-02, which is made of modified PVA gel and which has a higher efficiency for adsorbing rheumatoid factor and immune complex from the patients' plasma than does protein A sepharose CL4B.

In order to evaluate its biocompatibility, hematological and biochemical investigations were carried out during *in vitro* and *ex vivo* plasma perfusions through I-02 columns. These basic studies are described in this chapter.

MATERIALS AND METHODS

In Vitro Studies

Plasma obtained from a patient with rheumatoid arthritis was mixed with I-02, and batchwise adsorption (ratio of gel to plasma 1:3) was carried out for 2 hr at 37°C.

Ex Vivo Plasma Perfusion Through I-02 Column

The blood was pumped from a dog at a flow rate of 80–100 ml/min and led into the plasma separator, where the plasma was separated at a flow rate of 15–20 ml/min. The separated plasma passed through the I-02 column (net volume 100 ml) and then rejoined the blood, which was returned to the dog. A circuit diagram is illustrated in Fig. 1. Sodium citrate solution (3.8%) was infused, as the anticoagulant, at 1/10th of the flow rate of the blood, into the out-flow of the blood line from the dog as close to the animal as possible. Calcium glucanate (Calcicol) was infused into the animal at 1/10th of the flow rate of sodium citrate solution, that is, regional citration was used for anticoagulation. Therefore it was possible to analyze accurately the clotting factors, which are otherwise influenced by heparin used in ordinary extracorporeal circulation. The blood samples for hematological and biochemical analysis were taken immediately before, and 15 and 30 min after the start of perfusion.

Method for Analysis of Coagulation and Fibrinolytic Factors

Prothrombin time and activated partial prothrombin time were determined by ordinary laboratory procedures; concurrently, platelet counts, Factors XII and XI, fibrinogen, fibrin/fibrinogen degradation products (FDP), α_2 plasmin inhibitor, and plasminogen activator were measured by Bull's method (8), Hardisty's one stage assay (9), thrombin time method, the latex aggregation procedure (FDPL test by Teikokuzoki, Ltd.), Testztm Antiplasmin (Kabi, Sweden), and S-2322 (Kabi, Sweden), respectively. Soluble fibrin multiple compound was quantified by the modified Fletcher's technique (10) and expressed in terms of hypercoagulability score. Platelet aggregation value was determined by the optic densitometry method developed by Born and Obreien.

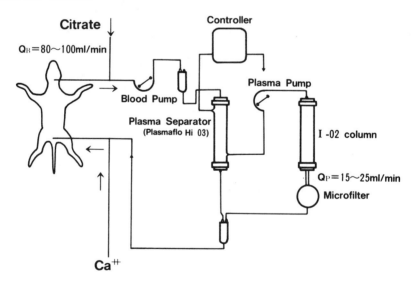

FIG. 1. Circuit diagram of I-02 plasma perfusion under membrane plasmapheresis with Plasmaflo and regional citration.

RESULTS

In Vitro Experiment

I-02 has a high efficiency for adsorbing rheumatoid factor and immune complexes as shown in Table 1. Plasma protein was reduced by 15%; this was mainly due to decreases in the globulin fraction which occurred because the plasma albumin level remained nearly constant during the experiment. Plasma fibrinogen was reduced by about 50%. No change in hypercoagulability score was noted.

Ex Vivo Plasma Perfusion Through I-02 Column

No changes in red blood cell counts or hematocrit were detected throughout the experiment. Very slight decreases in platelet counts were observed. White blood cell counts tended initially to decrease and then to revert to the preperfusion level.

Plasma biochemical components, such as electrolyte (sodium, potassium, chloride and calcium), glucose, urea-nitrogen, creatinine, lactic acid dehydrogenase, total cholestrol, glutamic oxaloacetic transaminase, and triglycerides remained nearly constant during the plasma perfusion through I-02 column.

Prothrombin time and activated partial prothrombin time had a tendency to be slightly prolonged. Figure 2 shows alterations of prothrombin time during perfusion through I-02 column under *ex vivo* membrane plasmapheresis in 11 dogs. Factor XII, α_2 plasmin inhibitor, and plasminogen decreased by a small amount. Changes in Factor XI and plasminogen activator were not significant after the initial slight decrease due to dilution effects of the priming solution in the extracorporeal circuit system. FDP was constant and remained at low levels. Fibrinogen decreased remarkably, as shown in Fig. 3.

Few variations of platelet aggregation were observed during I-02 plasma perfusion under *ex vivo* membrane plasmapheresis in 6 dogs, as shown in Fig. 4.

DISCUSSION AND CONCLUSION

It was clearly confirmed that I-02 is more efficient in adsorbing rheumatoid factor and immune complexes than the existing immunosorbent protein A sepharose. Before I-02 is applied to patients, the biocompatibility should be precisely examined.

TABLE 1. *Adsorbing capacity of immunosorbent*

	RF		IgG	ClqBA	Alb
Sample adsorbent	RAHA	RA	mg/dl	µg/ml	g/dl
Before	2,560	160	960	11.5	3.1
After					
I-02	40	20(−)	880	3.5	3.0
Protein A Sepharose CL4B	40	40	120	—	2.9

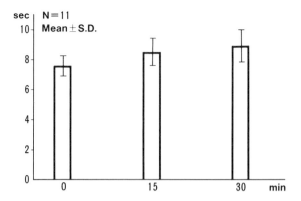

FIG. 2. Alteration of prothrombin time during I-02 plasma perfusion *ex vivo* under membrane plasmapheresis.

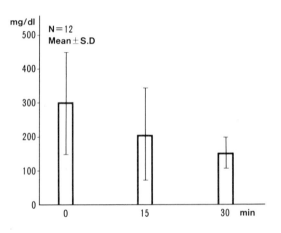

FIG. 3. Alteration of fibrinogen during I-02 plasma perfusion *ex vivo* under membrane plasmapheresis.

Therefore, these basic studies on hematological and biochemical parameters in dogs were carried out during *ex vivo* I-02 plasma perfusion with membrane plasmapheresis with Plasmaflo Hi modules and regional citration. It has been already ascertained that the Plasmaflo is safe (11) and it is now widely used. However, the sum of alterations of both Plasmaflo and I-02 in the various parameters had to be checked in our extracorporeal immunoadsorption system.

The platelet and contact factor (Factor XII) in the hypercoagulable system are extremely sensitive in contact with foreign bodies. Triggered by the activation of these factors, blood coagulation is accelerated rapidly, which induces the functional derangement of the organs, or hemostasis and thrombosis *in vivo*.

The purpose of the present investigation is to evaluate changes in platelet and the contact factors induced by contact of blood with foreign materials and to trace the resulting hypercoagulable changes using various indices. The initial slight decrease in these factors was considered to be caused by the presence of saline solution, which was used for priming the extracorporeal circuit (200 ml) and infused into

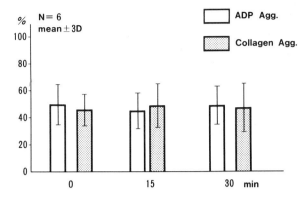

FIG. 4. Alteration of platelet aggregation during I-02 plasma perfusion *ex vivo* under membrane plasmapheresis.

the animal at the initial stage of the perfusion. Therefore, it is reasonable to conclude that the changes in these parameters, except for fibrinogen, were kept within acceptable ranges, and that there may be only minor decrements in the clotting factors due to contact-induced activation.

The marked decrease in fibrinogen (average 30%) was already noted (12) during membrane plasmapheresis with Plasmaflo Hi 03. Therefore, a significant decrease in fibrinogen (Fig. 3) during I-02 plasma perfusion is due to the membrane plasmapheresis alone. The decrease in fibrinogen is probably due to the adsorption of I-02 and the membrane, which is supported by the following facts: (a) no change in hypercoagulability score, (b) FDP is constant and remains at a low level, (c) Factor XI and plasminogen activator are kept almost constant, and (d) DIC phenomena are never observed. From these experimental results, it is concluded that I-02 has a promising future for the treatment of immune diseases.

REFERENCES

1. Inoue, N., Yamazaki, Z., Yoshiba, M., Okada, Y., Sanjo, K., Oda, T., and Wada, T. (1981): *Therapeutic Plasmapheresis, Vol 1*, edited by T. Oda, p. 57. Shattauer Verlag, Stuttgart, New York.
2. Rees, A. J., Lockwood, C. M., and Peters, D. K. (1980): *Plasma Exchange*, edited by H. G. Sieberth, p. 161. Shattauer Verlag, Stuttgart, New York.
3. Yamagata, J., and Shiokawa, Y. (1980): *Plasma Exchange*, edited by H. G. Sieberth, p. 265. Shattauer Verlag, Stuttgart, New York.
4. Sieberth, H. G. (1980): *Plasma Exchange*, edited by H. G. Sieberth, p. 29. Shattauer Verlag, Stuttgart, New York.
5. Agishi, T., Kaneko, Y., Hasuo, Y., Hayasaka, Y., Sanaka, T., Ota, K., Amemiya, H., and Sugino, N. (1980): *Plasma Exchange*, edited by H. G. Sieberth, p. 53. Shattauer Verlag, Stuttgart, New York.
6. Malchesky, P. S., Asanuma, Y., Zawicki, I., Blumenstein, M., Calabrese, L., Kyo, A., Krakauer, R., and Nosé, Y. (1980): *Plasma Exchange*, edited by H. G. Sieberth, p. 134. Shattauer Verlag, Stuttgart, New York.
7. Terman, D. S., Yamamoto, T., Mattioli, M., Cook, G., Tillquist, J., Henry, J., Poser, R., and Daskal, Y. (1980): Extensive necrosis of spontaneous canine mammary adenocarainoma after extracorporeal perfusion over staphyloccoccus aureus cowans. I. *J. Immunol.*, 124(2):795.

8. Bull, B. S., Scheiderman, M. A., and Brecher, G. (1965): Platelet count with Coulter counter. *Am. J. Clin. Pathol.*, 44:678.
9. Hardisty, R. M. (1962): A one stage factor VIII (antihemophilic globulin) assay and its use on venous and capillary plasma. *Diath. Haematol.*, 17:215.
10. Flecher, A. P., and Kaljaaersing, N. (1970): Blood hypercoagulability and thrombosis. *Clin. Res.*, 18:531.
11. Yamazaki, Z., Inoue, N., Fujimori, Y., Takahama, T., Wada, T., Oda, T., Ide, K., Kataoka, K., and Fujisaki, Y. (1980): *Plasma Exchange*, edited by H. G. Sieberth, p. 45. Shattauer Verlag, Stuttgart, New York.
12. Kazama, M., Morioka, M., Abe, T., Yamazaki, Z., Fujimori, Y., Wada, T., Ichikawa, K., Ichikawa, H., Inoue, N., Imamiya, T., Ozaki, R., Ide, M., and Fujisaki, Y. (1982): Effect of experimental plasmapheresis on platelet, coagulation and fibrinolysis using hollow fiber PF-02. *Art. Organs* (in Japanese), 11(1):53.

Plasmapheresis, edited by Y. Nosé, P. S.
Malchesky, J. W. Smith, and R. S. Krakauer.
Raven Press, New York © 1983.

Detoxification Using a Technically Simplified Plasma Filtration System

R. Bambauer, G. A. Jutzler, D. Stolz, and *P. Doenecke

*Departments of Nephrology and *Cardiology, University of Saarland,
D-6650 Homburg/Saar, Federal Republic of Germany*

Over the past few years plasma exchange (PE) in conjunction with conservative therapy has provided a useful addition to the range of therapeutic approaches available to remove antibodies circulating in the blood as well as larger molecular toxic substances released by immunological diseases and neoplasia. This method is also effective in quickly removing toxins caused by exogenous intoxications by substances with high protein binding. This chapter describes a technically simplified system, which, with a large degree of certainty, meets the requirements for effective detoxification through plasma filtration.

METHODS

Our simplified plasma filtration treatment procedure requires, apart from the membrane filter, only a double pump (BL760 Bellco, Freiberg, FRG), a substitution pump (BL705, Bellco, FRG), and a heater (Gambro, Munich, FRG) (Fig. 1). We use a cellulose diacetate (Plasmaflo 01 and 02, Asahi, Tokyo, Japan) or a polypropylene (Plasmaflux, Fresnius, D-6380 Bad Homburg, FRG) membrane with pore sizes of 0.2 μm, which allow molecules of up to about 3 million daltons to permeate (1,4,5). This is connected to the patient's vascular system according to the Seldinger technique with a Shaldon catheter (S 580, Avon Medicals, D-6057 Dietzenbach, FRG) placed in the internal jugular vein (6,7).

Both pumps of the double pump system are pressure controlled. The substitution pump is connected to the air trap of the double pump via a system of tubes, and the pumps deliver exact doses of the substitution solution into this chamber. The filtrate itself is also pumped out with the substitution pump through a further system of tubes. The amount of fluid substituted is equal to the amount of filtrate being pumped off.

The filtrate flow itself can be controlled (a) by changing the speed of the roller type pumps, and (b) by varying the transmembrane pressure (up to 300 mmHg for Plasmaflo and up to 150 mmHg for Plasmaflux). In this way the system can be individually controlled and adjusted to any specific situation. As a general rule, the filtrate flow at the beginning of plasmapheresis is between 70 and 80 ml/min and

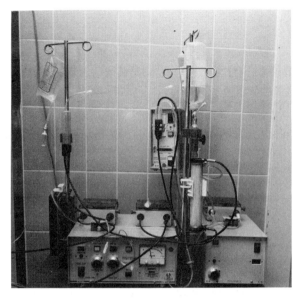

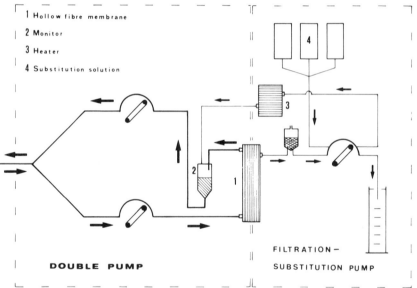

1 Hollow fibre membrane
2 Monitor
3 Heater
4 Substitution solution

DOUBLE PUMP

FILTRATION—
SUBSTITUTION PUMP

FIG. 1. Plasma filtration system with double pump, subsitution pump, heater, and hollow fiber membrane filter.

is somewhat decreased towards the end of the treatment. A normal electrolyte solution serves as a continual substitution of the filtrate, which is, according to the circumstances, enriched with human albumin solution to 1–6 g/100 ml and mostly 3 g/100 ml. This solution is warmed to between 35 and 39°C depending on the rate at which the substitution solution runs through the heater. As an anticoagulant the patient is initially given 2,000–3,000 U heparin and only 2,000 U is added to the substitution solution (3 liters).

RESULTS

A total of 24 plasma filtrations were carried out on 8 patients suffering from severe exogenous intoxications. The clinical reports and the case histories are summarized in Table 1. The intoxication symptoms could be rapidly eliminated or reduced in all 8 patients with plasma filtration.

The 50-year-old male patient suffering from Parathion intoxication died, however, 22 days after taking the poison following respiratory insufficiency during artificial respiration and mycopneumonia (Table 2). Apart from a decrease in blood pressure during three treatments of this patient, no complications during or after plasma-

TABLE 1. *Therapy and progress of intoxications treated with PE*

Patient No./age/sex	Diagnosis	Vascular access	PE	Healing/progress
1/60/M	Acetic acid intoxication Attempted suicide: approx. 120 g 25% acetic acid; intubation; artificial respiration	V. jug. int.	1	+
2/50/M	Parathion intoxication Suicide: alcohol in blood, 2.5 mg%, intubation; artificial respiration	V. jug. int.	10	22 Days later exitus letalis following artificial respiration and mycotic pneumonia
3/20/F	Digitalis intoxication Attempted suicide: 80–100 tablets Lanitop	V. jug. int.	2	+
4/19/F	Digitalis intoxication Attempted suicide: 50 tablets Novodigal	V. jug. int.	1	+
5/15/M	Phenytoin intoxication Attempted suicide: 30 tablets Zentropil; epileptic	V. jug. int.	3	+
6/56/F	Barbiturate intoxication Attempted suicide during known endogenous depression; intubation; artificial respiration	V. subcl.	1	+
7/18/M	Barbiturate intoxication Attempted suicide: unknown quantity Melidorm; intubation; artificial respiration	V. subcl.	3	+
8/53/F	Very severe meprobamate/ promazine intoxication Attempted suicide: 90 tablets Clindorm; intubation	V. subcl.	3	+

TABLE 2. *Parathion intoxication (E-605) (suicide)[a]*

PE no.	Parathion serum conc. before PE (mg/liter)	Vol. exchanged (liters)
1	0.7	6
2	0.3	6
3	0.1	3
4	0.16	6
5	0.3	5
6	0.05	4
7	0.05	4
8	0.03	3
9	0.01	3
10	0.01	3

Further course
Exitus letalis 13 days after last PE following mycotic pneumonia after artificial respiration.

[a]Fifty-year-old male. Intake of poisonous substance not known, additional alcohol level in blood 2.5 mg%. Intubation, artificial respiration (22 days).

pheresis were recorded. The addition of protein solution rapidly cured the hypotension. Hemorrhage complications were not observed.

DISCUSSION

Our simplified plasma filtration procedure has proved to be a very effective method of treatment particularly for exogenous intoxications caused by substances with high protein binding.

Our 60-year-old female patient with acetic acid intoxication manifested, apart from typical necrosis in the digestive tract, a pronounced hemolysis (8). With the aim of eliminating the free hemoglobin before it became settled, especially in the kidney, 3 liters of plasma were exchanged. The free hemoglobin, together with other hemolytic substances, could be significantly reduced (Table 3).

The insecticide Parathion is a highly toxic substance for humans. To date attempts to treat the intoxication showed that this toxin is hardly dialyzable (9), as it is not soluble in water but lipophilic. We were able to noticeably reduce the serum level of the toxin with the help of plasma filtration in the case of our 50-year-old patient with Parathion poisoning (Table 2, Fig. 2). Apart from Parathion the endogenous acetylcholine intoxication is no doubt also favorably influenced. This was demonstrated by a noticeable clinical improvement of the patient during and after each plasmapheresis. The patient died, however, 13 days after the last plasmapheresis following artificial respiration and mycopneumonia.

Also in the two cases of digoxin intoxication a rapid detoxification was possible with plasma exchange (Tables 4 and 5, Fig. 3). Digoxin has a high molecular

TABLE 3. *Acetic acid intoxication (attempted suicide)*[a]

Component	Serum concentrations		% Toxin elimination	Vol. exchanged	Filtrate
	Before PE	After PE			
Free Hgb	183 mg/liter	104 mg/liter	43.2	3 liters	116 mg/liter
LDH	2,430 U/liter	1,010 U/liter	58.4		
HBDH	1,230 U/liter	387 U/liter	68.5		
Hgb	10.8 g/dl	10.5 g/dl			

Further course
1 day later: abdominal crisis. Op: hemorrhagic infarction of the jejunum. Placing of a Braun-anastomose. Subsequently postoperative acute renal failure, 6 × hemodialysis. Full restitution of renal function.

Hgb, hemoglobin; LDH, lactic acid dehydrogenase; HBDH, hydroxybutyric dehydrogenase.
[a]Sixty-year-old male. Intake of poisonous substance: approximately 120 g of 25% acetic acid. Intubation, artificial respiration. Most severe hemolysis. PE exchange volume: 3.1 liters.

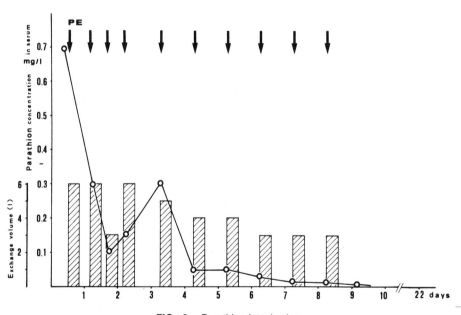

FIG. 2. Parathion intoxication.

weight and is bound to protein to 30–40%. Glöckner and Sieberth (10) assessed that only a small part of the total incorporated quantity of digoxin is eliminated with a plasma exchange of 3–5 liters because of the high binding to tissue. This is also illustrated by the increase of the serum concentration after the first plasmapheresis, due to rebound. Nevertheless, the acute reduction of the serum level by plasma exchange is of greatest importance, as the circulating amount of digitalis is critical for the course of the cardial intoxication because of its influence on the cell membrane.

TABLE 4. *Digitalis intoxication (attempted suicide)*[a]

PE no.	Digoxin concentration in serum		% Toxin elimination	Vol. exchanged (liters)
	Before PE (ng/liter)	After PE (ng/liter)		
1	14.1	9.9	29.8	2
2	14.4	6.4	55.6	3

Further course
After 2 PE: sinus rhythm, frequency 56/min. Conservative therapy with forced diuresis.

[a]Twenty-year-old female. Tablet intake: 80–100 Lanitrop tablets. Nausea, severe vomiting. Bipolar pacemaker caused by AV block II degree, bradycardia at 30/min.

TABLE 5. *Digitalis intoxication*[a]

1st day (min)	Digoxin concentration		Vol. exchanged (liters)
	Serum (ng/ml)	Filtrate (ng/ml)	
0	7.9		4
15	7.6		
30	7.3		
45	3.9	3.1	
60	5.9		
75	5.1	5.1	
90	4.8		
		6.2 Total filtrate	

Clearance digoxin = 36.84 ml/min

2nd day: 2.9

Further course
After PE: sinus rhythm, frequency 54/min.

[a]Nineteen-year-old female. Tablet intake: 50 Novodigal tablets. Nausea, severe vomiting. Bipolar pacemaker because of total AV block, bradyarrhythmia.

Plasma filtration for the phenytoin intoxication was especially impressive. Apart from a large affinity to tissue, phenytoin has a protein binding of 90–95%. With our 15-year-old patient complete consciousness was achieved and after the third treatment, the level was so low that conservative therapy was sufficient (Table 6, Fig. 4).

Cyclobarbital is also a medium-acting barbiturate and is bound to protein to 25%. A plasma exchange of 4 liters reduced the serum level by 71%. Propallylanol and hexobarbital are short-acting barbiturates and are rapidly eliminated by the kidney and are barely protein bound (Table 7).

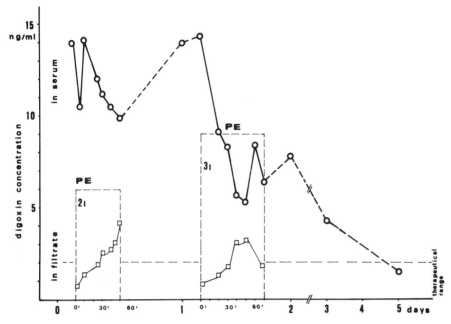

FIG. 3. Digoxin intoxication in a 20-year-old female.

TABLE 6. *Phenytoin intoxication*[a]

PE no.	Phenytoin conc. in serum[b]		% Toxin elimination	Vol. exchanged (liters)	Filtrate conc. (µg/liter)
	Before PE (µg/liter)	After PE (µg/liter)			
1	98	48	51	3	122
2	69	52	24.6	2.5	
3	64	38	40.6	2.5	

Phenytoin clearance = 43.93 ml/min

Further course
   During each PE patient fully awake; later renewed somnolence. After third PE, patient awake; therefore conservative therapy.

[a]Fifteen-year-old male. Patient suffers from epilepsia. Following family argument, took 30 Zentropil tablets. Two days in other hospital: deeply comatose. Referral for PE. Somnolent, only reacted to pain stimuli.
[b]Toxic level = 20 µg/liter.

The crotyle barbituric acid is regarded as a medium-acting barbiturate and has a protein binding of 30–40%. Following a plasma exchange totaling 9 liters over 2 days, the symptoms cleared and we were able to extubate the patient (Table 8).

Most severe signs of intoxication were shown by the 53-year-old female patient who had taken 90 Clindorm tablets (meprobamate 400 mg, promazine 10 mg) with

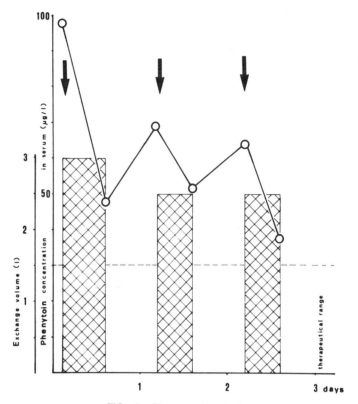

FIG. 4. Phenytoin intoxication.

TABLE 7. *Barbiturate intoxication (attempted suicide)[a]*

	Serum level		
	Before PE (mg/dl)	After PE (mg/liter)	Vol. exchanged (liters)
Propallylanol	33.4	15.0	4
Cyclobarbital	13.8	4.4	
Hexobarbital	11.2	0	
Further course During PE: complete consciousness, 3 hr after extubation.			

[a]Fifty-six-year-old female. Endogenous depressions. Tablet intake: unknown. Intubation, artificial respiration.

suicidal intentions. Although meprobamate is dialyzable and is only bound to protein to 15%, promazine is bound to albumin by 91–99% (11). The patient reacted to pain stimuli after 2 PE (7 liters) and after three treatments was responsive so that a few hours later she was extubated (Table 9).

TABLE 8. *Barbiturate intoxication (attempted suicide)*[a]

Time	Serum level of crotyle barbituric acid		Vol. exchanged (liters)
	Before PE (mg/liter)	After PE (mg/liter)	
1st day			
10 a.m.	74	11.4	3
6 p.m.	63.8	10.9	3
2nd day			
8 a.m.	36.8	2.5	3
Further course			
Complete consciousness during 3rd PE; extubation after 2 days.			

[a]Eighteen-year-old male. Melidorm intake (unknown quantity). Intubation, artificial respiration.

TABLE 9. *Very severe meprobamate–promazine intoxication (attempted suicide)*[a]

PE no.	Meprobamate conc.		Vol. exchanged (liters)
	Before PE (mg/liter)	After PE (mg/liter)	
1	402	302	4
2	216	168	3
3	112	75	3
Further course			
Continued forced diuresis.			

[a]Fifty-three-year-old female. Endogenous depressions. Tablet intake: 90 Clindorm tablets. Intubation, blood pressure 60/40 mmHg. Deeply comatose, no reaction to pain.

Our results show that with the technically simplified system, which consists of only a hollow fiber membrane, a double pump, a substitution pump, and a heater, similar results can be obtained as with the usual elaborate systems. Our treatment procedure works safely and effectively. A 3-liter plasma exchange takes about 45–60 min. Our system can be set up without extensive technical effort in any department in which the other conditions for such a treatment are met.

REFERENCES

1. Inoue, N., Yamazaki, Z., Sakai, T., Kanai, K., Oda, T., Yoshiba, M., Fujiwara, K., Sanjo, K., Wada, T., Miake, A., and Matsueda, K. (1979): A new method for plasmapheresis using cellulose-acetate hollow fiber as a plasma separator. ASAIO Proceedings, Vol. III. *Trans. Am. Soc. Artif. Intern. Organs*, 25.
2. Malchesky, P. S., Asanuma, Y., Smith, J., Zawicki, I., and Nosé, Y. (1979): Membrane plas-

mapheresis and its potential applications. *International Symposium on Hemoperfusion, Kidney and Liver Supports and Detoxification*, Haifa/Israel.

3. Tilz, G. P., Teubl, I., Kopplhuber, Ch., Vollmann, H., and Lanzer, G. (1976): Therapeutische Plasmapherese: Eine neue Form der symptomatischen Therapie. *Med. Klin.*, 71:1952.
4. Inoue, N., Yamazaki, Z., Oda, T., Sugiura, M., Wada, T., Fujisaki, Y., and Hayano, F. (1977): Treatment of intractable ascites by continuous reinfusion of the sterilized, cell-free and concentrated ascitic fluid. *Trans. Am. Soc. Artif. Intern. Organs*, 23:698.
5. Yamazaki, Z., Fujimori, Y., Sanjo, K., Kojima, Y., Sugiura, M., Wada, T., Inoue, N., Sakai, T., Oda, T., Kominami, N., Fujisaki, U., and Kataoka, K. (1976): New artificial liver support system (plasma perfusion detoxification) for hepatic coma. *Artif. Organs (Japan), Suppl.*, 5:227.
6. Bambauer, R., and Jutzler, G. A. (1980): Jugularis-interna-Punktion zur Shaldon-Katheterisierung. Ein neuer Zugang für akute Hämodialysen. *Nieren- und Hochdruckkrankheitin*, 9:109.
7. Bambauer, R., and Jutzler, G. A. (1980): Lagekontrolle grosslumiger zentraler Venenkatheter mittels intrakardialer Elektrokardiographie. *Intensivmedizin*, 17:317.
8. Moeschlin, S., and Bodmer, A. (1951): Urethane-caused blood and bone marrow changes in agranulocytosis and panmyelopathy of the cat. *Blood*, 5:242.
9. Gal, G., Simon, L., Rengel, B., Mindszenty, L., and Ember, M. (1970): Hemodialysis in the treatment of poisoning by methylparathion. *Res. Commun. Chem. Pathol. Pharmacol.*, 1:553.
10. Glöckner, W. M., and Sieberth, H. G. (1981): Plasmaaustausch bei Digitalis-Intoxikation. In: *Treatment Plasma-Exchange*, edited by H. J. Gurland, V. Heinze, and H. E. Lee, 105. Springer-Verlag, Berlin, Heidelberg, New York.
11. Curry, S. H. (1970): Plasma protein binding of chlorpromazine. *J. Pharm. Pharmacol.*, 22:193.

Plasmapheresis, edited by Y. Nosé, P. S. Malchesky, J. W. Smith, and R. S. Krakauer. Raven Press, New York © 1983.

Plasma Sorption: An Alternative Treatment for Intoxications?

D. Falkenhagen, E. Schmitt, P. Schneider, E. Behm, W. Tessenow, and H. Klinkmann

Department of Medicine, W. Pieck University, Rostock, GDR-2500 Rostock, German Democratic Republic

Plasma sorption is defined as a combination of plasma filtration and plasma perfusion over suitable adsorbents. Using this treatment it is possible to avoid the substitution of albumin or plasma solution necessary in plasma filtration. In comparison to hemoperfusion, plasma sorption does not strongly influence the behavior of blood cells. Therefore plasma sorption was recently used in the treatment of hepatic coma (1–3). In combination with hemodialysis using higher permeable membranes, plasma sorption could be advantageous especially in hepatic coma. Also plasma sorption should be preferred in the treatment of exogenous intoxications if the efficiency of this method can be increased to get an equivalent efficacy compared to hemoperfusion. Therefore we investigated *in vitro* the optimal conditions for the application to plasma sorption.

METHODS AND MATERIALS

In Vitro Investigations

The investigations were carried out on the resin "Wofatit Y 56" used in hemoperfusion columns in the GDR. Y 56 is a macroreticular resin based on polystyrene divinylbenzene (produced by Chemiekombinat, Bitterfeld, GDR), with a pore size of 8 nm and an active surface area of 450–500 m^2/g. The Y 56 resin was supplied in the mean particle sizes: 0.3, 0.48, 0.59, and 0.73 mm.

The behavior of platelets and leukocytes was investigated using a closed test circuit as described earlier (4). Also the adsorption rate of fibrinogen, albumin and vitamin B_{12} was estimated in a closed test circuit using ^{125}I-fibrinogen, ^{131}I-human serum albumin (20 mg/100 ml), and [58]Co-vitamin B_{12} (4). The vitamin B_{12} clearance was calculated for 5 min after the start of perfusion for 100 g resin Y 56 (wet weight) and for a blood flow of 1 liter/hr.

In Vivo Investigations

For the *in vivo* investigations we used two dogs (beagles, 15 kg). A blood flow of 200 ml/min was obtained from catheters inserted in the femoralis vein and in the femoralis artery. Investigations were made regarding the behavior of the filtrate flow in relation to the TMP (transmembrane pressure). The mean hematocrit of the dogs was 50%. We also investigated the platelet counts in the filtrate. In all estimations we used a TMP regulation monitor which maintained a constant TMP.

Patient Investigations

Investigations were carried out during five plasma sorptions combined with hemodialysis (Fig. 1) on a 25-year-old woman, who was hospitalized with an acute hepatic coma 3 days after bearing a jaundiced baby. The cause of the hepatic coma was supposed to be an acute steatosis in pregnancy. The time of each treatment was 5 hr. The combined plasma sorption–hemodialysis was performed using the Plasmaflux as a plasma filter, a CD 3500 as the hemodialyzer, and a Hemosorba 300 C as an adsorption column.

RESULTS

In Vitro Investigations

Regarding blood compatibility, the smaller the particle size of the Y 56 resin the higher the platelet drop (Table 1). The fall of platelets seems to be a function of the outer surface, which nearly correlates with the second power of the diameter of the resin particles.

Leukocyte counts were not affected by the particle size (Table 1). Fibrinogen adsorption also related to resin particle size (Table 1) and correlated with the drop in platelet count. Therefore, the fibrinogen adsorption should exhibit a dependence on the outer surface similar to that of albumin adsorption (Figs. 2 and 3). The adsorption rate of fibrinogen is higher in comparison to albumin. The smallest particles of the resin Y 56 (0.3 mm) absorb 55% of the fibrinogen in the test circuit, but only 15% of the albumin.

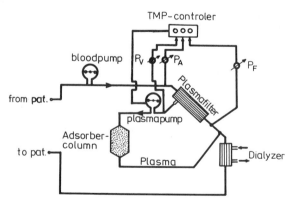

FIG. 1. Combined plasma sorption and dialysis including TMP regulation for treatment of liver coma.

TABLE 1. *Influence of the particle size of the resin Y 56 on the drop of platelets and leukocytes as well as the adsorption of fibrinogen*

Mean particle size (mm)	Decrease of platelets	Decrease of leukocytes (%)	Adsorption of fibrinogen (mg/g)
0.3	90.3	56.1	0.261
0.48	84.3	58.4	0.097
0.59	67.2	54.2	0.121
0.79	58.0	57.8	0.089

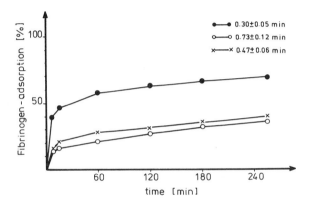

FIG. 2. Adsorption rate of fibrinogen on resin Y 56 using different particle sizes (10 g wet weight, $N = 3$).

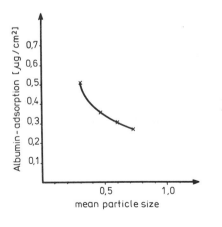

FIG. 3. Albumin adsorption on the surface of resin Y 56 with different particle sizes.

The vitamin B_{12} clearances, which varied as a function of the resin particle size, are given in Fig. 4. The results show that the efficiency for vitamin B_{12} can be increased about 60–70% using a particle size of about 0.1 mm.

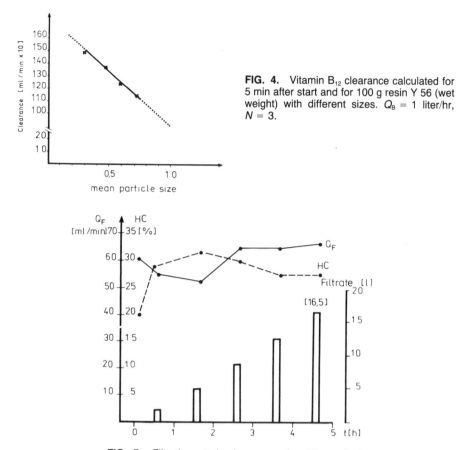

FIG. 4. Vitamin B_{12} clearance calculated for 5 min after start and for 100 g resin Y 56 (wet weight) with different sizes. $Q_B = 1$ liter/hr, $N = 3$.

FIG. 5. Filtration rate in plasma sorption (Plasmaflux).

In Vivo Investigations

The results of our investigations in dogs show very high filtration rates using the Plasmaflux. Also for a hematocrit of 50%, the filtration rate was nearly 90 ml/min using a blood flow of 200 ml/min. Over a TMP of 40 mmHg there was no increase of the filtration rate. The platelet count was 15–25 × $10^3/\mu l$ in the filtrated plasma, at a TMP of 40 mmHg.

The patient investigations (Fig. 5) clearly demonstrate the possibilities of plasma sorption using suitable plasma filters. During 5 hr, 17 liters of plasma could be purified by the adsorption column. The sieving coefficient of IgM and β-lipoprotein did not show a remarkable decrease during the treatment time (Table 2). In the case of the patient with the hepatic coma, the serum bilirubin level decreased from 11 mg/dl to 5 mg/dl during 5 days. Within 4 days the patient became reoriented, was able to converse, and was released from the hospital in good condition.

TABLE 2. *Decrease of sieving coefficients (S) in plasma sorption (N = 4) during 5-hr treatment with Plasmaflux*

Time (min)	S_{IgM}	$S_{\beta\text{-lipoprotein}}$
15	0.85	0.88
60	0.85	0.90
120	0.83	0.88
180	0.80	0.89
240	0.76	0.88
300	0.75	0.87

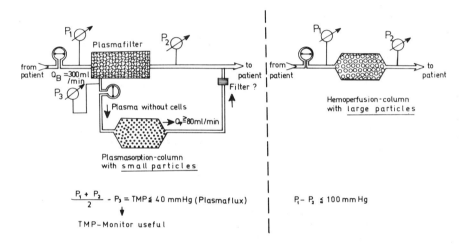

FIG. 6. Pressure drops in plasma sorption *(left)* and hemoperfusion *(right)*.

DISCUSSION AND CONCLUSIONS

The drop of platelets in hemoperfusion using the resin Y 56 is a function of the outer surface of the resin. The smaller the particle size the higher the drop of platelets. From this point of view, hemoperfusion columns filled with the resin Y 56 (similar to XAD 4) should not have too small a particle size. The size of the resin particles should be about 0.9–1.0 mm in diameter to have an optimal blood compatibility for these particles. The smaller adsorption rate should be compensated for by the prolongation of the treatment time of about 1–2 hr.

The leukocytes are not influenced by the different particle sizes. On the basis of these findings, it is suggested that the fall in platelet level and the fall in leukocyte level are caused by different mechanisms. The same conclusion could be suggested by the investigations of the fall of leukocytes using different albumin coatings (5).

Fibrinogen and albumin adsorption appear to be a function of the outer surface of resin Y 56. Therefore, very small particles (about 0.01 mm) of this adsorbent should be able to adsorb quantities of proteins. The fibrinogen adsorption was found to be much higher than the albumin adsorption. Because of the correlation between fibrinogen and γ-globulin adsorption (6), there is a basis to develop unspecific immunoadsorbents with a prevalence for γ-globulins in comparison to albumin.

The vitamin B_{12} clearance is a linear function of the particle size. Therefore we assume that also the adsorption rate of other substances is influenced by this effect. We thus recommend that a plasma sorption column with resin particles of about 0.1 mm be used for intoxications. This size ensures a reasonable pressure drop in plasma sorption combined with a reasonable efficiency in comparison to hemoperfusion (Fig. 6). The plasma filters used should guarantee a high filtration rate (≥ 100 ml/min) of long duration without decreasing sieving for IgM and β-lipoprotein as well as other proteins. Regarding these conditions, plasma sorption should also be of high value in the treatment of acute hepatic failure, especially in combination with high flux dialysis.

TMP regulation in plasma sorption seems to be reasonable as described in plasma filtration (7). Because the TMP regulation is able to keep the TMP constantly at a level as low as possible, blood cells will not be damaged.

REFERENCES

1. Smith, J. W., Asanuma, Y., Malchesky, P. S., and Nosé, Y. (1981): Treatment of hepatic dysfunction using membrane plasmapheresis with sorptive plasma detoxification. *Artif. Organs*, 5 (A):66.
2. Ouchi, K., Piatkiewicz, W., Malchesky, P. S., Carey, W. D., Herman, R. E., and Nosé, Y. (1978): An efficient, specific and blood compatible sorbent system for hepatic assist. *Trans. Am. Soc. Artif. Intern. Organs*, 24:246.
3. Inoue, N., Yoshiba, M., Yamazaki, Z., Sakai, T., Sanjo, K., Okada, K., Oda, T., Wada, T., and Inoue, T. (1981): Continuous flow membrane plasmapheresis utilizing cellulose acetate hollow fiber in hepatic coma. In: *Artificial Liver Support*, edited by G. Brunner and F. W. Schmidt, p. 175. Springer-Verlag, Berlin, Heidelberg, New York.
4. Falkenhagen, D., Esther, G., Ahrenholz, P., Holtz, M., Schmitt, E., and Klinkmann, A. H. (1980): Blood compatibility and efficiency of different hemoadsorbents. *Proc. Eur. Soc. Artif. Organs.*, 7:137.
5. Falkenhagen, D., Gottschall, S., Esther, G., Courtney, J. M., and Klinkmann, H.: *In vitro* assessment of charcoal and resin hemoadsorbents. *Contrib. Nephrol.*, 29(6): *(in press)*.
6. Mason, R. G., Chuan, H. Y. K., Mohammed, S. F., and Sharp, O. A. (1978): Extracorporeal thrombogenis and antikoagulation. In: *Replacement of Renal Function by Dialysis*, edited by W. Drukker, F. M. Parsons, J. M. Maher, and M. Nijhoff, p. 199. Medical Division.
7. Schmitt, E., Ahrenholz, P., Bukowski, J., Judicki, W., Klinkmann, H., Nalecz, M., and Piatkiewicz, W. (1981): Clinical application of an automated control system for plasmafiltration. *Artif. Organs*, 5(A):62.

Plasmapheresis, edited by Y. Nosé, P. S.
Malchesky, J. W. Smith, and R. S. Krakauer.
Raven Press, New York © 1983.

Clinical Experience with Cryofiltration in Japan

*†§Mitsuru Suzuki, *Nakanobu Azuma, *Takuo Nobuto,
§Shigeru Shinagawa, *§Takao Matsugane, §Paul S. Malchesky,
†Masatoshi Takahashi, †Tatsuo Suzuta, and †§Yukihiko Nosé

*Tokyo Tokatsu Clinic, Matsudo City, Chiba, Japan; †Tokyo Medical College,
Shinjuku-ku, Tokyo, Japan; §Cleveland Clinic, Cleveland, Ohio 44106*

A possible role of immune complexes (IC) in the pathogenesis of rheumatoid arthritis (RA) has been suspected (1). In fact, studies with analytical ultracentrifugation (2) and detection of IC in RA sera (3) have provided evidence that rheumatoid factor (RF) forms complexes with autologous IgG as the reactant, and activates complement, which plays a major role in the process of inflammation (4). It is therefore likely to be of therapeutic value to remove such immune complexes from the circulating blood. The plasma exchange treatment developed for this particular purpose (5,6) has been used in some institutions with good results. This procedure, however, has disadvantages because plasma preparations are not readily available in large quantitites, and also, it involves risks such as allergic reactions, infections, and adverse effects on cardiopulmonary hemodynamics (7,8). These considerations led Malchesky, Nosé, and the Cleveland Clinic group to develop the continuous cryofiltration (CCF) technique (9) based on the principle of plasmapheresis combined with cryoprecipitation. The usefulness of the new technique has been reported (10).

PATIENTS WITH RA

Nineteen patients with RA, 4 male and 15 female, were involved in this study (Table 1). They ranged in age from 31 to 66 years. According to the system of staging and classification proposed by Steinbrocker et al., 7 patients in this series were categorized at the time of first examination as having stage 4, class 4 disease; 5 as having stage 4, class 3 disease; 1 as having stage 3, class 3 disease; 1 as having stage 3, class 2 disease; 1 as having stage 2, class 3 disease; and 4 as having stage 2, class 2 disease. By the diagnostic criteria of ARA, 18 were diagnosed as having classical RA and the remaining 1 as having definite RA.

Anticoagulant heparin was administered intravenously in a dose of 5,000 units initially and in subsequent doses of 3,000 units/hr by continuous infusion. After

TABLE 1. *Patient population (RA)*

Class	Stage	Cases	Sex M	Sex F	Age (yrs)
4	4	7	1	6	31–68
3	4	5	1	4	36–63
3	3	1	1	—	49
3	2	1	—	1	45
2	3	1	1	—	66
2	2	4	—	4	46–64

TABLE 2. *Summary of cryofiltration at Tokyo-Tokatsu Clinic*

Total sessions of CCF	470 sessions/19 cases
Treated plasma vol./CCF	5,072.2 ml/CCF
Dose of FFP or albumin/CCF	260.4 ml/CCF
Time required for treatment	3–4 hr
Blood flow	Approx. 100 ml/min

the termination of CCF therapy, 5,000 units of protamine was administered by intravenous drip infusion.

The CCF procedure was performed three times a week for the initial 2 weeks, twice a week for the next 2–4 weeks, and then once every week or 10 days for the subsequent 1–11 months.

RESULTS

The 19 RA patients underwent CCF a total of 470 times. The total volume of blood plasma treated amounted to 2,383,950 ml and plasma preparations were used in the total amount of 122,400 ml. The volumes of blood plasma treated and plasma preparation used per CCF session were 5,072.2 ml and 260.4 ml, respectively (Table 2). In the initial stages of the study fresh frozen plasma was used for the replacement of plasma, but because there actually was a case in which its use was followed by the supervention of hepatitis, 4.4 wt/vol % albumin solution was later used instead.

Hematological Data

Comparison of hematological data obtained before and after CCF therapy showed a 5% reduction of the hemoglobin content, 22.4% increase of the white cell count, and 3% decrease of the platelet count as a result of this therapeutic procedure.

Serological Data

The serum total protein, albumin, and plasma fibrinogen decreased by 32, 28, and 49%, respectively, after CCF from their pretreatment levels.

Viscosity and ESR

As for changes in the viscosity of blood and plasma before and after CCF, an 11.2% decrease in viscosity of blood was noted after the treatment (Fig. 1). Measurements of plasma viscosity obtained at the inlet and outlet of and within the macromolecule filter were 1.581, 1.394, and 2.848 centipoise, respectively (Fig. 2). The decrease in blood viscosity resulted in a marked improvement of erythrocyte sedimentation rate. Thus, when compared to pre-CCF values, the mean of values obtained before the second and subsequent sessions was lower than the value prior to the first session in all 9 cases studied. By way of example, one patient gave a mean pre-CCF value of 52.2 mm as compared with a corresponding post-CCF value

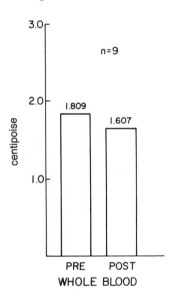

FIG. 1. Whole blood viscosity measured before and after CCF procedures. An 11% decrease in viscosity was found.

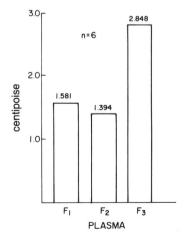

FIG. 2. Plasma viscosity measured on plasma samples obtained during a CCF procedure. F_1 is the viscosity of the plasma entering the cryofilter, F_2 is the viscosity of the plasma leaving the cryofilter, and F_3 is the viscosity of the plasma returned in the cryofilter.

of 8.8 mm for the second and ensuing sessions. Improvement rates of ESR (1-hr value) in 9 cases ranged from 77.1 to 91.2% (Fig. 3).

Immunological Data

Serum IgA levels were elevated in all 19 patients before treatment. Three of the 4 males in the series also had elevated IgE levels. Clinical symptoms were improved to a greater extent by CCF therapy in cases with higher pretreatment IgM levels. However, because of the difficulty of quantitative assay of aggregated immunoglobulins, no conclusive statement can be made as to the efficacy of CCF therapy on the basis of quantitative data concerning immunoglobulins. In a 68-year-old male patient (K. T.), RAHA, IC, CH_{50}, IgG, IgA, IgM, IgE, IgD, C3, and C4 were removed from the circulating blood by 83.4 ± 18.8, 56.9 ± 17.4, 50.0 ± 3.7, 36.2 ± 6.5, 29.9 ± 12.4, 29.2 ± 12.4, 33.9 ± 16.4, 29.0 ± 11.9, 38.9 ± 13.7, and 48.4 ± 15.0 %, respectively, per session during an 11-month period of CCF therapy (Table 3).

Immune Complexes

Prior to CCF therapy, 9 of the 19 patients had elevated IC. In 6 of these 9, clinical symptoms were improved as IC were depressed. Of 10 patients in whom the IC levels were within the normal limits before treatment, there was a marked improvement of clinical symptoms while on CCF. It seems therefore that the higher the pre-CCF IC levels, the more marked was the degree to which clinical manifestations were improved by the therapeutic procedure.

Effect of CCF

A total of 19 RA patients (18 classical RA and 1 definite RA) were treated with CCF. Remission was attained in 4 (21.0%); the treatment was evaluated as re-

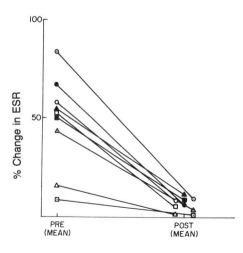

FIG. 3. Changes in erythrocyte sedimentation rate (ESR) during CCF procedures.

TABLE 3. *Immunological data of patient K. T. (male age 68)*

Parameter		CCF data (mean ± SD)		Reduction ratio/CCF
		Pre	Post	
RAHA	−x	2048 ± 627	288 ± 288	83.4 ± 18.8
IC	μg/ml	13.4 ± 7.5	4.9 ± 1.3	56.9 ± 17.4
CH_{50}	U/ml	27.9 ± 2.6	13.9 ± 1.5	50.0 ± 3.7
IgG	mg/dl	1426 ± 72	911 ± 107	36.2 ± 6.5
IgA	mg/dl	513 ± 29	359 ± 52	29.9 ± 12.4
IgM	mg/dl	179 ± 24.7	124 ± 26.0	29.2 ± 12.4
IgE	IU/ml	3650 ± 1297	2262 ± 470	33.9 ± 16.4
IgD	mg/dl	6.0 ± 1.7	4.2 ± 1.2	29.0 ± 11.9
C3	mg/dl	68.8 ± 10.8	42.6 ± 13.1	38.9 ± 13.7
C4	mg/dl	29.2 ± 2.8	15.2 ± 5.3	48.4 ± 15.0

TABLE 4. *Effect of CCF*

Remission	4 cases	21.0%
Remarkable	4 cases	21.0%
Effective	8 cases	42.1%
Poor	3 cases	15.9%
Total	19 cases	100%

markably effective in 4 (21.0%), effective in 8 (42.1%), and poor in 3 (15.9%) (Table 4). CCF-associated clinical improvement was appraised in terms of (a) grip power, (b) 25-meter walking time, (c) morning stiffness, (d) pain index, and (e) disease class. The results are described below.

Clinical Improvement

Grip Power

CCF therapy brought about improvement of grip power of both hands in all but 1 of the 19 of the patients (Table 5). The 4 patients who were brought to a state of remission after the treatment showed a 22.2–48.0% increment of the grip power of the right hand and a 35.7–252.6% increment in the left hand. Those who were labeled as having a remarkable therapeutic response had a −3 to 79.3% increase in the grip power of the right hand and a 32–102.2% increase in the left hand.

25-Meter Walking Time

Of the 19 patients, 15 (78.9%) showed a shortening of 25-meter walking time after receiving CCF. The remaining 4 patients did not benefit at all from the treatment, even though 3 of them had a value within the normal limits prior to the therapy (it takes 20 sec for healthy individuals to walk 25 meters). Of the 2 patients who were unable to walk initially, one was able to walk that distance in 130 sec after receiving CCF 59 times, and the other in 21 sec after receiving CCF 46 times.

TABLE 5. *Clinical improvement of remission and remarkable cases*

	G.P. (mmHg) R	L	25-m W.T. (sec)	M.S.	P.I.	Class/Stage Pre	Post
Remission	150	168	23	5' ↓	44		
	222	228	17	5' ↓	19	2/2	2
	48.0%	35.7%	26.1%	±	56.9%		
Remission	50	50	47	5' ↓	100		
	64	70	23	5' ↓	33	4/4	2
	28.0%	40.0%	51.1%	±	67.0%		
Remission	90	38	—	5'–2 hr	100		
	110	134	21	5' ↓	17	4/4	2
	22.2%	252.6%	100%	+ + +	83.0%		
Remission	34	18	58	4 ~ 8 hr	135		
	50	38	28	5' ↓	0	3/4	2
	47.0%	111.1%	51.8%	+ + +	100%		
Remarkable	58	76	86	30'	83		
	104	154	57	20'	49	3/2	2
	79.3%	102.2%	33.8%	33.3%	41.0%		
Remarkable	84	34	—	5–2 hr	100		
	114	58	130	5' ↓	117	4/4	3
	35.7%	70.5%	+ + +	+ + +	−17.0%		
Remarkable	78	50	46	5–2 hr	100		
	76	66	35	5–2 hr	57	3/3	2
	−3.0%	32.0%	24.0%	—	43.0%		
Remarkable	56	32	45	' 2 hr	95		
	72	60	45	5' ↓	64	4/4	2
	28.5%	87.5%	0%	+ + +	32.7%		

G.P.; grip power; 25-m W.T., 25-meter walking time; M.S., morning stiffness; P.I., pain index.

+ + +: Significant improvement.

Morning Stiffness

Of 11 patients who had morning stiffness of more than 5 min duration prior to treatment, 8 (72.7%) showed improvement of the symptom after CCF (Table 5). Of the 8 patients in whom CCF therapy brought about remission or produced a remarkable effect, 2 had morning stiffness of less than 5 min duration invariably before and after the therapy, while the other 6 obtained a marked improvement of the symptom with CCF.

Pain Index

When the effect of CCF on pain was evaluated in terms of pain index (on the basis of the pre-CCF intensity of pain as 100%), 3 (15.8%) of the 19 patients worsened with treatment and the remaining 16 (84.2%) improved. The degree of improvement of this symptom achieved in 8 patients categorized as having remission or remarkable response ranged widely from −17–100%.

Therapeutic Results Related to Disease Class

In 1 patient with class 2 RA, total freedom from pain was achieved after receiving CCF nine times; in another the disease improved from class 3 to class 2 after 11 sessions of CCF; in 2 others the disease improved from class 4 to class 2 after 46 or 59 sessions of CCF. These 4 patients, or 21.0% of the entire 19 patients, were described as having remission. The CCF therapy was evaluated as remarkably effective in 4 other patients (21.0%) experiencing a lesser degree of improvement in disease class and as effective in another 8 (42.1%) in whom there was noted a favorable clinical effect but without noticeable improvement in disease class.

Complications of CCF

CCF therapy in the present series was complicated by hepatitis in 1 case (5.3%) and also by fever, anemia, troubles with blood access, and hypoproteinemia in 27 of 470 treatments (5.7%), 11 (57.9%), 8 (42.1%), and 19 (100%) cases, respectively. In addition to these complications, 2 patients (10.5%) had one or more episodes of shock during CCF (Table 6).

DISCUSSION

Wallace et al. (11) state "A patient was said to be in 'remission' if three of the following four clinical observations were made: (1) a reduction of morning stiffness of more than 50%, (2) a decrease in 2 mm in the mean circumference of a target proximal interphalangeal joint, (3) 30% improvement in 50-feet walking time, and (4) a decrease in synovitis as evaluated by the examiner." In accordance with these authors we established the criteria of remission in which the criterion (2) above was excluded and pain index and grip power were included instead. However, in evaluating the decrease in synovitis resulting from CCF, one should recognize that the return of walking capacity to RA patients or increased range of movement in involved joints due to reduction of pain can adversely result in the causation of joint deformity with consequent aggravation of rheumatoid synovitis.

An increase in the number of leukocytes following CCF was noted. Thus, in 5 of 8 patients in whom serial white cell counts were performed, the white cell count was higher at the termination of CCF than its pre-CCF value, and returned to the pre-CCF level within 6 hr of the end of the treatment (Fig. 4).

TABLE 6. *Complications of CCF in 19 RA cases*

Hepatitis caused by fresh frozen plasma	1 case	5.3%
Anemia (iatrogenic)	11 cases	57.9%
Blood access problems	8 cases	42.1%
Hypoproteinemia	19 cases	100%
Fever (>38°C)	27/470 treatments	5.7%
Shock	6/470 treatments	1.2%

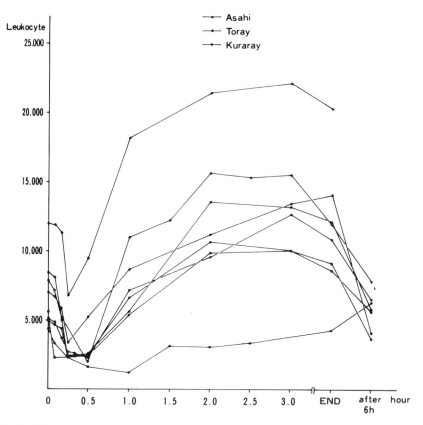

FIG. 4. Changes in leukocyte counts during CCF procedures, including a 6-hr post-procedure follow-up. Typical changes of initial leukopenia followed by leukocytosis are seen during the procedure, with return to pre-CCF levels by 6-hr post procedure.

The hepatitis which supervened in 1 patient was apparently associated with the use of fresh frozen plasma. When albumin solution was used instead, this complication did not occur in a single instance.

Of the 19 patients, fever, defined as temperature above 38°C, occurred in 27 of 470 procedures (5.7%). Possible causes of this elevation of temperature are contamination of handmade CCF circuits with pyrogen and the presence of pyrogen in membranes of the plasma separator and macromolecule filter (which are thicker than those of a dialyzer). This consideration led us to conduct tests of plasma separators of three different manufacturers for endotoxin by the Pyrodick method (normal: 0.04 ng/dl) and Pregel test (Table 7). Although the three devices were negative on both tests with physiological saline, two of them gave endotoxin levels in excess of the normal range in the contents of hollow fibers. Both of the products gave a negative Pregel test however. It was of interest to determine at what time interval fever tended to occur after the initiation of CCF. A review of temperature

TABLE 7. *Endotoxin test*

Filter type	Pyrodick method (ng/ml)			Pregel test	
A	Inside[a]	<0.04	<0.04	–	–
	Outside[a]	<0.04	<0.04	–	–
B	Inside	0.10	0.21	–	±
	Outside	0.07	0.08	–	–
C	Inside	<0.04	<0.04	–	–
	Outside	0.07	<0.04	–	–
N/S		<0.04		–	
Distilled water for i.v.		<0.04		–	

[a]Inside and outside fiber in plasma separator.

records at regular 30-min intervals after the beginning of the therapeutic procedure disclosed that temperature elevation above 38°C occurred at 60 min or later (Fig. 5). If pyrogen is present in the plasma separator, the fever must occur right after the start of CCF. The formation of yellow, cellular, clot-like aggregate deposits at the inlet of the plasma separator was noted in 21 sessions with fever. Subsequent microscopic study of the deposits revealed that they were composed of neutrophils, red cells, and platelets. Based on this evidence, we suspect that the CCF-associated fever may be caused by the destruction of leukocytes and a resultant release of enzymes, although this is yet to be verified (12–14).

In the present series blood access was gained by superficialization of the brachial artery in 4 patients and by an A-V fistula in the other 15 patients, both surgical procedures being done as a first operation. Of these 15 A-V fistulas, 8 became occluded later, since patients with RA usually have associated vasculitis and maintaining patency of A-V fistulas is difficult. To cope with the occulusion of A-V fistulas, reoperation was performed in those 8 patients, superficializing the brachial artery in 6 and reconstructing the A-V fistula in the other 2 patients.

One complication of CCF was shock, which 2 patients experienced in a total of 6 episodes; they received CCF a total of 96 times.

CONCLUSION

CCF was performed a total of 470 times on 19 patients with RA, 18 classical RA, and 1 definite RA. Improvement of clinical symptoms was achieved in 16 (84.1%) of these 19, with 4 of them having attained remission. The study indicates that CCF, unlike plasma exchange, has the advantage of being capable of treating 5,072.2 ml of plasma per session while requiring no more than 260.4 ml of albumin solution per session.

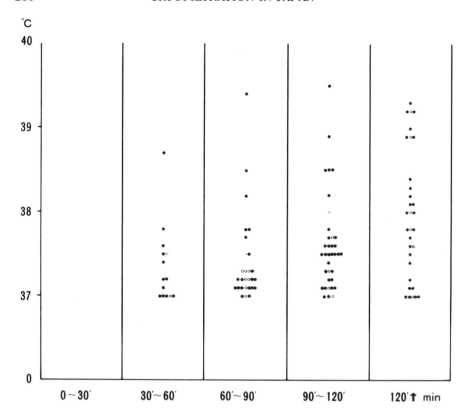

FIG. 5. A study of patient temperatures during CCF procedures. Most temperature elevations were noted to occur at 60 min or later during CCF.

Even though plasma exchange and CCF have nearly the same percentage of effectiveness, it is our opinion that CCF is much more useful, economical, and effective because CCF uses only 4.4% albumin solution as a substitution fluid. We therefore feel that there is a definite advantage to using CCF in place of plasma exchange because of the savings in plasma, and because of the decrease in certain risks, reactions, and adverse effects.

ACKNOWLEDGMENTS

The authors wish to express their thanks and cooperation to Dr. Nosé and the Cleveland Clinic group. A part of this study was supported by Asahi (Hibiya Mitsui Bldg., 1-1-2, Yurakucho, Chiyodaku, Tokyo, Japan) Kuraray (Shin-Nihonbashi Bldg., 3-8-2, Nihonbashi, Chou-ku, Tokyo, Japan), and Toray (Toyo Bldg., 3-7, Nihonbashihoncho, Chou-ku, Tokyo, Japan).

REFERENCES

1. Winchester, R. J., Agnello, V., and Kunkel, H. G. (1970): Gammaglobulin in complexes in synovial fluids of patients with rheumatoid arthritis. Partial characterization and relationship to lowered complement levels. *Clin. Exp. Immunol.*, 6:689.
2. Kunkel, H. G., Mueller-Eberhard, H. J., Fudenberg, H. H., et al. (1961): Gammaglobulin complexes in rheumatoid arthritis and certain other conditions. *J. Clin. Invest.*, 40:117.
3. Suzuta, T., and Shimo, K. (1981): Quantitation of complex and free rheumatoid factor in each immunoglobulin class by absorption of Fc-receptor bearing cell. In: *New Horizons in Rheumatoid Arthritis*, edited by Y. Shiokawa, T. Abe, and Y. Yamauchi, p. 22. Excerpta Medica, Amsterdam.
4. Jasin, H. E. (1981): Mechanism of trapping to immune complexes in joint collagenous tissues. *Clin. Exp. Immunol.*, 22:473.
5. Branda, R. F., Moldas, C. F., McCullough, J. J., et al. (1975): Plasma exchange in the treatment of immune disease. *Transfusion*, 15:570.
6. Calabrese, L., Clough, J. D., Krakauer, R. S., et al. (1980): Plasmapheresis therapy of immunologic diseases. *Cleve. Clin. Q.*, 47:53.
7. Lockwod, C. M., Rees, A. J., Perrson, T. A., et al. (1976): Immunosuppression and plasma exchange in the treatment of Goodpasture's syndrome. *Lancet*, 1:711.
8. Goldman, J. A., Casey, H. L., McIlwain, H., et al. (1979): Limited plasmapheresis in rheumatoid arthritis with vasculitis. *Arthritis Rheum.*, 22:1146.
9. Malchesky, P. S., Asanuma, Y., Zawicki, I., et al. (1980): On line separation of macromolecules by membrane filtration with cryogelation. *Artif. Organs*, 3:205.
10. Asanuma, Y., Malchesky, P. S., Suzuki, M., et al. (1981): Continuous cryofiltration (CCF) of plasma for rheumatoid arthritis. *Artif. Organs Jpn.*, 10:110.
11. Wallace, D. J., Goldfinger, D., Gatti, R., Lowe, C., Fan, P., Bluestone, R., and Klinenberg, J. R. (1979): Plasmapheresis and lymphoplasmapheresis in the management of rheumatoid arthritis. *Arthritis Rheum.*, 22:703.
12. Fehr, J., Craddock, P. R., and Jacob, H. S. (1975): *Blood*, 46:1054.
13. Craddock, P. R., Fehr, J., Brigham, K., and Jacob, H. (1975): *Clin. Res.*, 23:402.
14. McCullough, J., Weiblem, B. J., Amos, R. D., et al. (1976): *Blood*, 48:315.

Plasmapheresis, edited by Y. Nosé, P.S.
Malchesky, J. W. Smith, and R. S. Krakauer.
Raven Press, New York © 1983.

Effect of Cryofiltration on Immunologic and Clinical Parameters in Rheumatoid Arthritis

Arjeh J. Wysenbeek, Randall S. Krakauer, James W. Smith,
Paul S. Malchesky, *John V. Jones, †Bruce McLeod,
Richard Greenstreet, and Yukihiko Nosé

*Cleveland Clinic Foundation, Cleveland, Ohio 44106; *Dalhousie University Medical
Center, Halifax, Nova Scotia, Canada B3H 4H7; and †Rush–Presbyterian–St. Luke's
Medical Center, Chicago, Illinois 60612*

Rheumatoid arthritis is associated with circulating immune complexes including but not limited to rheumatoid factor (1) which is believed to be involved in the immunopathogenesis of disease symptoms. If so, their therapeutic removal might result in amelioration of disease. This has led to interest in various forms of apheresis or plasma exchange including lymphopheresis (2), plasmapheresis (3), and lymphoplasmapheresis (4). Although controversy continues in this regard, the preponderance of evidence appears to suggest efficacy for this approach, though cost effectiveness remains a debatable point (5).

Conventional plasmapheresis is relatively inefficient in depletion of macromolecules including immune complexes in that it requires plasma exchange and replacement blood proteins. We have taken advantage of the size and cryoprecipitability of immune complexes to design an extracorporeal cryopheresis circuit for selective removal of plasma macromolecules described elsewhere in these proceedings. Briefly, formed blood elements are separated from plasma by a hollow fiber filter, the formed elements are returned directly to the patient, and the plasma is cooled to 4°C and passed through a macromolecular cryofilter. This filter prevents the passage of large macromolecules and cryoprecipitable proteins by retaining them in the cryofilter. The treated plasma is rewarmed and returned to the patient. In this circuit (6), we can substantially deplete large macromolecules and cryoprecipitable protein without depletion of volume and with very little loss of total plasma protein. We evaluated this approach in 10 patients with rheumatoid arthritis at two centers.

METHODS AND PATIENTS

Patient selection: Ten adult patients with active seropositive rheumatoid arthritis, not functional class four, were selected for the study. All were on stable medical regimens for 3 months prior to and throughout the study period. All remained outpatients throughout the study period.

Laboratory evaluation: Erythrocyte sedimentation rates were done by Westergren technique. Immune complexes were determined by soluble phase Clq binding (7) and rheumatoid factor by laser nephelometry.

Patient observations: The following parameters were followed weekly on all patients studied: proximal interphalangeal joint circumference; grip strength; morning stiffness; 50-foot walk time; and Ritchie Index, an articular index of disease activity.

Protocol: All patients had 5 liters of plasma treated by this procedure twice weekly for 5 weeks.

RESULTS

Adverse effects: Two episodes of clotting of the primary filter occurred in the same patient. One episode of transient hypotension occurred which was believed to be due to volume changes rather than to complement activation, and one incident of infection at the venous access site was experienced.

Serologic parameters: Cryoprecipitable protein essentially disappeared early and completely in all patients studied. Concurrently with this, there was a reduction of mean circulating immune complexes from 847 ± 50 units/ml (nl < 69) to 107 ± 61 units/ml ($p < 0.01$ Friedman's test for comparison of nonparametric grouped data) (8). Rheumatoid factor likewise decreased from 206 ± 21 RLS (nl < 10) to 88 ± 32 RLS ($p < 0.01$ by Friedman's test) and Westergren sedimentation rate from 47 ± 15 mm/hr to 22.7 ± 5 mm/hr (difference not significant).

Clinical parameters: Morning stiffness decreased from a mean of 5.2 ± 1.6 hr to 1.2 ± 1.0 hr ($p < 0.01$ by Friedman's test) and 50-foot walk time from 37.8 ± 21 sec to 31 ± 14 sec ($p < 0.01$ by Friedman's test). Right grip strength increased from a mean of 49.5 ± 17 mmHg to 64 ± 28 mmHg (not significant) and Ritchie Index improved from a mean of 32.2 ± 5.6 to 17.3 ± 4.3 ($p < 0.01$ by Friedman's test). There was no depletion of formed blood elements, but transient leukocytosis was frequently noted subsequent to procedures.

DISCUSSION

This study represents a total of 10 patients and 100 procedures. The lack of significant evidence of toxicity in this series combined with similar reports from Japan (M. Suzuki, *personal communication*) and West Germany (M. Blumenstein, *personal communication*) indicates that this procedure is reasonably safe. Although the possibility of complement activation and/or depletion of cryoprecipitable materials such as clotting factors does exist, these potential problems do not appear serious enough to preclude the safe application of this technology. The immunochemical results are most dramatic, that is, there is a very substantial clearance of circulating immune complexes without loss of volume and with very little loss of other plasma proteins. In our previous single case report of this technology, we noted that improvement of immunochemical parameters appeared to be associated subsequently with impressive clinical improvement in that patient's disease activity

(9). The same appeared to be the case in these 10 patients. Clinical improvement over baseline, in virtually all cases, occurred subsequent to immunochemical improvement. The possibility that this is due either to placebo effect or to spontaneous remission in such large numbers of patients who had had active uncontrolled, unremitting disease we believe is remote, and although this study does not represent comparison to a control group and does not involve sham procedures, we believe that the evidence for clinical efficacy in this situation is quite substantial.

We feel that on-line cryofiltration is safe and effective in selective removal of plasma macromolecules, and is probably of clinical efficacy in rheumatoid arthritis and perhaps in other immune complex diseases as well. It does not require replacement plasma proteins and additionally, has the advantage over centrifugal devices of not depleting formed elements such as platelets. It does however require filters whose present costs are comparable to that of blood proteins. We have therefore not achieved cost effectiveness at this stage. Were this procedure to become more widely available, it is likely that the cost of these filters could decrease to approximately those of dialysis filters, which would result in a substantial cost advantage over conventional plasma exchange.

REFERENCES

1. Burnett, E. V. (1979): Circulating immune complexes: Their immunochemistry, detection, and importance. *Ann. Intern. Med.*, 91:430.
2. Karsh, J., Klippel, J. H., Plotz, P. H., Decker, J. L., Wright, D. G., and Fly, M. W. (1981): Lymphapheresis in rheumatoid arthritis: A randomized trial. *Arthritis Rheum.*, 24:867.
3. Calabrese, L. H., Clough, J. D., Krakauer, R. S., et. al. (1980): Plasmapheresis therapy of immunologic disease: Report of nine cases and review of the literature. *Cleve. Clin. Q.*, 47:53.
4. Wallace, D. J., Goldfinger, D., Gatti, R., et al. (1979): Plasmapheresis and lymphoplasmapheresis in the management of rheumatoid arthritis. *Arthritis Rheum.*, 22:703.
5. Wallace, D. J., Goldfinger, D., Lowe, C., Nichols, S., Weiner, J., Brachman, M., and Klinenberg, J. R. (1982): A double-blind, controlled study of lymphoplasmapheresis versus sham apheresis in rheumatoid arthritis. *N. Engl. J. Med.*, 306:1406.
6. Malchesky, P. S., Asanuma, Y., Zawicki, I., Blumenstein, M., Calabrese, L., Kyo, A., Krakauer, R., and Nosé, Y. (1980): On-line separation of macromolecules by membrane filtration with cryogelation. In: *Plasma Exchange*, edited by H. G. Sieberth, p. 113. Schattauer-Verlag, Stuttgart, New York.
7. Zubler, R. H., Lange, G., Lambert, P. H., et al. (1976): Detection of immune complexes in untreated sera by a modified ^{125}I-Clq binding test: Effect of heating on the binding of Clq by immune complexes and application of the test to systemic lupus erythematosus. *J. Immunol.*, 116:232.
8. Hollander, M., and Wolfe, D. A. (1973): *Nonparametric Statistical Methods*. Wiley, New York.
9. Krakauer, R. S., Asanuma, Y., Zawicki, I., Calabrese, L., Malchesky, P., and Nosé, Y. (1982): Circulating immune complexes in rheumatoid arthritis: Selective removal by cryogelation with membrane filtration. *Arch. Intern. Med.*, 142:395.

Plasmapheresis, edited by Y. Nosé, P. S. Malchesky, J. W. Smith, and R. S. Krakauer. Raven Press, New York © 1983.

Plasma Exchange in Systemic Lupus Erythematosus

John Verrier Jones

Section of Rheumatology, Rush-Presbyterian-St. Luke's Medical Center, Chicago, Illinois 60612

In cases of active systemic lupus erythematosus (SLE), there is substantial evidence for the presence in the circulation of high levels of circulating immune complexes (1,2). There is also evidence that levels of antibody to DNA and nucleoprotein antigens often correlate with clinical activity in SLE (3–6). It was therefore logical to consider that the exchange of plasma, by removing an excess of deleterious substances, might be a useful therapeutic intervention in the treatment of severe SLE.

The first application of plasmapheresis for the treatment of SLE, however, was dictated more by desperation than by rational planning. In July 1974, we admitted to Southmead Hospital, Bristol, England, a 45-year-old woman whose severe SLE had failed to respond to prednisolone, given in a dose of 80 mg/day for 1 month. On admission, she was profoundly leukopenic (WBC 0.6×10^9/liter; neutrophils 0.4×10^9/liter) with a reduced platelet count (80×10^9/liter). The low WBC clearly made the use of cytotoxic drugs extremely hazardous. In searching for alternative therapy we chose, because of our experience with plasmapheresis in the management of patients with hyperviscosity, to introduce this as the next stage of treatment. The patient showed a gratifying clinical response, with a reduction of antibodies to DNA, reduction of immune complexes, and a gradual return to normal of C3, C4, and hemolytic complement.

On the basis of this encouraging result, we studied the effect of plasmapheresis in another 14 cases of SLE: the results have been reported in detail elsewhere (7,8). In summary, 8 out of 14 patients showed evidence of either clinical improvement or clinical and immunochemical improvement at the time of plasmapheresis. In 3 patients with high levels of circulating immune complexes before treatment there was a sudden fall in the level of complexes which was quantitatively greater than could be explained by the amount removed. This suggested that in some patients with SLE, clearance of complexes by the mononuclear phagocyte system is initially

---

Present address: Head, Division of Rheumatology, Department of Medicine, Dalhousie University, Halifax Civic Hospital, 5938 University Avenue, Halifax, Nova Scotia B3H 2Y9 Canada.

blocked by high levels of circulating complexes, and that one effect of plasmapheresis may be to reverse this blockade.

Kater and his colleagues (9) from Utrecht, in the Netherlands, have reported the results of plasmapheresis in 8 patients with active SLE. Half of the patients underwent 5 sessions in 2 weeks, with removal of 1.5 liters of plasma at each session, while the other half continued plasmapheresis for a more prolonged period, with diminishing frequency, to a total of 20 exchanges. In 4 patients who had detectable circulating immune complexes, and who were resistant to prednisone, plasmapheresis was followed by a complete clinical remission. In 2 others, there was an improvement of arthritis, and in 1 patient, thrombocytopenia disappeared. One of the patients (no. 7) was initially treated with plasmapheresis alone for 12 weeks, with no detectable clinical or immunochemical response.

In a study of 8 patients with SLE initiated in Chicago, we have attempted to study the short-term fluctuations of immune complexes and antibodies following plasmapheresis, and to determine the duration of the effect (10). Drug treatment was maintained at a constant level for at least 4 weeks before plasmapheresis was introduced and all patients were either stable or deteriorating clinically. Levels of circulating immune complexes were measured by a Raji-cell radioimmunoassay and by a solid-phase Clq-binding assay. Antibodies to dsDNA and ssDNA were measured by the Farr assay. In all cases immune complexes and antibodies were lowered by plasmapheresis. In 5 cases, plasmapheresis was followed by a rapid rebound of complexes and antibodies to pretreatment levels. In 3, in whom plasmapheresis was followed by treatment with cyclophosphamide for 1 month, a sustained immunochemical and clinical improvement followed, lasting in 2 cases for up to 3 years. Since in the future, plasmapheresis is likely to be used in combination with drugs in the management of SLE, it is instructive to review the data available worldwide on the interaction of plasmapheresis and drugs.

INTERACTIONS OF PLASMAPHERESIS AND DRUGS

Plasmapheresis Alone

Concomitant drug therapy appears to have an important impact on the duration of the effect of plasmapheresis. In 2 patients from our most recent series who were treated with plasmapheresis alone before the use of corticosteroids or cytotoxic drugs, there was a return of immune complexes to pretreatment levels within 10 days, followed by an overshoot in the material detected by the Raji-cell assay. In both cases this was accompanied by an exacerbation of clinical signs and symptoms. This suggests that plasmapheresis alone is unlikely to have a role in the management of SLE. Schlansky and his co-workers (11) came to a similar conclusion. They reported a study of 4 patients with SLE in whom plasmapheresis was used as the only form of treatment. One patient showed rapid deterioration of renal disease and recurrence of cerebral manifestations of SLE within 1 month of plasmapheresis. Two patients experienced some relief of arthritis, malaise, and vasculitis during plasmapheresis, but also deteriorated within 1 month of the conclusion of exchange therapy. One patient with thrombocytopenia was unchanged during plasmapheresis, but became worse 2 months later. In our initial report (8) we also described 2 patients who were treated with plasmapheresis alone. One (A. G.), showed no clinical response over 3 weeks, while the other (M. M.) showed a rapid improvement of his skin rash and mucosal ulcers, but developed a transient dysphasia and hemiparesis after two exchanges of 1.5 liters of plasma. It is reasonable to conclude that plasmapheresis used as the sole therapy for patients with SLE may be transiently helpful, but is likely to be followed rapidly by a relapse and possibly by a clinical and immunological exacerbation.

There are four published reports in which patients with SLE have been treated with plasmapheresis alone (8–11). Of 12 patients, 6 (50%) in this group are judged to have improved clinically as a result of plasmapheresis, but in most the response was brief, lasting between 10 days and 1 month. Taking the term "rebound" to indicate the clinical or immunological deterioration occurring within 1 month of plasmapheresis, it is striking that 5 out of 12 (42%) patients in this group showed evidence of a post-exchange rebound.

Plasmapheresis with Corticosteroids

If plasmapheresis alone is unlikely to be therapeutically important, are there any indications of what drug or combination of drugs is likely to potentiate or prolong the effects of plasmapheresis? Before considering the evidence, we should recognize clearly the limitations of anecdotal discussions of small numbers of patients. A patient with SLE can be treated once. There is no guarantee that when the treatment is repeated the patient will be in a comparable state. It is reasonable to argue that when plasmapheresis is combined with therapeutic drugs, the changes seen are as likely to be due to the drugs as to the plasmapheresis. Ultimately, a clear determination of whether plasmapheresis changes the outcome of a disease, compared with available drug therapy, will only be made as a result of randomized studies, in which groups of patients treated with plasmapheresis and drugs are compared with similar groups treated with drugs alone. Such studies are in progress (12), but until their results are available it is reasonable to draw what information we can from the uncontrolled studies which have so far been published. It is also obvious that no randomized, controlled trial can be designed with any likelihood of success, unless the results of available anecdotal studies are analyzed as closely as possible.

There are 13 published accounts of patients treated with plasmapheresis and corticosteroids (8–10,13–21). Of 42 patients, 34 (81%) are said to have improved clinically, or clinically and immunochemically, for a period of at least 2 weeks. The duration of improvement was very variable, ranging between 2 weeks and 2 years. No investigators reported a rebound following plasmapheresis in this group.

Ten publications describe the effect of plasmapheresis combined with corticosteroids and cytotoxic drugs (8,10,12,15–17,21–24). Of the 16 patients, 12 (75%) are said to have improved for a period of at least 2 weeks. The best results are seen in the 7 cases treated with cyclophosphamide, where 7 out of 7 showed clinical improvement. When the proportion of 6 out of 7 with a prolonged (>20 weeks) response is compared with the 13/70 prolonged responses in the whole group, the difference, applying the null hypothesis and using exact binomial probability, is highly significant ($p < 0.0003$). Some of the responses in this group are remarkably prolonged. Two of the Chicago patients (10) are controlled on a small dose of prednisone after 4 years. One patient reported by Lockwood et al. (21) and one reported by Schilderman et al. (22) remained in remission for at least 18 months.

In general, then, the results of plasmapheresis alone, or with concomitant drug therapy can be summarized as follows: (a) Plasmapheresis alone may produce a transient improvement in joint pain and skin rash, but the effect is short-lived, and a number of reports have drawn attention to a rapid worsening of clinical and immunochemical manifestations of SLE between 1 and 4 weeks after plasmapheresis is discontinued. (b) Plasmapheresis with corticosteroids was associated with clinical improvement in 80% of patients reported. The duration of the response was variable, but usually rather short. (c) Plasmapheresis with corticosteroids and azathioprine was associated with improvement in 5 out of 8 patients, but was again brief. The most prolonged responses were reported in the group treated with plasmapheresis, corticosteroids, and cyclophosphamide, where 7 out of 7 patients showed a clinical improvement, lasting between 4 years and not less than 4 months.

REFERENCES

1. Koffler, D., Agnello, V., Thoburn, R., and Kunkel, H. G. (1971): Systemic lupus erythematosus: Prototype of immune complex nephritis in man. *J. Exp. Med.*, 134:169s.
2. Clough, J. D., and Calabrese, L. H. (1981): Theoretical aspects of immune complex removal by plasmapheresis. *Plasma Therapy Transfusion Technol.*, 2:73.
3. Schur, P. H., and Sandson, J. (1968): Immunologic factors and clinical activity in systemic lupus erythematosus. *N. Engl. J. Med.*, 278:533.
4. Pincus, T., Schur, P. H., Rose, J. A., Decker, J. R., and Talal, N. (1969): Measurement of serum DNA-binding activity in systemic lupus erythematosus. *N. Engl. J. Med.*, 281:701.
5. Mattioli, M., and Reichlin, M. (1974): Heterogeneity of RNA protein antigens reactive with sera of patients with systemic lupus erythematosus. *Arthritis Rheum.*, 17:421.
6. Notman, D. D., Kurara, N., and Tan, E. M. (1975): Profiles of antinuclear antibodies in systemic rheumatic diseases. *Ann. Intern. Med.*, 83:464.
7. Jones, J. Verrier, Cumming, R. H., Bucknall, R. C., Asplin, C. M., Fraser, I. D., Bothamley, J., Davis, P., and Hamblin, T. J. (1976): Plasmapheresis in the management of acute systemic lupus erythematosus? *Lancet*, i:709.
8. Jones, J. Verrier, Cumming, R. H., Bacon, P. A., Evers, J., Fraser, I. D., Bothamley, J., Tribe, C. R., Davis, P. G., and Hughes, G. R. V. (1979): Evidence for a therapeutic effect of plasmapheresis in patients with systemic lupus erythematosus. *Q. J. Med.*, 48:555.
9. Kater, L., Derksen, R. H. W. M., Houwert, F. A., Hene, R. J., Struyvenberg, A., Gmelig Meyling, R. J. H., and Verroust, P. (1981): Effect of plasmapheresis in active systemic lupus erythematosus. *Neth. J. Med.*, 24:209.
10. Jones, J. Verrier, Robinson, M. F., Parciany, R. K., Layfer, L. F., and McLeod, B. (1981): Therapeutic plasmapheresis in systemic lupus erythematosus: Effect on immune complexes and antibodies to DNA. *Arthritis Rheum.*, 24:1113.
11. Schlansky, R., Dehoratius, R. J., Pincus, T., and Tung, K. S. K. (1981): Plasmapheresis in systemic lupus erythematosus. A cautionary note. *Arthritis Rheum.*, 24:49.
12. Parry, H. F., Moran, C. J., Snaith, M. L., Richards, J. D. M., Goldstone, A. H., Nineham, L. J., Hay, F. C., Morrow, W. J. W., and Roitt, I. M. (1981): Plasma exchange in systemic lupus erythematosus. *Ann. Rheum. Dis.*, 40:224.

13. Dequeker, J., Geusens, P., and Wielands, L. (1980): Short and long-term experience with plasmapheresis in connective tissue diseases. *Biomedicine*, 32:189.
14. Wei, N., Huston, D. P., Lippel, J. H., Balow, J. E., Dawley, T. J., Hall, R. P., Plotz, R. M., Steinberg, A. D., and Decker, J. L. (1981): A randomized trial of plasmapheresis in systemic lupus erythematosus. *Arthritis Rheum.*, 24:299 *(abstr. suppl.)*.
15. Abdou, M. I., Lindsley, H. B., Pollock, A., Stechschulte, D. J., and Wood, G. (1981): Plasmapheresis in active systemic lupus erythematosus: Effects on clinical serum, and cellular abnormalities. Case report. *Clin. Immunol. Immunopathol.*, 19:44.
16. Moran, C. J., Parry, H. F., Mowbray, J., Richards, J. D. M., and Goldstone, A. H. (1977): Plasmapheresis in systemic lupus erythematosus. *Br. Med. J.*, i:1573.
17. Wallace, D. J., Goldfinger, D., Thompson-Breton, R., Martin, V., Lowe, C. M., Bluestone, R., and Klinenberg, J. R. (1980): Advances in the use of therapeutic pheresis for the management of rheumatic diseases. *Sem. Arthritis Rheum.*, 10:81.
18. Rossen, R. D., Hersh, E. M., Sharp, J. T., McCredie, K. B., Gyorkey, F., Suki, W. N., Eknoyan, G., and Resiberg, M. A. (1977): Effect of plasma exchange on circulating immune complexes and antibody formation in patients treated with cyclophosphamide and prednisone. *Am. J. Med.*, 63:674.
19. Hubbard, H. C., and Portnoy, B. (1979): Systemic lupus erythematosus in pregnancy treated with plasmapheresis. *Br. J. Dermatol.*, 101:87.
20. Young, D. W., Thompson, R. A., and Mackie, P. H. (1980): Plasmapheresis in hereditary angioneurotic edema and systemic lupus erythematosus. *Arch. Intern. Med.*, 140:127.
21. Lockwood, C. M., Pussel, B., Wilson, C. B., and Peters, D. K. (1979): Plasma exchange in nephritis. *Adv. Nephrol.*, 8:383.
22. Schilderman, B., Dequeker, J., and Van De Putte, I. (1979): Plasmapheresis combined with corticosteroids in uncontrolled active systemic lupus erythematosus. *J. Rheum.*, 6:687.
23. Hamilton, W. A. P., Vergani, D., Bevis, L., Tee, D. E. H., Zilkha, K. H., and Cotton, L. T. (1980): Plasma exchange in SLE. *Lancet*, i:1249.
24. Calabrese, L. H., Clough, J. D., Krakauer, R. S., and Hoeltge, G. A. (1980): Plasmapheresis therapy of immunologic disease. *Cleve. Clin. Q.*, 47:53.

Plasmapheresis, edited by Y. Nosé, P. S.
Malchesky, J. W. Smith, and R. S. Krakauer.
Raven Press, New York © 1983.

Membrane Plasma Filtration for Treatment of Plasma Cell Disease

Matthias Blumenstein, Walter Samtleben, David H. Randerson, Rupert Habersetzer, and Hans J. Gurland

Nephrology Division, Medizinische Klinik I, Klinikum Grosshadern, University of Munich, D-8000 Munich 70, Federal Republic of Germany

Plasma cell neoplasms constitute a group of related disorders in which a single clone of plasma cells produces large quantities of an immunoglobulin molecule. The most important entity is multiple myeloma with an annual incidence of 3 per 100,000 of population. Other related conditions include Waldenström's macroglobulinemia, primary amyloidosis, and the heavy chain diseases. There is a wide spectrum of clinical symptoms resulting from the damage produced by plasma cell tumors in the bone marrow and from the effects of abnormal proteins. The mean survival time of patients with multiple myeloma who receive combinations of alkylating agents, steroids, and vincristine is about 30 months. The prognosis for Waldenström's macroglobulinemia is slightly better. The most common clinical complications due to abnormal high protein concentrations include hyperviscosity syndrome, progressive renal failure, and bleeding disorders. Rapid removal of the excess protein by means of plasma exchange (PE) is the treatment of choice to control these life-threatening situations. In paraproteinemic patients, this mode of treatment has proved to be an effective tool, as reported in the literature on about 100 patients who were treated between 1952 and 1981. The main indication for plasmapheresis was hyperviscosity syndrome, followed by renal failure and bleeding tendencies. The overall benefit of the patients treated was 80% (Table 1).

TABLE 1. *Plasmapheresis therapy in paraproteinemia (literature review, 1952–1981)*

Diagnosis	Patients treated	Benefit (%)
Multiple myeloma	40	83
Waldenström's macroglobulinemia	44	91
No classification	15	100
Total	99	81

PE treatments have been carried out by centrifugal methods for the most part, with membrane systems recently entering into this field. In general, the automated centrifugal PE machines are costly and too bulky to be mobile, whereas membrane plasma filtration is a relatively simple procedure which can be performed in any institution where there is experience with extracorporeal circulation. In addition, with centrifugal techniques the separation of the plasma and blood cells is not complete, and the plasma contains a significant amount of blood cells, particularly platelets. This limits the application of centrifugal techniques in disease states associated with severe bone marrow dysfunction.

In addition to a short review of indications for PE in plasma cell disease, our own experience with treatment of paraproteinemic patients using the membrane technique will be discussed in this chapter.

REVIEW OF THE LITERATURE

Hyperviscosity Syndrome

Several factors contribute to hyperviscosity including the serum concentration of monoclonal immunoglobulins, polymer or aggregate formation, cryoprecipitation, antibody activity against serum proteins, and red cells. Hyperviscosity is common in Waldenström's macroglobulinemia due to IgM in its pentameric form, but may be found in multiple myeloma also. Cardiovascular, neurological, and ocular complications cause most of the clinical manifestations. Hyperviscosity syndrome was one of the first therapeutic applications for PE reported by Skoog et al. in 1959 (1).

The beneficial effects of plasmapheresis in this complication have been demonstrated in many patients since that time, suggesting PE as the treatment of choice (2–10). A review of the literature reveals that successful results were obtained in all of 20 patients with Waldenström's macroglobulinemia, and in 78% out of 23 patients with multiple myeloma. Moreover, repeated PEs on a long-term basis may be effective in maintaining an acceptable quality of life in patients whose problems are due to paraprotein and where chemotherapy is complicated due to side effects (10) (Table 2).

Progressive Renal Failure—Myeloma Kidney

Besides factors such as hypercalcemia, hyperuricemia, and amyloidosis, glomerular filtration of abnormal proteins is believed to play a pathogenic role in producing the typical renal lesions of myeloma kidney. Immunoglobulin light chains are normally filtered at the glomerulus and then catabolized in the proximal tubule epithelium (11). In case of high light chain concentration, Bence Jones proteinuria occurs, indicating that the capacity of the proximal tubule to reabsorb and catabolize light chains is exceeded.

Damage of the kidney is caused either through precipitation of proteins within tubules leading to intrarenal obstruction or through toxic damage to tubule cells

TABLE 2. *Plasmapheresis therapy in paraproteinemia. Indications for plasmapheresis: Hyperviscosity syndrome (literature review, 1952–1981)*

Diagnosis	Patients treated	Benefit (%)	Authors
Multiple myeloma	23	78	Powles et al. (2) 1971 Cohen and Rundles (3) 1975 Isbister et al. (4) 1978 Rosenbaum et al. (5) 1978 Iwamoto et al. (6) 1980
Waldenström's macroglobulinemia	20	100	Reynolds (7) 1956 Solomon and Fahey (8) 1963 Schwab and Fahey (9) 1964 Powles et al. (2) 1971 Buskard et al. (10) 1977 Isbister et al. (4) 1978

TABLE 3. *Plasmapheresis therapy in paraproteinemia. Indications for plasmapheresis: Progressive renal failure (literature review, 1952–1981)*

Diagnosis	Patients treated	Benefit (%)	Authors
Multiple myeloma	11	91	Powles et al. (2) 1971 Feest et al. (13) 1976 Isbister et al. (4) 1978 Misiani et al. (14) 1979 Jako et al. (15) 1981

(12). Therefore, progressive renal failure might be avoided by a decrease of serum light chain concentration. In comparison to chemotherapy and peritoneal dialysis, plasmapheresis is the most effective therapeutic tool in removing those abnormal proteins. Eleven patients were treated with PE as reported by several different authors. Normal function of the kidney was restored in about 90% (2,4,13–15). However, in most of the cases combined therapy was used to overcome renal failure. Consequently, it is difficult to evaluate the beneficial role of plasmapheresis treatment alone in myeloma kidney, indicating the need for further investigations (Table 3).

Bleeding Defects

Hemostatic impairment is common in association with paraproteinemia and seems to be caused by several pathogenic mechanisms. Abnormalities of platelet function have been documented as well as inhibition of coagulation factors and impairment of fibrin polymerization (16). Patients treated for bleeding tendencies are reported to respond well to plasmapheresis (2,4,8,17,18). It might be expected that bleeding stops during the exchange procedure despite systemic anticoagulation with heparin or citrate (Table 4).

MEMBRANE PLASMA FILTRATION FOR TREATMENT OF PARAPROTEINEMIA

After this review of the literature I would like to report on our own experience with PE using the membrane filtration technique. In our institution, 7 patients were treated by membrane plasma filtration for paraproteinemia. Indications for PE were coronary microangiopathy (3 patients), cryoglobulinemia (1 patient), renal failure (1 patient), hyperviscosity syndrome (1 patient), and coma (1 patient). Plasma was separated from whole blood using commercially available plasma separators of a membrane hollow fiber design (Plasmaflo 01 and 02, Asahi Medical Co., Japan, and Plasmaflux P2, Fresenius-MTS, FRG). Sieving of plasma proteins is in the range of almost 100% for these devices. In one session, about 2 liters of the patient's plasma was exchanged. The total volume exchanged varied from 4 to 20 liters. For substitution of the discarded plasma, 3% albumin solution was used. Anticoagulation consisted of an initial bolus injection of 5,000 units of heparin followed by continuous heparinization (60 U/min heparin). Technical aspects of the procedure have been discussed in detail elsewhere (19). All patients were under concomitant chemotherapy during the time of plasma therapy.

RESULTS

By means of membrane plasma filtration, abnormal proteins were removed to a significant extent in all cases depending on molecular weight and volume exchanged. Treatments were tolerated well by all patients. No serious complications due to plasmapheresis were observed. Reduced paraprotein concentration was followed by clinical improvement in 5 out of 7 patients. One patient with coma and another one with renal failure died from heart failure. Both cases had already been in critical condition before plasma treatment was started. In a patient with multiple myeloma, serum IgG concentration was reduced from 6,600 mg/dl to 1,340 mg/dl after a total exchange of 9 liters of paraproteinemic plasma. The efficacy of membrane plasma

TABLE 4. *Plasmapheresis therapy in paraproteinemia. Indications for plasmapheresis: Bleeding disorders (literature review, 1952–1981)*

Diagnosis	Patients treated	Benefit (%)	Authors
Multiple myeloma	2	100	Powles et al. (2) 1971
			Isbister et al. (4) 1978
Waldenström's macroglobulinemia	7	100	Conway and Walker (17) 1962
			Soloman and Fahey (8) 1963
			Powles et al. (2) 1971
			Messmore et al. (18) 1978
			Isbister et al. (4) 1978

filtration in the removal of high molecular weight proteins is demonstrated in case of 2 patients suffering from Waldenström's macroglobulinemia. The first patient, a 72-year-old male, was treated for hyperviscosity syndrome. Total volume exchanged in 5 sessions was 12.2 liters. By means of these treatments serum IgM concentration fell from 6,800 to 1,700 mg/dl. Increased serum viscosity tended to normal range. The second patient with Waldenström's macroglobulinemia, a 52-year-old female, was treated by PE for angina pectoris at normal coronary arteriogram. Three treatments reduced the IgM concentration as well as plasma and blood viscosity parameters followed by improvement of coronary blood flow and coronary vascular reserve. The patient was free of angina symptoms afterward.

These results demonstrate membrane plasma filtration to be as effective as centrifugal techniques in the removal of highly concentrated abnormal protein. However, to obtain optimum results, the following facts must be observed. Concerning selection of membranes, high porosity and sufficient surface area should be taken into consideration. The second generation of hollow fiber membranes characterized by enlarged porosity offers improved sieving for high molecular weight proteins. In any case of membrane plasma filtration, the sieving of macromolecules highly depends on the proper selection of operating conditions. To gain optimum clearance of proteins and to avoid complications such as hemolysis, plasma flux should be controlled for operating at low transmembrane pressure. In cryoglobulinemia, attention should be paid to the temperature of the extracorporeal circuit. Depending on cryoprotein concentration, cryoprecipitation often occurs already at temperatures in the range of 35°C, causing irreversible blocking of the hollow fibers. Working at 37°C by placing the plasma separator in a warming bath prevents this problem.

CONCLUSIONS

Plasmapheresis should be considered as an additional therapeutic tool for treatment of paraproteinemia in case of complications, such as hyperviscosity syndrome, renal failure, and bleeding tendencies. PE alone is effective in controlling the disease state when conventional chemotherapy fails or temporary side effects limit its application.

Membrane filtration for therapeutic PE in paraproteinemia offers the following advantages: (i) It is effective in removing abnormal proteins, (ii) it is a safe and simple procedure, and (iii) there is no loss of blood cells.

REFERENCES

1. Skoog, W. A., Adams, W. S., and Coburn, J. W. (1962): Metabolic balance study of plasmapheresis in a case of Waldenström's macroglobulinemia. *Blood*, 19:425.
2. Powles, R., Smith, C., Kohn, J., and Hamilton Fairley, G. (1971): Method of removing abnormal protein rapidly from patients with malignant paraproteinaemias. *Br. Med. J.*, 3:664.
3. Cohen, H. J., and Wayne Rundles, R. (1975): Managing complications of plasma cell myeloma. *Arch. Intern. Med.*, 135:177.
4. Isbister, J. P., Biggs, J. C., and Penny, R. (1978): Experience with large volume plasmapheresis in malignant paraproteinaemia and immune disorders. *Aust. N.Z. J. Med.*, 8:154.

5. Rosenbaum, E. H., Thompson, H. E., and Glassberg, A. B. (1978): Priapism and multiple myeloma. Successful treatment with plasmapheresis. *Urology*, 12:201.
6. Iwamoto, H., Nakagawa, S., Matsui, N., Yoshiyama, N., Shinoda, T., Shibamoto, T., and Takeuchi, J. (1980): An experience of plasma exchange by membrane separator for IgA myeloma. In: *Plasma Exchange. Plasmapheresis—Plasmaseparation*, edited by H. G. Sieberth, p. 377. Schattauer, Stuttgart.
7. Reynolds, W. A. (1981): Late report of the first case of plasmapheresis for Waldenström's macroglobulinemia. *J.A.M.A.*, 245:606.
8. Solomon, A., and Fahey, J. L. (1963): Plasmapheresis therapy in macroglobulinemia. *Ann. Intern. Med.*, 58:789.
9. Schwab, P. J., and Fahey, J. L. (1960): Treatment of Waldenström's macroglobulinemia by plasmapheresis. *N. Engl. J. Med.*, 263:574.
10. Buskard, N. A., Galton, D. A. G., Goldman, J. M., Kohner, E. M., Grindle, C. F. J., Newman, D. L., Twinn, K. W., and Lowenthal, R. M. (1977): Plasma exchange in the long-term management of Waldenström's macroglobulinemia. *C.M.A. J.*, 117:135.
11. Mogielnicki, R. P., Waldmann, T. A., and Strober, W. (1971): The renal handling of low molecular weight proteins: L chain and metabolism in experimental renal disease. *J. Clin. Invest.*, 25:280.
12. Clyne, D. H., Pesce, A. J., and Thompson, R. E. (1979): Nephrotoxicity of Bence Jones protein in the rat. *Kidney Int.*, 16:345.
13. Feest, T. G., Burge, P. S., and Cohen, S. L. (1976): Successful treatment of myeloma kidney by diuresis and plasmapheresis. *Br. Med. J.*, 1:503.
14. Misiani, R., Remuzzi, G., Bertani, T., Licini, R., Levoni, P., Crippa, A., and Mecca, G. (1979): Plasmapheresis in the treatment of acute renal failure in multiple myeloma. *Am. J. Med.*, 66:684.
15. Jako, J., Virágh, S., Schopper, J., and Sebók, Juhász (1981): Nierenerkrankungen bei monoklonalen Gammopathien—eine klinisch-pathologische Studie. *Immun. Infekt.*, 9:60.
16. Lackner, H. (1973): Hemostatic abnormalities associated with dysproteinemias. *Semin. Hematol.*, 10:125.
17. Conway, N., and Miles Walker, J. (1962): Treatment of macroglobulinemia. *Br. Med. J.*, 11:1296.
18. Messmore, H. L., Fareed, J., Silberman, S., Gawlik, G. M., and Bermes, E. W. (1978): Macroglobulinemia of Waldenström. Diagnosis and managment. *Ann. Clin. Lab. Sci.*, 8:310.
19. Gurland, H. J., Nosé, Y., Asanuma, Y., Blumenstein, M., Malchesky, P. S., Samtleben, W., Schmidt, B., and Zawicki, I. Membrane plasma filtration. In: *Plasma Exchange in Immunology and Oncology*, edited by G. A. Nagel and J. H. Beyer. Karger, Munich *(in press)*.

Plasmapheresis, edited by Y. Nosé, P. S. Malchesky, J. W. Smith, and R. S. Krakauer. Raven Press, New York © 1983.

Effects of Various Immunosuppressive Regimens on the "Rebound Phenomenon" Induced by Plasma Exchange in Pemphigus

J. C. Roujeau, *C. Andre, J. Revuz, and R. Touraine

*Departments of Dermatology and Immuno-Hematology, *Hôpital Henri Mondor 94 010 Creteil, France*

The growing popularity of plasma exchange (PE) in the management of autoimmune diseases (1) has been hampered by the "rebound phenomenon", a phenomenon first observed more than 10 years ago by Bystryn et al. (2,3) in rabbits. The removal of a serum antibody (by exchange transfusion) was followed by a specific reaccumulation of this antibody, reaching peak titers higher than the initial level, an average of 8 days later. These experiments suggested a feedback regulation of antibody production in relation to serum antibody levels.

Such rebounds in antibody synthesis have already been observed in human autoimmune diseases treated by PE, sometimes with dramatically noxious effects (4,5). As a result of that risk most authors use immunosuppressive (IS) therapy in conjunction with PE, treating patients concurrently by an association of adrenal steroids and cytotoxic drugs (6).

However, rebounds had been observed despite the IS regimen in some patients with lupus erythematosus (7), myasthenia gravis (8), or pemphigus vulgaris (9–11).

Pemphigus vulgaris is a suitable model for the search for an IS regimen capable of suppressing autoantibody rebound after PE. This severe disease, characterized by bullous eruptions of the skin and mucous membranes, results from acantholysis, that is, the disruption of epidermal cells. There is growing evidence suggesting the pathogenic role of IgG autoantibodies directed against epidermal cell membranes, usually called intercellular antibodies (IC Ab). Ic Ab may be easily detected in the perilesional skin by direct immunofluorescent staining and in the serum by indirect immunofluorescent staining. In individual patients, IC Ab serum levels fluctuate with and reflect the disease activity, easily estimated by the daily count of new blisters (12).

For several years we have used PE as a rational approach to the management of severe pemphigus (9). Various regimens of adrenal steroids and cytotoxic drugs have been employed with PE to determine the drug regimen that best suppresses rebound.

PATIENTS AND METHODS

Patients

Eleven patients with pemphigus entered the study from November 1977 to March 1981. The clinical data have been reported elsewhere (10,13,14). Briefly, 7 patients had previously been treated by adrenal steroids, but their diseases were either resistant to high doses (3 cases) or relapsing at low doses (4 cases); in the other cases PE was a part of the initial therapy.

Drugs Given During the PE Course

Daily oral cytotoxic drugs were given to 9 patients: 7 received cyclophosphamide (CY), 2–3 mg/kg/day; 1 received chlorambucil, 0.1 mg/kg/day; and 1 received azathioprine, 2 mg/kg/day. Daily oral prednisolone was given to 10 patients: 3 received low doses (0.1, 0.1, and 0.15 mg/kg/day) and 7 received high doses (0.5–2 mg/kg/day). Thus, PE was performed with oral CY for 1 patient, with oral CY and low prednisolone doses for 3 patients, with oral cytotoxic drugs and high prednisolone doses for 5 patients, and with high prednisolone doses for 2 patients.

Plasma Exchanges

PE was performed two or three times a week with a discontinuous flow blood processor, Haemonetics H 30 (Haemonetics, 400 Wood Road, Braintree, MA 02184). Each procedure removed 150% of the theoretical plasma volume, replaced isovolumetrically by fresh frozen human plasma. The mean number of PE for each patient was 9.8 (range 3–20) over 4 weeks (range 1–10).

IC Ab

Serum levels of IC Ab were determined before and after each PE by indirect immunofluorescence microscopy using fluorescein conjugated goat antibody globulins to human IgG, IgA, and IgM (Hyland Diagnostics, Travenol Laboratories, Deerfield, IL 60015). Rat esophagus and normal human skin were used as substrates. The Ab titer was defined as the highest serum dilution still giving a positive immunofluorescence test on rat esophagus. For reliable evaluation of changes in titers, old and new sera were tested simultaneously in each patient. For studying long-term evolution of IC Ab, we considered only the titers determined before each PE or 2 days or more after the last PE in order to avoid the short-term fluctuation induced by each exchange.

The "rebound" was defined as a reaccumulation of IC Ab level, even of one dilution, above the minimal level observed after a few PE (considering always the preexchange titers).

Geometric means of IC Ab titers were compared with the Mann–Whitney nonparametric test.

RESULTS

Effect of One PE

Immediately after each procedure the mean decrease of IC Ab was of two dilutions. Iterative determinations of IC Ab titers during the hours following a PE in 1 patient showed a reaccumulation to only one dilution below the initial level 3 hr after the end of the PE (Fig. 1).

Effect of Further PE

As PE was repeated every other day, IC Ab titer dropped again, decreasing by two dilutions each time and then rising again before the next procedure, thus producing a stepwise lowering.

If we consider only the titer determined before each procedure, discarding the fluctuations following each PE, the IC Ab curve shows a regular decrease reaching a nadir after three or four PE (mean 3.7, range 3–7) in a mean of 7.6 days (range 4–16) (Fig. 2).

A rebound in IC Ab level was then observed in 6 out of 11 patients (Fig. 2). This rebound was greatly variable in amplitude and in delay. The top level occurred 7–24 days after the first PE (mean 14 days). IC Ab titers rose above their initial level in 1 patient, to their initial level in 2 patients, and remained below the initial level in 3 patients. There was no rebound at all in 5 patients. After the rebound (if any), and proceeding with the same PE regimen, the antibody level lowered again (Fig. 2). Two months after the first PE, IC Ab were no longer detectable in the serum of 7 patients (including the 5 without rebound). Table 1 shows IC Ab fluctuations for each patient during the PE course.

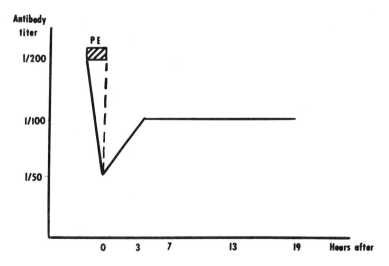

FIG. 1. Evolution of Ab titer after one PE.

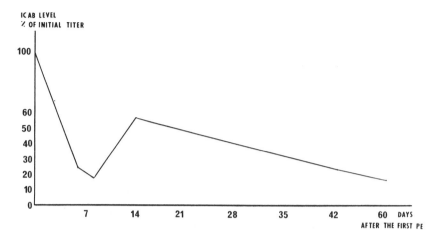

FIG. 2. Evolution of IC Ab levels (pre-PE titers) during PE course for 11 pemphigus patients.

TABLE 1. *Evolution of IC Ab titers for each patient*

		IC Antibody titers			
Case	Associated therapy[b]	Before PE	Minimal level (after 3 or 4 PE)	Rebound level	End of PE	2 Mos after first PE
1[a]	CY(2)	1/200	1/50	1/500[a]	1/50	1/50
2[a]	CY(2) P(0.1)	1/100	1/20	1/50[a]	1/20	1/20
3[a]	CY(2) P(0.1)	1/50	1/20	1/50[a]	1/20	1/20
4[a]	CY(3) P(0.15)	1/200	1/50	1/200[a]	1/200	1/200
5[a]	CY(2) P(2)	1/100	0	1/20[a]	1/20	0
6	AZA(2) P(2.5)	1/200	0	0	0	0
7	CHL(0.1) P(1)	1/500	1/100	1/100	1/10	0
8	CY(3) P(0.5)	1/50	1/10	1/10	1/10	0
9	CY(2) P(0.5)	1/200	1/50	1/50	1/50	0
10	P(0.5)	1/20	0	0	0	0
11[a]	P(1)	1/100	1/20	1/50[a]	1/10	0

[a]Cases who experienced a rebound.
[b]P, prednisone; CY, cyclophosphamide; AZA, azathioprine; CHL, chlorambucil. The numbers in parentheses indicate the daily dose in mg/kg.

Effects of Drugs on the Rebound Phenomenon

Table 2 shows the relationship between the various drug regimens given to our 11 patients during their PE and the magnitude of the serum IC Ab fluctuations. While the initial decrease was quite similar, the rebound was quite variable. It was high for the patient given only oral cyclophosphamide and for the 3 patients treated by oral cyclophosphamide and low doses of prednisolone. Conversely, the rebound was low among the 7 patients given more than 0.5 mg/kg/day of prednisolone; there was no difference between the 5 patients who received oral cytotoxic drugs in addition to prednisolone and the 2 patients who received only prednisolone.

TABLE 2. *Magnitude of the rebound in relation to the therapeutic regimen[a]*

Drug regimen	Minimal level (after 3 or 4 PE)	Rebound level
CY only (1 pt)	25	250
CY + low-dose prednisolone (3 pts)	27	83
CY + high-dose prednisolone (5 pts)	13	17
High-dose prednisolone (2 pts)	10	25

[a]Ab titers are expressed as mean percent of pretreatment level.

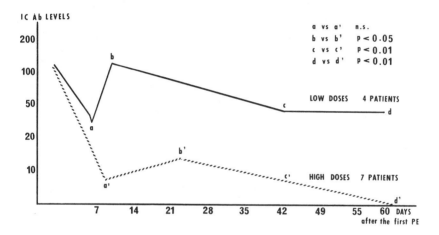

FIG. 3. IC Ab levels during PE with two steroid regimens.

To further specify the effect of adrenal steroids on the rebound, we compared the IC Ab kinetics of the 4 patients given very low doses of prednisolone (0, 0.1, 0.1, 0.15 mg/kg/day) with that of the 7 patients given 0.5–2 mg/kg/day of prednisolone (Fig. 3). The two groups of patients had a similar mean antibody titer before treatment (1/120 for the low-dose group vs 1/110 for the high-dose group), and a similar mean nadir level after three or four PE (1/32 for the low-dose group vs 1/7 for the high-dose group). However, the crest of the rebound occurred later (22 days, vs 9 days after the first PE) and was much weaker in the high-dose group (mean 1/13 vs 1/126, $p < 0.05$). In the high-dose group the IC Ab level dropped progressively and disappeared, while it remained at 1/45 in the low-dose group ($p < 0.01$).

DISCUSSION

The rise in serum antibody level observed during the hours following the first PE results from the redistribution of extravascular IgG autoantibodies (2), as IgG is distributed approximately equally in the intravascular and the extravascular compartments (15).

Following the first three PE, the observed stepwise decrease of serum IC Ab level was quite similar to the expected one, suggesting a very low rate of new antibody synthesis. However, 4–16 days after the first PE the IC Ab synthesis had increased enough to exceed removal by periodic PE and to cause increased serum level.

The maximum rebound occurred at a mean of 14 days after the first PE. This delay was shorter among the less immunosuppressed patients (with low doses or no adrenal steroids), with a mean of 9.5 days. This time course is close to the 8-day delay observed by Bystryn et al. (2) in rabbits for the maximum rebound in antibodies after their removal by a single exchange transfusion. These comparable delays suggest that the rebound in autoantibody synthesis in pemphigus results from the triggering of "educated" antibody forming cells immediately or soon after the first plasma exchange. Such an assumption may lead to clinical trials of pulse doses of immunosuppressive drugs during the few days following the first PE. With regard to the better immunosuppressive regimen, in our patients oral daily cyclophosphamide, alone or in association with low doses of adrenal steroids, provided insufficient suppression of the rebound. Conversely, high doses of adrenal steroids, with or without oral cyclosphosphamide, markedly or completely suppressed the rebound. The real usefulness of cyclophosphamide (in this dosage) is debatable, since adrenal steroids alone afforded the same efficiency as the combined regimen.

These results challenge the usual concepts about the effects of immunosuppressive drugs in man, cyclophosphamide being considered capable of impairing antibody synthesis, while adrenal steroids are not (16).

The effects of cytotoxic drugs may vary with species, drug doses, and timing of treatment in relation to immune stimulation (17). Immunosuppressive agents have a relatively small effect on established antibody response (18), and cyclophosphamide may even potentiate IgG production in secondary antibody response in rodents (19).

In experimental models of the rebound phenomenon cyclophosphamide was partially effective in mice (at 200 mg/kg, i.p.) (3), but only delayed the onset of rebound in dogs (at 5 mg/kg) (20) without reducing its amplitude. In the same experiments on dogs, combination chemotherapy was necessary to suppress the rebound. In man the suppressive effect of cyclophosphamide on antibody production had been demonstrated with intravenous daily doses of 3.5 and 7 mg/kg while oral daily doses of 1.7 mg/kg were ineffective (16). Our failure to reduce the rebound phenomenon in pemphigus with oral daily doses of 2–3 mg/kg does not preclude cyclophosphamide efficiency at higher doses, or in other situations.

The effectiveness of adrenal steroids on the rebound phenomenon is quite surprising inasmuch as the antibody response to many natural antigens is not impaired in man by steroids, even in high concentration (16,17,21,22). However, the same doses improve most autoimmune diseases, pemphigus among others, not only by an antiinflammatory effect but also by lowering the level of autoantibodies (16).

The triggering of antibody synthesis by lowering of the serum antibody level may be a more complex phenomenon than the stimulation by an antigenic challenge. Adrenal steroids may well interfere with the former phenomenon and not with the latter.

CONCLUSION

A rebound in autoantibody synthesis was observed in 6 of 11 patients undergoing plasma exchange for pemphigus, despite various immunosuppressive regimens. Oral daily cyclophosphamide at low doses (2–3 mg/kg) had no suppressive effect on the rebound, while adrenal steroids, at doses ≥0.5 mg/kg/day of prednisolone, had a far better immunosuppressive effect.

ACKNOWLEDGMENTS

The authors would like to give special thanks to Dr. J. C. Ansquer for statistical analysis. This work was supported by Grant 900 651 073 from Université Paris, Val de Marne.

REFERENCES

1. Wenz, B., and Barland, P. (1981): Therapeutic intensive plasmapheresis. *Semin. Hematol.*, 18:147.
2. Bystryn, J. C., Graf, M. W., and Uhr, J. W. (1970): Regulation of antibody formation by serum antibody. II. Removal of specific antibody by means of exchange transfusion. *J. Exp. Med.*, 132:1279.
3. Bystryn, J. C., Schenkein, I., and Uhr, J. W. (1971): A model for the regulation of antibody synthesis by serum antibody. In: *Progress in Immunology*, edited by B. Amos, p. 627. Academic Press, New York.
4. Barclay, G. R., Greiss, M. A., and Urbanlak, S. J. (1980): Adverse effect of plasma exchange on anti-D production in rhesus immunisation owing to removal of inhibitory factors. *Br. Med. J.*, 280:1569.
5. Schlansky, R., De Horatius, R. J., Pincus, T., and Tune, K. S. K. (1981): Plasmapheresis in systemic lupus erythematosus. A cautionary note. *Arthritis Rheum.*, 24:49.
6. Balow, J. E. (1981): Plasmapheresis therapy. Problems in the evaluation of clinical studies and in the definition of the role of immunosuppressive drug therapy. *Contemp. Dial.*, 3:9.
7. Jones, J. V., Robinson, M. F., Parciany, K., Layfer, L. F., and McLeod, B. (1981): Therapeutic plasmapheresis in systemic lupus erythematosus. Effect on immune complexes and antibodies to DNA. *Arthritis Rheum.*, 24:1113.
8. Carter, B., Harrison, R., Lunt, G. G., O'Behan, P. and Simpson, J. A. (1980): Anti-acetylcholine receptor antibody titers in the sera of myasthenia patients treated with plasma exchange combined with immunosuppressive therapy. *J. Neurol. Neurosurg. Psychiatr.*, 43:394.
9. Auerbach, R., and Bystryn, J. C. (1979): Plasmapheresis and immunosuppressive therapy. Effects on levels of intercellular antibodies in pemphigus vulgaris. *Arch. Dermatol.*, 115:728.
10. Roujeau, J. C., Revuz, J., Fabre, M., Andre, C., Akerman, C., Mannoni, P., and Touraine, R. (1980): Plasma exchanges in pemphigus vulgaris. In: *Plasma Exchange*, edited by H. G. Sieberth, p. 315. Schattauer Verlag, Stuttgart, New York.
11. Schiltz, J. R. (1980): Pemphigus acantholysis: A unique immunological injury. *J. Invest. Dermatol.*, 74:359.
12. Ahmed, R. A., Graham, J., Jordan, R. E., and Provost, T. T. (1980): Pemphigus: Current concepts. *Ann. Intern. Med.*, 92:396.
13. Roujeau, J. C., Kalis, B., Lauret, P., Flechet, M. L., Joneau-Fabre, M., Andre, C., Revuz, J., and Touraine, R. (1982): Plasma exchange in corticosteroid-resistant pemphigus. *Br. J. Dermatol.*, 106:103.

14. Roujeau, J. C., Andre, C., Joneau-Fabre, M., Lauret, P., Flechet, M. L., Kalis, B., Revuz, J., and Touraine, R. (1983): Plasma exchange in pemphigus. Uncontrolled study of 10 patients. *Arch. Dermatol.*, 119:215.
15. Waldmann, T. A., and Strober, W. (1969): Metabolism of immunoglobulins. *Progr. Allergy*, 13:1.
16. Berenbaum, M. C. (1975): The clinical pharmacology of immunosuppressive agent. In: *Clinical Aspects of Immunology*, edited by P. G. H. Gell, R. R. A. Loombs, and P. J. Lachmann, p. 689. Blackwell, Oxford.
17. Santos, G. W. (1967): Immunosuppressive drugs. *Fed. Proc.*, 26:907.
18. Gagnon, R. F., and MacLennan, I. C. M. (1979): Immunosuppression in established humoral responses. *J. Clin. Pathol.*, 13:126.
19. Gagnon, R. F., and MacLennan, I. C. M. (1979): Regulation of secondary antibody responses in rodents. I. Potentiation of IgG production by cyclophosphamide. *Clin. Exp. Immunol.*, 37:89.
20. Terman, D. S., Garcia-Rinaldi, R., Danneman, B., Moor, E. D., Crumb, C., Tavel, A., and Poser, R. (1978): Specific suppression of antibody rebound after extracorporeal immuno adsorption. I. Comparison of single versus combination chemotherapeutic agents. *Clin. Exp. Immunol.*, 34:32.
21. Parillo, J. E., and Fauci, A. S. (1979): Mechanisms of glucocorticoids action on immune processes. *Annu. Rev. Pharmacol. Toxicol.*, 19:179.
22. Tuchinda, M., Newcomb, R. W., and Devald, B. L. (1972): Effect of prednisone treatment on the immune response to keyhole limpet hemocyanin. *Int. Arch. Allergy Appl. Immunol.*, 42:533.

Plasmapheresis, edited by Y. Nosé, P. S.
Malchesky, J. W. Smith, and R. S. Krakauer.
Raven Press, New York © 1983.

Plasmapheresis in Active Systemic Lupus Erythematosus Resistant to Immunosuppressive Drugs

Conny Edenö, Mattias Aurell, Hans Herlitz, Henric Mulec, and
Gunnar Westberg

*University of Göteborg, Medical Department V, Sahlgren's Hospital,
S-413 45 Göteborg, Sweden*

We have used plasmapheresis (PP) as supplemental therapy in active cases of systemic lupus erythematosus (SLE) when conventional therapy with high dose prednisolone and immunosuppressive drugs has failed. The present chapter is a retrospective study of 9 patients with active SLE who were treated with PP. The study was performed to determine if PP is of any value as adjunctive therapy in patients with active SLE.

PATIENTS AND METHODS

Nine patients who met the ARA criteria (1) for SLE were studied. All had signs of active disease and predominant manifestations are shown in Table 1. All patients were treated with high dose prednisolone and immunosuppressive drugs (azathioprine in 8 cases, cyclophosphamide in 1 case) for at least 4 weeks prior to institution of PP.

PP was carried out manually in 1 case, with Haemonetics Model 30 blood-cell separator (Haemonetics Corp., Boston, MA) in 2 cases, and with a plasmafilter, Plasmaflo (Asahi Medical Co., Ltd., Tokyo, Japan), in 6 cases. With the former methods 1–2 liters of plasma was exchanged each time, with the latter method 4–

TABLE 1. *Predominant manifestation of disease*

Generalized disease symptoms and renal failure (RF)	2
Nephrotic syndrome and renal insufficiency	2
Rapidly progressive lupus nephritis	1
Fever and arthralgia/myalgia	2
Dermal symptoms	1
Perimyocarditis and left ventricular failure	1

5 liters was exchanged each time. PP was repeated 2–3 times per week for at least 3 weeks. A balanced salt solution with human albumin (40 g/liter) was used to substitute for the plasma removed. Vascular access was by A-V shunt in 7 cases and by femoral vein puncture in 2 cases.

CIC were analyzed by several methods: The Raji cell test (2), a Clq binding assay (3), and the platelet aggregating test (4). Antibodies to DNA were examined with a Farr assay (5).

RESULTS

The effect of PP was considered beneficial in 4 cases (Table 2), unevaluable in 4, and in 1 case there was no effect (Table 3). The course of 1 of the cases with fever and myalgia is illustrated in Fig. 1, and the patient with nephrotic syndrome and renal failure is shown in Fig. 2. The patient with dermal symptoms was relieved of his severe pruritus and the widespread erythema improved for 1 month following the last PP, but then deteriorated again.

The result of PP could not be properly evaluated in 4 cases. In 3, PP could not be performed as planned because the patients were terminally ill (2 cases), or there were problems with vascular access and bleeding tendency (1 case). In the fourth case, which was an adolescent with nephrotic syndrome and renal insufficiency, serological improvement occurred immediately before starting PP, followed by clinical improvement during PP and gradual normalization of renal function after PP. The course is illustrated in Fig. 3.

No Effect

In 1 patient with rapidly progressive lupus nephritis, therapy with PP had no discernible effect on the course, and the patient had to be started on hemodialysis. Renal biopsy showed endo- and extracapillary proliferation in all glomeruli, with

TABLE 2. *Beneficial effects of PP in 4 cases*

Fever and myalgia/arthralgia	2
Nephrotic syndrome and renal failure	1
Dermal symptoms	1

TABLE 3. *Immunological parameters*

Effect of PP *(N)*		Pts with positive tests for CIC	Pts with depressed serum levels of complement C3 and C4
Beneficial	4	2	2
Unevaluable	4	4	4
None	1	0	0

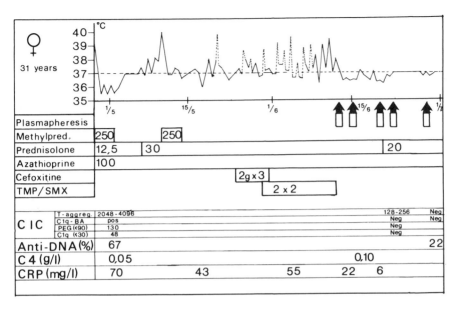

FIG. 1. Thirty-one-year-old woman who developed butterfly erythema, periarticular myalgia, oral ulcerations, proteinuria, and microscopic hematuria at the age of 30. Renal biopsy showed a diffuse proliferative lupus nephritis. In April 1980 the patient developed fever and myalgia. Azathioprine was added and she was treated with methylprednisolone pulses with only transient effect. After the first PP her fever and other symptoms vanished and she has since remained in excellent health for 1½ years without further exacerbations of SLE.

crescent formation in 80%. Among tests for CIC only the Raji cell test was positive, other methods were negative and serum levels of complement were normal.

DISCUSSION

In accordance with earlier studies (6,7) we have found PP to be of value in some patients with active SLE, when conventional therapy has failed. To make adequate evaluation of the effect of PP possible, the patients should be maintained on constant medication for a sufficiently long time and regularly assessed clinically and by immunological tests to detect changes in disease activity. This point is well illustrated in Fig. 3, where immunological tests showed signs of improvement on the very day that PP was started, making it unjustified to ascribe the ensuing clinical improvement to PP only. Another interesting point is that PP can produce rapid effects in certain cases of active SLE with symptoms of prolonged fever and aching joints and/or muscles (provided of course that an infectious etiology has been ruled out). Both cases who exhibited these symptoms had been treated for more than 1 month with high dose prednisolone and immunosuppressive drugs (azathioprine in 1 case, cyclophosphamide in the other) without effect, and responded rapidly to PP. It has been shown (8,9) that the Fc-receptor mediated clearance of CIC in the

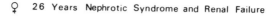

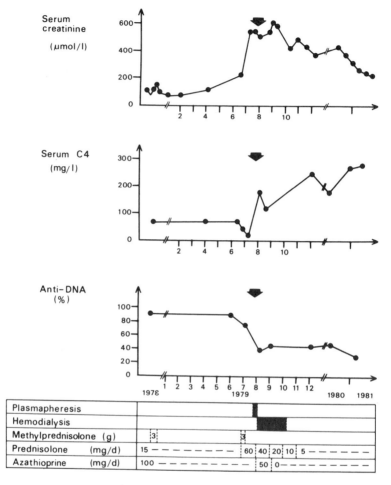

FIG. 2. Female patient born in 1953, developed migrating, nondestructive polyarthritis in 1971 and pericarditis and pleuritis in 1972. She was maintained on a low dose of prednisolone and had a rather quiescent course until nephrotic syndrome with ascites and pleural fluid developed in 1978. Azathioprine was added without effect, but after methylprednisolone pulse therapy, the nephrotic syndrome went into remission. In June 1979 the nephrotic syndrome relapsed. After PP her renal function improved gradually and she was taken off dialysis after 2 months. She has been maintained on a low dose of prednisolone every other day, and renal function has remained stable.

reticuloendothelial system is defective in active SLE, and it is suggested that PP works by "unloading" a saturated Fc-receptor function in the reticuloendothelial system (10). The rapid effects produced by PP in these two cases are in agreement with this concept.

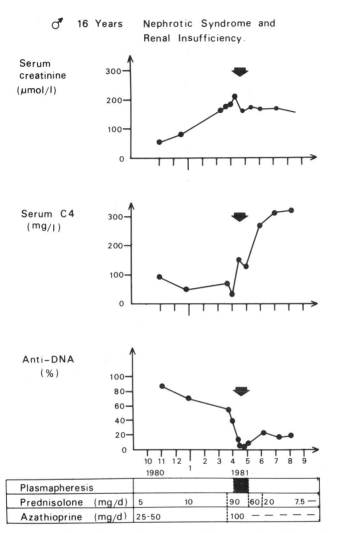

FIG. 3. Sixteen-year-old adolescent who developed fever, proteinuria, and microscopic hematuria at the age of 10. Renal biopsy showed a diffuse, proliferative lupus nephritis and the patient was treated with prednisolone and azathioprine. Severe nephrotic syndrome developed in 1975, with relapse in March 1981 that resisted treatment with high dose prednisolone p and azathioprine. After PP the proteinuria has persisted, but the renal function has gradually improved. The patient is now maintained on azathioprine + low dose prednisolone every other day. Because of severe hypertension that resisted treatment with furosemide + prazosin + metoprolol, the patient was treated with Captopril, which normalized the blood pressure.

CONCLUSIONS

Adjunctive PP therapy in cases of active SLE who have failed to respond to conventional therapy may be of definite value in some patients. It is not yet possible to predict which patient will respond to PP. To facilitate evaluation, PP should not be started in patients with active SLE unless they have been maintained on constant medication for sufficient time and can be closely monitored clinically and immunologically to allow criteria for optimal use of PP therapy to be defined.

REFERENCES

1. Cohen, A. S., Reynolds, W. E., Franklin, E. C., Kulka, J. P., Ropes, M. W., Schulman, L. E., and Wallace, S. L. (1971): Preliminary criteria for the classification of systemic lupus erythematosus. *Bull. Rheum. Dis.*, 21:643.
2. Theofilopoulos, A. N., Wilson, C. B., and Dixon, F. J. (1976): The Raji cell radioimmune assay for detection of immune complexes in human sera. *J. Clin. Invest.*, 57:169.
3. Nydegger, U. E., Lambert, P. H., Gerber, H., and Miescher, P. A. (1974): Circulating immune complexes in the serum in systemic lupus erythematosus and in carriers of hapatitis β antigen. *J. Clin. Invest.*, 54:297.
4. Penttinen, K. (1976): The platelet aggregation test. *Ann. Rheum. Dis.*, 36(Suppl.):55.
5. Pincus, T., Schur, P. H., Rose, J. A., Decker, J. L., and Talae, L. (1969): Measurement of serum DNA-binding activity in systemic lupus erythematosus. *N. Engl. J. Med.*, 281:701.
6. Abdou, N. I., Lindsley, H. B., Pollack, A., Stechschultze, D. J., and Wood, G. (1981): Plasmapheresis in systemic lupus erythematosus: Effects on clinical, serum, and cellular abnormalities. Case report. *Clin. Immunol. Immunopathol.*, 19:44.
7. Jones, J. V., Robinson, M. F., Parciany, R. K., Layfer, L. F., and McLeod, B. (1981): Therapeutic plasmapheresis in systemic lupus erythematosus. Effect on immune complexes and antibodies to DNA. *Arthritis Rheum.*, 24(9):1113.
8. Frank, M. M., Hamburger, M. I., Lawley, T. J., Kimberley, R. P., and Plotz, P. H. (1979): Defective reticuloendothelial system Fc-receptor function in systemic lupus erythematosus. *N. Engl. J. Med.*, 300:518.
9. Hamburger, M. I., Lawley, T. J., Kimberley, R. P., Plotz, P. H., and Frank, M. M. (1982): A serial study of splenic reticuloendothelial system Fc-receptor functional activity in systemic lupus erythematosus. *Arthritis Rheum.*, 25(1):48.
10. Lookwood, C. M., Worlledge, S., Path, F. R. C., Nicholas, A., Cotton, C., and Peters, D. K. (1979): Reversal of impaired splenic function in patients with nephritis or vasculitis (or both) by plasma exchange. *N. Engl. J. Med.*, 300(10):524.

Plasmapheresis, edited by Y. Nosé, P. S. Malchesky, J. W. Smith, and R. S. Krakauer. Raven Press, New York © 1983.

Effect of Plasma Exchange on the Course of Cryoglobulinemias

*E. Cassuto-Viguier, §**J. F. Quaranta, †J. P. Ortonne, §J. P. Cassuto, *H. Duplay, and §P. Dujardin

*Clinique Néphrologique et †Service de Dermatologie, Hôpital Pasteur, 06031 Nice; §Service de Médecine Interne A, Département d'Hématologie, Hôpital de Cimiez, 06031 Nice; **Laboratoire d'Immunologie, Hémobiologie, Faculté de Médecine, 06034 Nice, France*

According to Brouet and co-workers (1), cryoglobulins (CG) can be classified into three groups: type I, isolated monoclonal immunoglobulin (Ig); type II, a monoclonal component possessing antibody activity towards polyclonal Ig; and type III, one or more classes of polyclonal Ig, sometimes with non-Ig molecules. This classification allows correlations between biological findings, clinical features, and the underlying diseases.

Clinically, diseases associated with cryoglobulinemias (CGm) may vary widely and include infections, autoimmune phenomena, and lymphoproliferative, renal, or liver diseases, as well as a familial or essential form of CGm (2). There is a sharp contrast in prognosis between asymptomatic CGm and life-threatening forms.

Therapeutically, clinical improvement appears to be related to the antiinflammatory effects of immunosuppressive therapy and to the reduction in the concentration of CG, but such reductions do not occur quickly. Moreover, cytotoxic drugs may modify the antigen–antibody ratio and result in the precipitation of immune complexes (1). Thus, the time between institution of therapy and effective lowering of immune complexes may be sufficiently long as to lead to irreversible tissue damage. In contrast, plasma exchange (PE) with immunosuppressive therapy reduces both immune complex and CG levels and may prevent deposition (3,4).

Many investigations have proposed various combinations of PE and immunosuppressive therapy in the managment of CGm (5–16). The following report details the results of our studies of 6 cases treated with PE associated with immunosuppressive therapy.

CASE REPORTS

Case 1

C. R. is a 52-year-old Caucasian woman with a 25-year history of arthritis associated with cutaneous and renal vasculitis. Previous treatment included nonsteroidal antiinflammatory drugs as well as steroids.

In 1976, the occurrence of edema and ascites led to the diagnosis of cirrhosis, confirmed by biopsy. Immunochemical analysis of her plasma showed a kappa-type IgM monoclonal gammopathy. Proteinuria and hematuria were also present, without renal failure. In 1981, a mixed kappa-type IgM–IgG CG type II was discovered. Skeleton X-ray examinations and bone marrow biopsy were normal. Persisting hematuria and proteinuria led to a diagnosis of membranoproliferative glomerulonephritis (MPGN) confirmed by biopsy. Six PE within 2 weeks were then combined with cyclophosphamide (100 mg/day). Pancytopenia required stoppage of immunosuppressive therapy. Improvement of arthralgias and cutaneous vasculitis paralleled the disappearance of CG. However, hematuria and proteinuria persisted. The patient was discharged from hospital on betamethasone (1.5 mg/day). Three months later, arthralgias and cutaneous vasculitis recurred (Fig. 1), associated with congestive heart failure and pericarditis. At this time, however, CG could not be detected. Because of persistent clinical symptoms, the patient was rehospitalized and CG was found. Six PE were performed within 2 weeks associated with immunosuppressive therapy (chlorambucil, 4 mg/day and betamethasone, 1.5 mg/day). Clinical and biochemical improvements were observed. The patient was then discharged from hospital and maintained on immunosuppressive therapy. Her clinical status is satisfactory following 3 months of follow-up, but the hematuria remains unchanged.

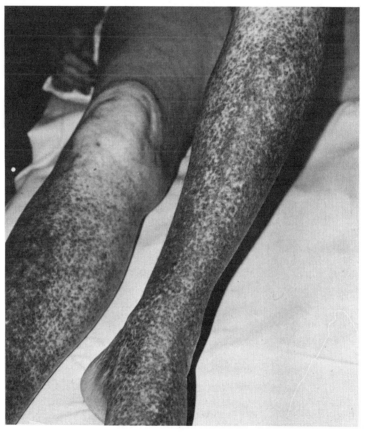

FIG. 1. Cutaneous vasculitis.

Case 2

R. D., a 66-year-old Caucasian man, was hospitalized for the treatment of a cutaneous ulcer of the left leg associated with purpura. Hematuria of recent onset was also present with azotemia, proteinuria, and creatininemia (200 mM/liter). Focal membranoproliferative changes were discovered by biopsy. Disturbances in atrioventricular conduction with congestive heart failure occurred during hospitalization, and a pacemaker was placed. Six PE were performed at a frequency of three times per week. Treatment with cyclophosphamide (125 mg/day) was started after the third exchange and was continued for 6 weeks (Fig. 2). Following PE, CG were no longer detectable, and this was paralleled by a marked clinical improvement, and disappearance of cutaneous vasculitis and hematuria. Following a 12-month follow-up, no clinical or biochemical evidence of worsening patient status was observed.

Case 3

A. M., a 39-year-old Tunisian woman, presented in October 1979 with cardiac insufficiency, cutaneous vasculitis, arthritis, and nephritic–nephrotic syndrome. Cutaneous and pericardial biopsies showed typical leukocytoclastic vasculitis. Type I membranoproliferative glomerulonephritis was diagnosed on renal biopsy (Fig. 3). Type II CG (IgG–IgM, kappa) was present. The monoclonal IgM kappa component was also observed by immunoelectrophoresis. Skeleton X-ray examinations, bone marrow biopsies, and liver biopsy were normal. PE with corticosteroid (0.25 mg/kg/day) and cyclophosphamide (50 mg/day) were then started. Clinical improvement was apparent 1 month later, but the rapid reappearance of CG after each exchange necessitated an increase of corticosteriod (0.5 mg/kg/day) and cyclophosphamide (100 mg/day) accompanied by maintenance PE (15 PE/26 weeks). This long-term PE therapy has been of no measurable effect.

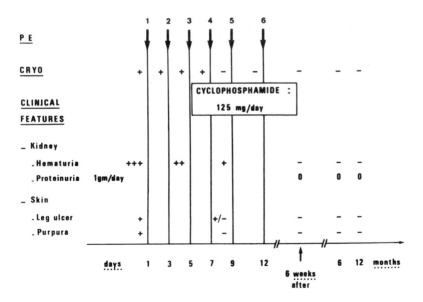

FIG. 2. Clinical and biological course with treatment including PE for a representative patient.

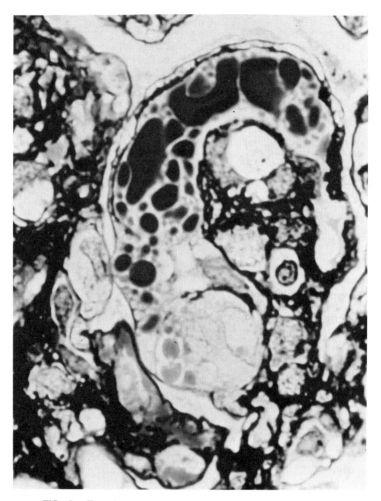

FIG. 3. Type I membranoproliferative changes in type II CGm.

Case 4

M. G., a 17-year-old Portuguese girl, was first hospitalized in July 1979 with arthritis and nephritic–nephrotic syndrome. Renal biopsy showed type I membranoproliferative glomerulonephritis without crescent formation. Type II CG (IgG–IgM, kappa) was also present. PE was started (six exchanges within 2 weeks) in combination with corticosteroid (0.6 mg/kg/day) and cyclophosphamide (100 mg/day). One month later, clinical improvement was evident and CG were not detectable, but an asymptomatic proteinuria persisted (1–2 g/day). M. G. was then discharged and was lost from follow-up for 10 months. She was admitted again in May 1981 for acute renal failure. Kidney biopsy showed membranoproliferative glomerulonephritis and many crescents, and CG were detected. Twelve PE with dialysis were performed within 2 weeks associated with corticosteroid (1 mg/kg/day), cyclophosphamide (100 mg/day), and heparin, resulting in a disappearance of CG and improvement of renal function. Tapering of corticosteroid and cyclophosphamide began 2 months later.

One year after this second episode, the patient still manifested renal insufficiency (creatininemia $\simeq$ 400 mm/liter) with a proteinuria of 1–2 g/day.

Case 5

F. V. was a 58-year-old Caucasian man with a 2-year history of chronic lymphoid leukemia treated by chlorambucil who presented with a sudden onset of polyneuropathy associated with arthritis. Type I CG was present with a lambda-type monoclonal IgG. PE was begun with a frequency of one treatment per week for 3 months. This therapy was combined with corticosteroid (1 mg/kg/day). An immediate disappearance of arthritis was noted. The CG was present until the tenth PE, but improvement of polyneuritis did not begin until the end of the PE series. Polyneuritis reappeared 6 months later, but was not accompanied by CG. The neuropathy disappeared again after five PE performed within 2 weeks. The patient died 3 weeks later due to fungal septicemia.

Case 6

S. V., a 58-year-old Spanish man, was hospitalized in October 1980 with polyneuritis. The immunoelectrophoresis of his plasma revealed a kappa-type IgM monoclonal component, and bone marrow biopsy revealed a massive infiltration of lymphoplasmacytoid cells, supporting a diagnosis of Waldenström's macroglobulinemia. This was accompanied by a type II CG (IgG–IgM, kappa). His renal function was normal but there was an asymptomatic proteinuria (0.25 g/liter), and Bence–Jones proteins were identified. A series of nine PE in 9 weeks was performed, combined with corticosteroid (0.75 mg/kg/day) and chlorambucil (4 mg/day). An improvement of neuropathy was observed in 2 months. The CG disappeared after the third PE and was no longer detectable after 2 months of follow-up. The patient has now returned to Spain and is lost from follow-up.

PATIENTS AND METHODS

Six patients (3 males and 3 females), ages 17–66 years, were studied. Their CG were classified as 5 type II and 1 type I. Clinical and biochemical features are summarized in Table 1.

PE consisted of continuous-flow centrifugation (IBM 2997), discontinuous-flow centrifugation (Haemonetics Pex 60), or plasma filtration (Asahi Plasmaflo) occasionally performed with dialysis. Blood access, exchanged volumes, substitution products, and the number and frequency of PE are shown in Table 2. All procedures were explained to each patient before therapy was begun.

RESULTS

PE resulted in the disappearance of CG in 5 out of 6 cases. A complete resolution of symptoms was noted in 2 of the 5 cases, and a partial resolution was obtained in 3 of the 5. In the sixth case, CG persisted but clinical improvement was obtained. These results are detailed in Tables 2 and 3. In our experience, clinical improvement and/or resolution of symptoms seem to be related to the disappearance of CG, and clinical relapses also seem to parallel the return of CG (Table 3).

TABLE 1. *Clinical and biochemical features of patients*

Case	Sex/age (yrs)	Type of cryoglobulin	Associated disease	Predominant organ involvement
1	F/52	II (IgM kappa–IgG)	Cirrhosis	Kidney, myocardium, skin, joints
2	M/66	II (IgG lambda–IgA)	Essential	Myocardium, kidney, skin
3	F/39	II (IgM kappa–IgG)	Essential	Kidney, myocardium, pericardium, skin, joints
4	F/17	II (IgM kappa–IgG)	Essential	Kidney, joints
5	M/58	I (IgG lambda)	Chronic lymphoid leukemia	Peripheral nervous system, joints
6	M/58	II (IgM kappa–IgG)	Waldenström's macroglobulinemia	Peripheral nervous system

DISCUSSION

A pathologic role of CG, which are in fact immune complexes, is their deposition in tissues which results in immunopathology, suggesting that their removal may be beneficial (4). In practice, removal can be accomplished in three ways: (a) by eliminating antibodies or inhibiting their synthesis (9); (b) by dissolving immune complexes after modifying the antigen–antibody ratio; or (c) by a combination of (a) and (b) (3). PE can also accomplish these objectives and in addition is thought to lead to an inhibition of the underlying inflammatory process (9).

While removal of immune complexes increases the functional effectiveness of the reticuloendothelial system (7), suppression of CG synthesis requires cytotoxic drugs. The onset of life-threatening complications directly related to CG is generally unexpected (6). High levels of CG seem to be mainly responsible for cutaneous vasculitis (6). More frequently, mixed CG are associated with glomerular lesions (1,2,17). The severity and prognosis of such glomerulopathies are unpredictable (17). In emergency conditions, PE might be used when high levels of monoclonal CG are identified, because these seem to be most often associated with acute accidents (1,6,8). It is difficult to predict the appropriate number and frequency of PE, and different reports have not yet resolved this problem (2,5,9–13,15,16,18,19). The results presented here do not resolve the problem either. Yet, our results and those of some authors do seem to suggest an induction treatment of six PE in 2 weeks followed by PE maintenance determined by the patient's clinical course and biochemical measurements. In addition to PE, the use of antiinflammatory and/or immunosuppressive drugs such as cyclophosphamide and chlorambucil seems to be reasonable therapy in type II symptomatic CGm. Immunosuppressive therapy alone does not seem to be adequate treatment, particularly for CGm with nephropathies, according to recent observations [Brouet et al. (1), Gorevic et al. (2,6), Grey et al. (8)].

TABLE 2. *Methodology of PE*

Case	Blood access	Technique	No. of PE/week	Volume	Temp. of procedure	Substitution products	Accidents-incidents	Immunosuppressive therapy
1	1 Femoral vein	12 Plasma filtration	1st: 6/2 2nd: 6/2	≥1.5 Plasma mass	37°C	1st: Cryoprecipitate supernatant, albumin 2nd: Albumin	1st: Femoro-femorous fistula, thrillings, pruritus, paresthesiae 2nd: Supraventricular tachycardia	1st: CS + CPM 2nd: CS + CLB
2	2 Forearm AV fistula	6 Plasma filtration	6/2	≥1.5 Plasma mass	37°C	Cryoprecipitate supernatant, albumin	Thrillings, papular erythema, fever	CPM
3	15 Forearm AV fistula	8 Continuous-flow centrifugation 7 Plasma filtration	1st: 6/2 2nd: 9/24	≥1.5 Plasma mass	37°C	1st: Cryoprecipitate supernatant 2nd: Cryoprecipitate supernatant	1st and 2nd: Pruritus, fever, thrillings, hypertension	1st: CS + CPM 2nd: CS + CPM
4	18 Forearm AV fistula	6 Continuous-flow centrifugation 12 Plasma filtration	1st: 6/2 2nd: 12/2	≥1.5 Plasma mass	37°C	1st: Fresh frozen plasma 2nd: Fresh frozen plasma, cryoprecipitate supernatant	1st and 2nd: Paresthesiae, hepatitis (HBs−)	1st: CS + CPM 2nd: CS + CPM
5	19 Superficial vein	19 Discontinuous-flow centrifugation	1st: 14/14 2nd: 5/2	≥1.5 Plasma mass	22–25°C	1st: Dessicated plasma, plasmion; cryoprecipitate supernatant, albumin 2nd: Albumin, dessicated plasma	1st: Paresthesiae, urticaria, hepatitis (HBs+) 2nd: Thrillings, shock	1st: CS 2nd: CS + CLB
6	9 Superficial vein	9 Discontinuous-flow centrifugation	9/9	≥1.5 Plasma mass	22–25°C	Dessicated plasma, plasmion; cryoprecipitate supernatant, albumin	Thrillings, paresthesiae, headaches, erythrodermia	CS + CLB

1st and 2nd: first and second treatment by PE. CS; corticosteroid; CPM, cyclophosphamide; CLB, chlorambucil.

TABLE 3. Results of PE

| Cases[a] | Clinical course: Symptoms[b] | | | | | Cryoglobulin | |
	Kidney	Myo- and pericardium	Skin	Joints	PNS	Disappearance	Recurrence and follow-up
1							
1st T	+ → +	+ → + +	+ → −	+ → −		Yes	Yes[1]
2nd T	+ → +	+ → + +	+ ↑[1]↓ −	+ ↓[1]↑ −		Yes	No (3 mos)
2	+ → −	+ → → −	+ ↑ −	+ → −		Yes	No (12 mos)
3	+ → + −	+ → + −	+ → + + −			No (18 mos)	No (12 mos)
4	+ → + −	+ → + −				Yes	
5							
1st T	+ → + −			+ → −	+ → −	Yes	Yes[2]
2nd T	+ + + →[2] + +			+ ↑[2]↓ −	+ →[3] −	Yes	No (10 mos)
6				+ → −	+ + → + −	Yes	No (2 mos)

[a]1st T and 2nd T: First and second treatment.
[b]+ → −: Overall view of the patient status including organ specific clinical, biological, and histological parameters. 1, 2, 3: 2, 10, and 6 months later.

There are several disadvantages to PE, including the risk of infections such as hepatitis and the cost of substitution products. [Cryoglobulinpheresis recently described by McLeod et al. (20) may be a more specific approach to this problem.] PE in patients with CGm is frequently a more complicated procedure (Table 2).

Finally, the associated diseases are heterogeneous, and this heterogeneity undoubtedly plays a role in response to treatment. Clearly, controlled, prospective, therapeutic trials are certainly needed in order to evaluate the effectiveness of PE in life-threatening CGm.

ACKNOWLEDGMENTS

We wish to thank Dr. J. C. Roujeau (C.H.U. Créteil, France) for his interest in this research and Pr. W. P. Faulk for the critique of this manuscript.

REFERENCES

1. Brouet, J. C., Clauvel, J. P., Danon, F., Klein, M., and Seligmann, M. (1974): Biological and clinical significance of cryoglobulins. A report of 86 cases. *Am. J. Med.*, 57:775.
2. Gorevic, P. D., Kassab, H. J., Levo, Y., Kohn, R., Meltzer, M., Prose, P., and Franklin, E. C. (1980): Mixed cryoglobulinemia: Clinical aspects and long-term follow-up of 40 patients. *Am. J. Med.*, 69:287.
3. Glassman, A. B. (1979): Immune responses—The rationale for plasmapheresis. *Plasmatherapy*, 1:13.
4. Nydegger, U. E., Kazatchkine, M. D., and Lambert, P. H. (1980): Involvement of immune complexes in disease. In: *Immunology 80: Progress in Immunology IV*, edited by M. Fougereau and J. Dausset, p. 1025. Academic Press, London.
5. Betourne, C., Buge, A., Dechy, H., Dorra, M., Dournon, E., and Rancurel, G. (1980): Neuropathies périphériques au cours d'un myélome à IgA et d'une cryoglobulinémie mixte. Traitement par plasmaphérèses itératives. *Nouv. Presse Med.*, 9:1369.
6. Brouet, J. C., Clauvel, J. P., and Seligmann, M. (1973): Cryoglobulinémie mixte et purpura hyperimmunoglobulinémique: Maladie avec complexes immuns circulants. In: *Problèmes Immunologiques en Médecine Interne. Les Maladies auto-immunes. Les transplantations d'organes*. Masson, Paris, p. 17.
7. Cordonnier, D., Vialtel, P., Jeannoel, P., Renversez, J. C., Chenais, F., Arvieux, J., and Denis, M. C. (1980): Plasma exchange (PE) in 3 cases of type II mixed IgM–IgG cryoglobulinaemia with severe membranoproliferative glomerulonephritis (MPGN). *International Symposium on Plasma Exchange*, Cologne, June 6–7, Abstr. 16.
8. Grey, H. M., and Kohler, P. E. (1973): Cryoimmunoglobulins. *Semin. Hematol.*, 10:87.
9. Houwert, D. A., Hene, R. J., Kater, L., and Struyvenberg, A. (1980): Study of the effects of plasma exchange (PE), corticosteroids and cyclophosphamide in essential mixed cryoglobulinaemia. *International Symposium of Plasma Exchange*, Cologne, June 6–7, Abstr. 38.
10. James, M. P., and Kingston, P. J. (1979): Essential monoclonal cryoglobulinaemia, the use of intermittent plasmapheresis to control cold-induced symptoms. *Clin. Exp. Dermatol.*, 4:209.
11. Lockwood, C. M., Worlledge, S., Micholas, A., Cotton, C., and Peters, D. K. (1979): Reversal of impaired splenic function of plasma exchange. *N. Engl. J. Med.*, 300:524.
12. Maggiore, Q., L'Abbate, A., Caccamo, A., Misefari, V., and Bartolomeo, F. (1980): Effects of cryoglobulin removal on the course of glomerulonephritis associated with essential mixed cryoglobulinemia (EMC). *International Symposium on Plasma Exchange*, Cologne, June 6–7, Abstr. 50.
13. Reumont, G., Hillemand, B., Godin, M., and Dero, M. (1980): Cryoglobulinémie mixte essentielle et néphropathie glomérulaire. *Semin. Hop. Paris*, 56:1531.
14. Rosenblatt, S. G., Knight, W., Bannayan, G. A., Wilson, C. B., and Stein, J. H. (1979): Treatment of Goodpasture's syndrome with plasmapheresis. A case report and review of the literature. *Am. J. Med.*, 66:689.
15. Vandelli, L., Gaiani, G., Furci, L., Baldini, E., and Lusvarghi, E. (1980): Control of clinical

symptoms in mixed essential cryoglobulinemia with plasma exchange alone. *International Symposium on Plasma Exchange*, Cologne, June 6–7, Abstr. 74.

16. Vialtel, P., Colomb, H., Arvieux, J., Chenais, F., Cordonnier, D., Dubos, G., Renversez, J. C., and Vila, A. (1981): Neuropathie périphérique et cryoglobulinémie. Efficacité des échanges plasmatiques. *Nouv. Presse Méd.*, 10:427.

17. Habib, R., and Levy, M. (1979): Contribution of immunofluorescent microscopy to classification of glomerular diseases. In: *Progress in Glomerulonephritis*, edited by P. Kincaid-Smith, A. J. F. D'Apice, and R. C. Atkins, p. 119. Wiley, New York.

18. Cordonnier, D., Vialtel, P., Chenais, F., and Bayle, F. (1981): Plasmapheresis in 8 severe membranoproliferative GN with type II IgM–IgG cryoglobulinaemia. *8th International Congress of Nephrology*, Athens, June 7–12, Abstr. CN-153.

19. Maggiore, Q., L'Abbate, A., Caccamo, A., Misefari, V., and Bartolomeo, F. (1981): Cryopheresis in the treatment of essential mixed cryoglobulinemia (EMC) with glomerulonephritis (GN). Proc. Third Annu. Meet. Int. Soc. Artif. Organs, *Artif. Organs, (Suppl.)*, 5:47.

20. McLeod, B. C., and Sassetti, R. (1980): Plasmapheresis with return of cryoglobulin-depleted autologous plasma (cryoglobulinpheresis) in cryoglobulinemia. *Blood*, 55:866.

Plasmapheresis, edited by Y. Nosé, P.S.
Malchesky, J.W. Smith, and R.S. Krakauer.
Raven Press, New York © 1983.

Plasma Exchange in Idiopathic Inflammatory Myopathy

Paul A. Reuther, Reinhard Rohkamm, *Dieter Wiebecke, and Hans Georg Mertens

*Department of Neurology and *Transfusion Center, University of Würzburg, D-8700 Würzburg, Federal Republic of Germany*

Idiopathic inflammatory myopathy is a nonhereditary disease of voluntary muscle. Histologically, degenerative, regenerative, and often inflammatory changes are present together with vascular endothelial changes. The myositis may involve the striated muscle without any accompanying illness (polymyositis or dermatomyositis). In a minority of patients the myositis may be precipitated by external factors (malignancies, drugs, viral infections) or may be associated with other disorders such as connective tissue diseases and agammaglobulinemia (1–3).

The etiology of idiopathic inflammatory myopathy is still uncertain, but there is evidence for alterations of the immune system. Based on morphological (2,3) and immunocytological (4–6) observations, cellular immune processes seem to be the major event in causing myositis. However, there are some reports of alterations in humoral immune responses (7–12). For the treatment of idiopathic inflammatory myopathy, prednisone (13–16) and often immunosuppressive or cytotoxic drugs (17–21) are recommended. Plasma exchange therapy for long intervals has recently been reported as an additional measure in the management of idiopathic inflammatory myopathy (22–24).

We report our experience with the treatment of 12 patients with myositis by plasma exchange for brief intervals combined with immunosuppression for a long period.

PATIENTS AND METHODS

Our therapeutic trial with plasma exchange in patients with myositis began in 1979. The clinical data of the 12 patients, their treatment before plasma exchange therapy, and the criteria for initiating plasma exchange are listed in Table 1. All patients had severe, mainly proximally located muscular weakness. In 8 patients the weakness developed acutely or subacutely, and in 4 patients a chronic course of disease occurred. The diagnosis was established by typical clinical and laboratory findings (elevated creatine kinase, myopathic EMG findings, and histological features conclusive for myositis).

TABLE 1. *Clinical data on 12 myositis patients treated with plasma exchange and immunosuppressives*

Pt no./sex/age at onset	Type of myositis[a]	Duration of myositis	Drug treatment before plasma exchange[b]	Duration of pretreatment	Criteria for plasma exchange[c]
1/M/35	PM	9 yrs	P–A–M	3 yrs	A–B
2/F/16	PM	3 yrs	P–A	1 yr	A–B–D
3/M/54	PM	3 yrs	—	—	A–C
4/M/39	DM	1 yr	—	—	A–C
5/M/13	DM	11 mos	P	8 mos	A–B–C–D
6/F/24	DM	11 mos	P–A	4 mos	A–B–C
7/F/34	DM	1 yr	P–A	6 mos	A–B–C–D
8/M/51	DM	3 mos	P–A	3 mos	A–B–C
9/F/44	DM	6 mos	P–A	2 mos	A–B–C
10/F/54	DM + RA	16 yrs	P–A	2 yrs	A–B
11/F/20	DM + SLE	6 yrs	P–A	2 yrs	A–B–C
12/F/21	DM + Sarc	1 yr	—	—	A–C

[a]Type of myositis: PM, polymyositis; DM, dermatomyositis; RA, rheumatoid arthritis; SLE, systemic lupus erythematosus; Sarc, sarcoidosis.
[b]Immunosuppression: P, prednisone; A, azathioprine; M, methotrexate.
[c]Criteria for plasma exchange therapy: A, severity of myositis; B, resistance to drug therapy; C, progression of disease; D, side effects of immunosuppressives.

Of the 12 patients, 9 received prednisone (initially 100–150 mg daily with dosage reduced thereafter according to the clinical course) and azathioprine (2–3 mg/kg body weight daily) for at least several months before plasma exchange was performed. In only 1 of the pretreated cases was this regimen changed directly prior to plasma exchange. In all other cases the immunosuppressive therapy was unaltered before, during, and 4 weeks after plasma exchange. In 3 cases without any therapy prior to plasma exchange, immunosuppressive drug therapy was initiated with the beginning of exchange procedure.

Plasma exchange was performed by means of an IBM Bloodprocessor 2997. Each patient had one course of three to eight consecutive exchanges every other day, except 1 patient had two courses 4 weeks apart. Exchange volumes amounted to 5% of body weight per session. Isooncotic and isovolumetric plasma substitution was performed using human albumin (Behring, Marburg, FRG).

Before, during, and after plasma exchange the clinical status of each patient was evaluated according to the disability scale of Rose and Walton (13), by measuring quantitative muscular strength in certain muscle groups and by recording changes in other clinical signs such as skin rash or renal symptoms. The activity of serum creatine kinase (normal range up to 60 U/liter) and serum aldolase (normal range up to 3.0 U/liter) was monitored.

Follow-up after termination of plasma exchange extended from 8 to 32 months. During the whole period of time the patients were maintained on immunosuppressive therapy and regularly examined with respect to clinical state and activity of serum enzymes.

RESULTS

The effects of the combined therapeutic approach are summarized in Table 2. Of the 12 patients, 8 had a marked increase in muscular strength and a corresponding decline in serum activity of enzymes together with an improvement in accompanying diseases (proteinuria, oliguria, arthralgia) in relation to plasma exchange therapy. Definite improvement of clinical and laboratory parameters occurred only in patients with active disease manifested by rapid development of muscular weakness and manyfold increases in serum levels of creatine kinase and aldolase at time of plasma exchange. The clinical signs of acute inflammation, especially erythematous rash, edema, and myalgia, disappeared regularly within a few hours after the first or second plasma exchange. An increase in muscle strength was observed in most cases within several days after the onset of plasma exchange, reaching a maximum after the fourth or fifth exchange. The patients suffered no relapses during the period of time we were involved in their care. However, in 4 cases a transient increase in serum creatine kinase activity was noted during the tapering of prednisone. By increasing prednisone for a short period, the serum activity returned to normal values.

In 6 of these 8 responders the improvement could be attributed only to plasma exchange, since they had been refractory to immunosuppressive treatment prior to exchange procedures, and improved only after plasma exchange had been initiated while drug treatment remained unchanged. In the 2 other cases the clinical improvement could not be assigned to plasma exchange alone, since drug therapy had been started or altered with the initiation of plasma exchange.

TABLE 2. *Response to treatment: Short-term and long-term*

Pt. no.	Plasma exchange (no./days)	Follow-up (mos)	IS modification[a]	Clinical effects	Disability grade[b] Before	After	Last	Creatine kinase (U/liter) Before	After	Last
1	4/12	6	o	−	4	4	4	275	134	250
2	3/5	8	o	−	5	5	5	396	281	534
3	4/12	7	+	−	5	5	5	630	13	320
4	4/6	22	+	+ +	5	4	2	1,390	390	42
5	a) 7/14		+	+ +	6	5		246	114	
	b) 3/7	19	o	+	5	4	2	23	20	21
6	6/14	16	o	+	4	3	2	508	25	48
7	5/10	19	o	+ +	4	3	2	72	60	35
8	8/14	24	o	+ +	5	4	2	2,370	184	74
9	6/14	24	o	+ +	5	4	2	254	224	100
10	6/14	8	+	−	4	4	4	100	82	96
11	5/21	32	o	+ +	5	3	1	3,290	75	43
12	5/20	16	+	+ +	5	3	2	1,668	981	49

[a]Modification of immunosuppression during plasma exchange. o, drug doses unchanged; +, drug therapy intensified or initiated with onset of plasma exchange.
[b]Rose and Walton, 1966 (ref. 13).

In the remaining 4 patients plasma exchange together with long-lasting immunosuppressive therapy did not alter the course of the disease. These patients had a chronic and/or inactive myositis manifested by long-standing weakness, proximal muscular atrophy, only slightly elevated serum enzyme activity, and no signs of acute inflammatory myopathy in EMG.

Plasma exchange was uncomplicated except for two mild anaphylactoid episodes. Two patients had minor side effects of long-standing steroid application.

Case Reports

The following two cases are reported in detail to illustrate our observations.

Beneficial Effect of Plasma Exchange

This 44-year-old woman complained of facial and acral rash in October 1978 together with aching and progressive weakness of proximal upper and lower extremities. A diagnosis of dermatomyositis was made in January 1979 on grounds of the clinical signs and the biochemical, neurophysiological, and histological changes (Fig. 1). At that time the patient was severely disabled, being unable to walk without assistance (Grade 5 according to Rose and Walton, ref. 13). A course of prednisone (100 mg/day) and azathioprine (150 mg/day) for 8 weeks did not affect the disease activity, and muscle weakness increased despite a slight fall in serum enzyme activity of creatine kinase.

Plasma exchange was performed without changing immunosuppressive therapy (six exchanges within 14 days equal to 17 liters of total volume). After the first exchange the skin rash, muscle tenderness, and myalgia improved significantly. After the second exchange an increase in muscle strength was noted, and this continued to improve during the following exchanges (Fig. 2). Ten days after termination of plasma exchange the patient was discharged showing only mild residual signs of disease activity. She was able to move freely and perform her housework. With maintenance drug therapy the muscle function continued to improve gradually. While tapering prednisone a transient increase in creatine kinase occurred without

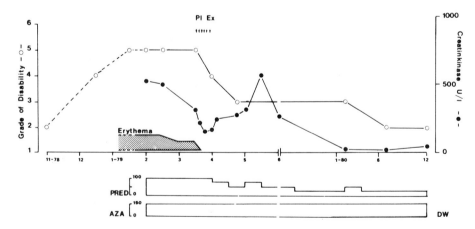

FIG. 1. Long-term course of subacute dermatomyositis in case 9 (responder to plasma exchange). See case report for details. PRED, prednisone; AZA, azathioprine; Pl Ex, plasma exchange.

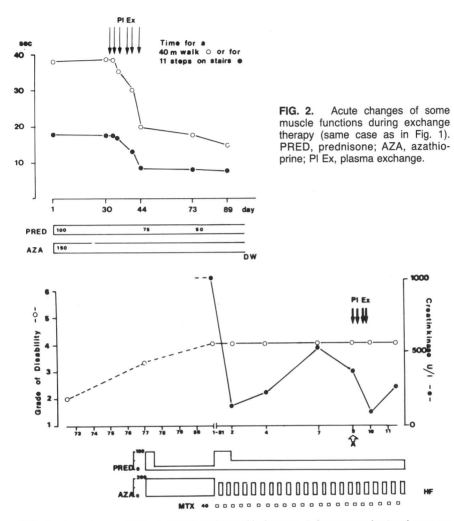

FIG. 2.   Acute changes of some muscle functions during exchange therapy (same case as in Fig. 1). PRED, prednisone; AZA, azathioprine; Pl Ex, plasma exchange.

FIG. 3. Long-term course of chronic polymyositis in case 1 (nonresponder to plasma exchange). See case report for details. PRED, prednisone; AZA, azathioprine; Pl Ex, plasma exchange.

other signs of deterioration. An increase of prednisone caused the enzyme activity to return to normal values. One year thereafter muscle strength is approximately normal without signs of active disease.

No Effect of Plasma Exchange

This 40-year-old man complained of increasing muscular weakness since 1972. The disease ran a slowly progressive course over several years with weakness and marked atrophy of proximal muscles of the extremities. Muscle biopsy, EMG, and moderately elevated serum creatine kinase levels suggested a diagnosis of chronic polymyositis in 1977 (Fig. 3). Prednisone (20 mg/day over 3 years after initial 100 mg/day) and azathioprine (150 mg/day) were unable to prevent disease activity and progression of weakness. The first examination at our department revealed a moderately disabled patient (Grade 4). There was general muscular atrophy and contractures. Muscle biopsy showed degeneration of muscle fibers together with an increase of connective tissue but failed to demonstrate signs of inflammatory changes. Creatine kinase was elevated to 1,000 U/liter. Immunosuppressive treatment with high dose prednisone (100 mg/day) and weekly alternating azathioprine (200 mg/day) and methotrexate (50 mg/week) caused a decrease in serum creatine kinase activity but did not affect the patient's muscular weakness. Four plasma exchanges in 12 days (total 13.8 liters) and continuous immunosuppressive treatment thereafter did not alter the clinical state.

DISCUSSION

Most patients with polymyositis and dermatomyositis improve with treatment using prednisone and cytotoxic drugs within a couple of months (13–20). Spontaneous remissions of disease activity are rare (2,3,15,16). Some patients, however, do not respond to drug therapy and have persistent muscular weakness (2,3,13–16,19,20).

In 1977 the first reports on a successful combination of immunosuppressive drug therapy together with plasma exchange in myositis were published (22). Therapeutic regimens have since been presented that differ from each other with respect to acute or chronic application of plasma exchange (23–25). The largest series reports results of combined therapy with plasma exchanges in weekly intervals over a long period of time and intensified immunosuppression in most of 35 cases (24). The cumulative results of the published reports show a beneficial effect of combined therapy in 35 patients and no effect in 3.

Our experience with plasma exchange combined with immunosuppressive treatment in polymyositis and dermatomyositis confirms these reports, and shows that short courses of plasma exchange can produce a rapid and striking improvement in some patients. As is demonstrated by our results, plasma exchange alters the clinical course of disease activity only in acutely active polymyositis/dermatomyositis—even in cases resistant to drug therapy prior to plasma exchange. Chronic forms of the disease are not affected by plasma exchange. Beneficial effects of plasma exchange are suggested by the strong relation of clinical improvement to the therapeutic exchanges without changes in the drug treatment regimen in most of the responders. It is noteworthy that we observed the beneficial long-lasting effects of plasma exchange as early as the first two to four exchanges.

The efficacy of short courses of plasma exchange in idiopathic inflammatory myopathy is a strong argument for the involvement of circulating factors in the pathogenesis of the disease. The type of serum factor(s) is yet unidentified. They could be specific or unspecific, immunological or biochemical mediators of inflammatory lesions in voluntary muscle.

The role of plasma exchange in the treatment of idiopathic inflammatory myopathy is still unclear. Its observed efficacy in active disease offers additional possibilities in the management of the disease. However, no prospective clinical trials have been published to date to answer the many open questions. The understanding of basic principles of plasma exchange therapy in idiopathic inflammatory myopathy requires further studies.

REFERENCES

1. World Federation of Neurology Research Group on Neuromuscular Disorders (1968): Classification of the neuromuscular disorders. *J. Neurol. Sci.*, 6:165–177.
2. Hudgson, P., and Walton, J. N. (1981): Polymyositis. In: *Handbook of Clinical Neurology: Vol. 41*, edited by P. J. Vinken and G. W. Bruyn, pp. 59–93. Elsevier, Amsterdam.
3. Currie, S. (1981): Polymyositis and related disorders. In: *Disorders of Voluntary Muscle*, edited by J. N. Walton, p. 525. Churchill Livingstone, Edinburgh.
4. Saunders, M., Knowles, M., and Currie, S. (1969): Lymphocyte stimulation with muscle homogenates in polymyositis and other muscle wasting disorders. *J. Neurol. Neurosurg. Psychiatr.*, 32:569.
5. Currie, S., Saunders, M., Knowles, M., and Brown, A. (1971): Immunological aspects of polymyositis. *Q. J. Med.*, 40:63.
6. Esiri, M. M., MacLennan, I. C. M., and Hazleman, B. L. (1973): Lymphocyte sensitivity to skeletal muscle in patients with polymyositis and other disorders. *Clin. Exp. Immunol.*, 14:25.
7. Whitaker, J. N., and Engel, W. K. (1972): Vascular deposits of immunoglobulin and complement in idiopathic inflammatory myopathy. *N. Engl. J. Med.*, 286:333.
8. Reichlin, M., and Mattoli, M. (1976): Description of a serological reaction characteristic of polymyositis. *Clin. Immunol. Immunopathol.*, 5:12.
9. Judge, D. M., McGlynn, T. J., and Abt, A. B. (1977): Immunologic myopathy: Linear IgG deposition and fulminant terminal episode. *Arch. Pathol. Lab. Med.*, 101:362.
10. Oxenhandler, R., Adelstein, E. H. and Hart, M. N. (1977): Immunopathology of skeletal muscle. *Human Pathol.*, 8:357.
11. Heffner, R. R., and De Jong, R. N. (1979): Skeletal muscle in polymyositis: Immunohistological study. *Arch. Pathol. Med. Lab.*, 103:310.
12. Ringel, S. P., Thorne, E. G., Panuphah, P., Lava, N. S., and Kohler, P. S. (1979): Immune complex vasculitis, polymyositis and hyperglobulinemic purpura. *Neurology*, 29:682.
13. Rose, A. L., Walton, J. N. (1966): Polymyositis: A survey on 89 cases with particular reference to treatment and prognosis. *Brain*, 89:747.
14. Riddoch, D., and Morgan-Hughes, J. A. (1975): Prognosis of adult polymyositis. *J. Neurol. Sci.*, 25:71.
15. Devere, R., and Bradley, W. G. (1975): Polymyositis: Its presentation, morbidity and mortality. *Brain*, 98:637.
16. Bohan, P., Peter, J. B., Bownan, R. L., and Pearson, C. M. (1977): A computer assisted analysis of 153 patients with polymyositis and dermatomyositis. *Medicine*, 56:255.
17. Currie, S., and Walton, J. N. (1971): Immunosuppressive therapy in polymyositis. *J. Neurol. Neurosurg. Psychiatr.*, 34:447.
18. Haas, D. C. (1973): Treatment of polymyositis with immunosuppressive drugs. *Neurology*, 23:55.
19. Mertens, H. G., and Lurati, M. (1975): Immunsuppressive Behandlung der Polymyositis. *Dtsch. Med. Wochenschr.*, 100:45.
20. Niakan, E., Pitner, S. E., Whitaker, J. N., and Bertorini, T. E. (1980): Immunosuppressive agent in corticosteroid-refractory childhood dermatomyositis. *Neurology*, 30:286.
21. Bunch, T. W. (1981): Prednisone and azathioprine for polymyositis: Long-term followup. *Arthritis Rheum.*, 24:45.
22. Rossen, R. D., Hersh, E. M., Sharp, J. T., McCredie, K. B., Gyorkey, F., and Suki, W. N. (1977): Effect of plasma exchange on circulating immunecomplexes and antibody formation in patients treated with cyclophosphamide and prednisone. *Am. J. Med.*, 63:674.
23. Brewer, E. J., Giannini, E. H., Rossen, R. D., Patten, B., and Barkley, E. (1980): Plasma exchange of a childhood onset dermatomyositis patient. *Arthritis Rheum.*, 23:509.
24. Dau, P. C. (1981): Plasmapheresis in idiopathic inflammatory myopathy. *Arch. Neurol.*, 38:544.
25. Rohkamm, R., Przuntek, H., Röckel, A., and Reuther, P. (1981): Effect of plasma exchange in SLE with severe myopathy. In: *Plasma Exchange Therapy*, edited by H. Borberg and P. Reuther, p. 197. Thieme, Stuttgart, New York.

Plasmapheresis, edited by Y. Nosé, P. S.
Malchesky, J. W. Smith, and R. S. Krakauer.
Raven Press, New York © 1983.

Reduction of Anti-Acetylcholine Receptor Antibodies by Plasmapheresis in Myasthenia Gravis

R. Lenzhofer, W. Graninger, Ch. Dittrich, *B. Mamoli, and
*J. Zeitelhofer

*Departments of Chemotherapy and *Neurology, University of Vienna,
A-1090 Vienna, Austria*

In the past decades myasthenia gravis (MG) was established as an autoimmune disease associated with disorders of humoral and cellular immunity. Antistriate muscle antibodies were found to be present in the serum of 30 and 95% of patients with MG and MG associated with concomitant thymoma, respectively (1). Using immunofluorescence techniques, Van der Geld et al. (2) showed these skeletal muscle antibodies to cross-react with thymic tissue. On electronmicroscopy, the thymic cells were found to contain myofilaments which were indistinguishable from those of skeletal muscle (3). About 20% of MG patients have antinuclear antibodies (4–6), which may belong to the IgA, IgM, or IgG class (5). In 30% of myasthenic sera at least one antithyroid antibody was found to be present (4,6,7). A small percentage of cases was shown to have antigastric mucosa antibodies (7) and rheumatoid factor positivity (4,6,7), while complement activities were found to be reduced in the majority of MG patients (8). The identification of circulating antibodies against nicotinic acetylcholine receptors (AChR) (9) furnished evidence of the pathophysiologic mechanisms involved in MG and shed some light on the factors underlying the functional reduction of AChR. When assaying anti-AChR-antibodies, 9% of MG patients are, however, missed (10). This may be explained by the poor sensitivity of the test system for borderline antibody concentrations. Alternatively, it may be due to the presence of a special variant of MG in which humoral antibodies do not play a major pathogenetic role.

The current treatment of MG consists of numerous supportive measures, including the administration of cholinesterase inhibitors, steroids, and cytostatics as well as thymectomy. In sporadic cases thoracic duct lymphocyte depletion substantially improved the muscle weakness (11,12). Recently, plasmapheresis has been introduced into the treatment program for acutely reducing the circulating anti-AChR-antibody titers (13–15). Our studies served the purpose of monitoring changes in anti-AChR-antibody concentrations and several other immunological parameters in patients with MG and of correlating them with the clinical course.

PATIENTS AND METHODS

Between 1978 and 1980 11 patients with generalized MG and 1 patient with ocular MG underwent plasmapheresis. Of the total series, 8 were females aged between 24 and 72 years, while 4 were males between 39 and 74 years of age. Prior to plasma exchange, 6 patients had been thymectomized. In 1 case the thymus had been irradiated, as both pneumomediastinoscopy and computer tomography were suggestive of thymoma and surgery was contraindicated for medical reasons. Immunosuppressive therapy (azathioprim, 100 mg daily) was received by 2 patients, another 2 were pretreated with steroids (aprednisolon, 100 mg every other day), while 1 received both azathioprim and steroids. A total of 46 plasma exchanges were performed, with patients undergoing between 1 and 11 treatments.

For plasmapheresis a continuous flow cell separator (Aminco) was used. The plasma withdrawn (total volume/exchange, 2,000 ml) was replaced by 5% human albumin (Sero, Vienna, Austria) at equal volumes. Prior to plasmapheresis patients received heparin sodium intravenously, 5,000 IU, for anticoagulation. In addition, heparin, 1,500 IU/hr, was continuously administered during the procedure. The blood was centrifuged at 1,500 rpm. Before and after plasmapheresis electrolytes, total protein, albumin, and globulin were determined by an autoanalyzer technique (Technicon). For evaluating hematologic parameters, that is, red blood count (RBC), hematocrit, hemoglobin, white blood count (WBC), and platelets, the "Hämalog" autoanalyzer system was used. Immunoglobulins were assayed on Partigen plates (Behring) with the Mancini technique.

Anti-AChR-Antibody Determination

Serum anti-AChR-antibodies were assayed according to Lindström (16) and with the Toyka modification (10) of the technique by Monnier and Fulpius (17).

Antinuclear Antibody and Antistriate Muscle Antibody Determination

Rat liver and rat muscle cryostat sections were incubated with patient serum (dilution, 1:10 with PBS) at 20°C for 20 min, washed, and covered with FITC-conjugated anti-human-rabbit globulin (Hyland, F/P = 5.3 µg/mg). After 20-min incubation, sections were washed and evaluated by direct fluorescence microscopy (Ortholux, Leitz).

Circulating Immune Complex Determination

This was done by polyethyleneglycol precipitation according to Riha et al. (18). Serum samples of patients with exacerbating systemic lupus erythematosus or acute hepatitis served as positive controls.

RESULTS

A positive response to plasmapheresis was observed in 9 of our 12 cases. No response was seen in our single case with strictly ocular symptoms, where anti-

AChR-antibodies were not demonstrated, and in another 2 patients with cardiac arrest, which ruled out more than one plasmapheresis. Cardiac arrest occurred 12 and 15 hr after plasma exchange so that a causal relation is unlikely. In these 3 cases a final assessment of the therapeutic effects is, obviously, impossible.

Figure 1 details the pre- and post-exchange anti-AChR-antibody concentrations of 6 patients with MG. The severity of the disease was not found to correlate with the anti-AChR-antibody concentrations. In fact, the lowest antibody titer (11.0×10^{-9} M ^{125}I-bungarotoxin binding/liter serum) was recorded in a female patient on artificial respiration. By contrast, the individual clinical course was found to correlate well with the anti-AChR-antibody concentrations.

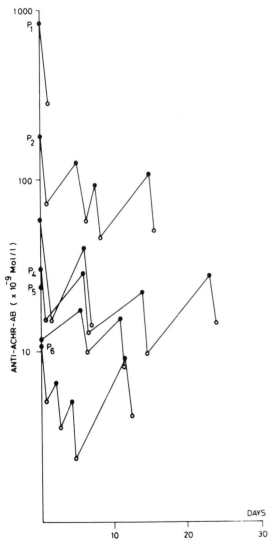

FIG. 1. Anti-AChR-receptor antibody titers in 6 patients with MG before and after plasmapheresis.

Figure 2 exemplifies anti-AChR-antibody and IgG concentrations as well as circulating immune complexes in a female patient over a period of 1 year. After every plasmapheresis both the antibody titer and the IgG concentration were found to drop substantially. Clinically, the first series of three exchanges produced excellent results. While the patient had been unable to keep her arms extended for more than 5–7 sec, she succeeded in doing so for 65 sec after the first series of exchanges. Anti-AChR-antibody concentrations dropped from 384.9×10^{-9} to 116×10^{-9} M ^{125}I-bungarotoxin binding/liter serum. As her condition deteriorated again after 50 days, the patient was scheduled for another series of exchanges. At that time she kept her arms extended for 10–35 sec. After no more than two exchanges her performance improved to 150 sec. As after the first course, anti-AChR-antibody titers dropped from 551.3×10^{-9} to 110.8×10^{-9} M ^{125}I-bungarotoxin/liter serum. Three months later the symptoms became worse again so that alternating high-dose cortisone therapy was instituted. As this failed to improve her condition, the patient underwent a third series of plasmapheresis 240 days after her initial course. This enabled her to keep her arms extended for 57 sec versus 8 sec before treatment.

As in the previous exchange series, the clinical improvement was associated with a clear-cut reduction in anti-AChR-antibody titers. This was paralleled by a reduction in immunoglobulin concentrations, which were assayed before and after plasmapheresis. Positive circulating immune complexes coincided with clinical exacerbations and disappeared after plasmapheresis.

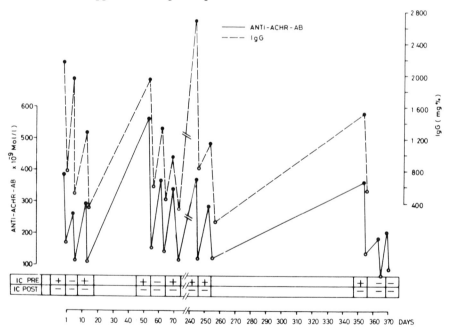

FIG. 2. Anti-AChR-antibody titers and IgG concentrations in a myasthenic patient before and after plasmapheresis over a period of 1 year.

The total percentage of antibodies removable on plasmapheresis is shown in Fig. 3. As can be seen, antibody titers can be effectively reduced (to about 20% of the preexchange concentration) during the first three exchanges, while no further reduction is obtained, when plasmapheresis is continued.

In Fig. 4 the percentage reductions of anti-AChR-antibodies, IgG, and globulin obtained in 28 exchanges (6 patients) are correlated. This correlation clearly shows that anti-AChR-antibody determinations cannot be replaced by IgG or globulin assays for monitoring the course of MG. Overall, 7 of our 10 patients had positive immune complexes, 6 had antistriate muscle antibodies, and 5 had antinuclear antibodies. Antimitochondrial antibodies and anti-smooth muscle antibodies were identified in 2 and 5 cases, respectively.

Plasmapheresis was not associated with any serious side effects. The effects of plasma exchange on serum electrolytes in MG patients are shown in Table 1. In some instances ($N = 13$) potassium concentrations decreased to subnormal levels without producing clinical signs of hypopotassemia. Patients affected had low normal preexchange potassium levels throughout. Hematologic changes produced by plasmapheresis in myasthenic patients are reproduced in Table 2. Plasmapheresis was associated with a substantial reduction in platelet count [($\overline{X} = 66.69 \pm 38.37 \times 10^3$ platelets/μl) and with a minor decrease in RBC] ($\overline{X} = 0.59 \pm 0.37 \times 10^6/\mu$l).

DISCUSSION

As elevated anti-AChR-antibody titers are demonstrable in 90% of all myasthenic patients (9,19), their determination can be used in doubtful cases to confirm the diagnosis. Generally, the correlation between absolute antibody titers and the severity of the disease is poor (19,20). However, the relative intraindividual antibody titer changes in myasthenic patients correlate well with the symptoms present (19).

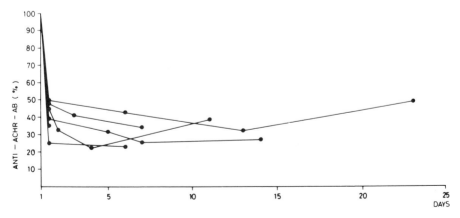

FIG. 3. Anti-AChR-antibody titers after plasmapheresis in percentage of the preexchange concentrations (6 patients).

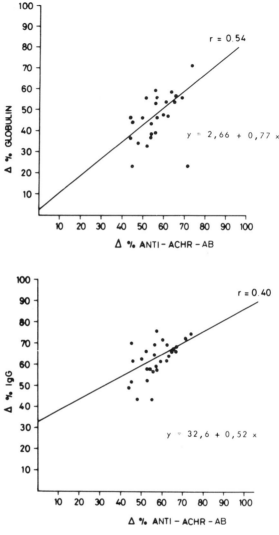

FIG. 4. Correlation between reduction of anti-AChR-antibody titers and globulin ($N = 25$) and IgG ($N = 28$) depletion by plasmapheresis (in percent).

Our data support both the poor correlation between the absolute antibody titer and the patient's condition (Fig. 1) and the good agreement between these parameters in intraindividual comparisons (Fig. 2). Preexchange titers ranged from 11.0×10^{-9} to 820×10^{-9} M ^{125}I-bungarotoxin binding/liter serum. The lowest titer was found in a female on intensive care. Both the generally good agreement of repeatedly determined anti-AChR-antibody titers with the clinical course of the disease and the absence of a correlation with the severity of the disease may have a dual explanation: They may be due to an individually variable sensitivity to the antibody-

TABLE 1. Electrolyte changes after
plasmapheresis in myasthenic
patients expressed as mean of
difference between pre- and
postexchange values ± SE (N = 47)

Electrolyte	mmoles/liter
Sodium	−2.66 ± 2.62
Potassium	−0.50 ± 0.44
Chloride	+4.40 ± 3.65
Inorganic phosphate	−0.12 ± 0.09
Calcium	−0.24 ± 0.12

TABLE 2. Hematologic changes after
plasmapheresis in myasthenic patients
expressed as mean of difference between pre-
and postexchange levels ± SE (N = 47)

RBC	$-0.59 \pm 0.37 \times 10^6/\mu l$
Hematocrit	−5.32 ± 3.09%
Hemoglobin	−1.71 ± 1.09 g%
WBC	$+1.40 \pm 1.39 \times 10^3/\mu l$
Platelets	$-66.69 \pm 38.37 \times 10^3/\mu l$

related AChR dysfunction. Alternatively, the anti-AChR-antibodies currently assayed may not play a primary role in the etiology of MG (13). While various assaying techniques established the heterogeneity of anti-AChR-antibodies (21–24), attempts at identifying an anti-AChR-antibody subpopulation whose absolute concentrations would closely correlate with the clinical stage of MG have so far failed. Statistically, a close correlation of IgG and globulin concentrations with anti-AChR-antibodies is not demonstrable (Fig. 4). Consequently, anti-AChR-antibody cannot be replaced by determinations of the IgG and globulin concentrations for monitoring the course of MG.

CONCLUSIONS

Plasmapheresis has a limited place in the treatment of MG. It can be used as a short-term measure for rapidly obtaining transient clinical improvement in life-threatening situations requiring intensive care or artificial respiration. Frequently repeated exchanges accompanying immunosuppressive therapy can, however, not be expected to produce a cumulative reduction of anti-AChR-antibodies and persistent clinical improvement (15). Side effects were confined to measurable electrolyte and hematologic alternations. As a result, RBC, platelets, and electrolytes should be monitored after every exchange series. In view of the potential risks involved, for example, IgG depletion with resultant elevated risk of infections, thrombocytopenia with resultant hemorrhage and hypopotassemia, and in view of the high cost factor, plasmapheresis should be reserved for particularly severe cases.

ACKNOWLEDGMENT

We are indebted to the Department of Immunochemistry (Head: Prof. Dr. A. Fateh Mogadan) at Klinikum Grosshadern LMU, Munich (Director: Prof. Dr. M. Knedel) for performing the anti-acetylcholine receptor antibody assays.

REFERENCES

1. Strauss, A. J. L., Van der Geld, H. W. R., Kemp, P. G., Exum, E. D., and Godman, H. C. (1965): Immunological concomitants of myasthenia gravis. *Ann. N.Y. Acad. Sci.*, 124:744.
2. Van der Geld, H. W. R., Feltman, T. E. W., and Oosterhus, H. J. G. H. (1964): Reactivity of myasthenia gravis serum γ-globulin with skeletal muscle and thymus demonstrated by immunofluorescence. *Proc. Soc. Exp. Biol. Med.*, 115:782.
3. Strauss, A. J. L., Kemp, P. G., and Douglas, S. D. (1966): Myasthenia gravis: Immunological relationships between muscle and thymus, thymic myoid cells. *Lancet*, i:772.
4. Aarli, A. J. (1970): Binding of γ-globulin fragments to muscle tissue. *Clin. Exp. Immunol.*, 7:23.
5. McFarlin, D. E., and Johnson, J. S. (1971): Studies of antimuscle factor in myasthenia gravis: II. Reactions of fragments produced in enzymatic digestion. *J. Immunol.*, 106:292.
6. Vetters, J. M., Simpson, J. A., and Folkarde, A. (1969): Experimental myasthenia gravis. *Lancet*, ii:28.
7. Simpson, J. A. (1960): Myasthenia gravis: A new hypothesis. *Scott. Med. J.*, 5:419.
8. Nastuk, W. L., Plescia, O. J., and Osserman, K. E. (1960): Changes in serum complement activity in patients with myasthenia gravis. *Proc. Soc. Exp. Biol. Med.*, 105:177.
9. Lindstrom, J., Seybold, H. E., Lennon, V. A., Wittingham, S., and Duane, D. D. (1976): Antibody to acetylcholine receptor in myasthenia gravis: Prevalence, clinical correlates, and diagnostic value. *Neurology*, 26:1054.
10. Toyka, K. V., Becker, T., Fateh-Moghadem, A., Besinger, U. A., Brehm, G., Neumeier, D., Heininger, K., and Birnberger, K. L. (1979): Die Bedeutung der Bestimmung von Antikörpern gegen Acetylcholinrezeptoren in der Diagnostik der Myasthenia gravis. *Klin. Wochenschr.*, 57:937.
11. Bernstrom, K., Fransson, C., Matell, G., Nilsson, B. Y., Persson, A., Reis, G., and Stensman, R. (1975): Drainage of thoracic duct lymph in twelve patients with myasthenia gravis. *Eur. Neurol.*, 13:19.
12. Tindall, S. C., Peters, B. H., Sarles, H. E., Fish, J. C., and Caverley, J. R. (1973): Thoracic duct lymphocyte depletion in myasthenia gravis. *Arch. Neurol.*, 29:202.
13. Carter, B., Harrison, R., Lunt, G. G., Behan, P. O., and Simpson, J. A. (1980): Anti-acetylcholine receptor antibody titres in the sera of myasthenia patients treated with plasma exchange combined with immunosuppressive therapy. *J. Neurol. Neurosurg. Psychiatr.*, 43:397.
14. Dau, P. C. (1980): Plasmapheresis therapy in myasthenia gravis. *Muscle Nerve*, 3:468.
15. Newsom-Davis, J., Vincent, A., Wilson, S. G., and Ward, D. (1979): Long-term effects of repeated plasma exchange in myasthenia gravis. *Lancet*, i:464.
16. Lindstrom, J. (1977): An assay for antibodies to human acetylcholine receptor in serum from patients with myasthenia gravis. *Clin. Immunol. Immunopathol.*, 7:36.
17. Monnier, V. M., and Fulpius, B. W. (1977): A radioimmunoassay for the quantitative evaluation of antihuman acetylcholine receptor antibodies in myasthenia gravis. *Clin. Exp. Immunol.*, 29:16.
18. Riha, I., Haskova, V., Kaslik, J., Maierova, M., and Stransky, J. (1979): The use of polyethyleneglycol for immune complex detection in human sera. *Mol. Immunol.*, 16:489.
19. Lefvert, A. K., Bergström, K., Matell, G., Osterman, P. O., and Pirshauen, R. (1978): Determination of acetylcholine receptor antibody in myasthenia gravis: Clinical usefulness and pathogenic implications. *J. Neurol. Neurosurg. Psychiatr.*, 41:394.
20. Barkas, T., Harrison, R., Lunt, G. G., Stephenson, F. A., Behan, P. O., and Simpson, J. A. (1979): Acetylcholine receptor antibody titres in myasthenia gravis. In: *Progress in Neurological Research with Particular Reference to Motor Neurone Disease*, edited by P. O. Behan and R. Clifford, p. 169. Pitman Medical Press, London.
21. Mittag, T. W., Tormay, A., and Marsa, T. (1978): Heterogeneity of acetylcholine receptors in denervated muscle: Interactions of receptors with immunoglobulin from patients with myasthenia gravis. *Mol. Pharmacol.*, 14:60.

22. Savage-Marengo, T., Harrison, R., Lunt, G. G., and Behan, P. O. (1980): Patient-specific anti-acetylcholine receptor antibody patterns in myasthenia gravis. *J. Neurol. Neurosurg. Psychiatr.*, 43:316.
23. Vincent, A., and Newsom-Davis, J. (1979): Bungarotoxin and anti-acetylcholine receptor antibody binding to the human acetylcholine receptor. *Adv. Cytopharmacol.*, 3:269.
24. Weinberg, C. B., and Hall, Z. W. (1979): Antibodies from patients with myasthenia gravis recognise determinants unique to extrajunctional acetylcholine receptors. *Proc. Natl. Acad. Sci. USA*, 76:504.

Plasmapheresis, edited by Y. Nosé, P. S. Malchesky, J. W. Smith, and R. S. Krakauer. Raven Press, New York © 1983.

Plasma Exchange Therapy of Immune Complex Mediated Vasculitis

D. Mandel, L. Calabrese, and J. Clough

Department of Rheumatic and Immunologic Disease, Cleveland Clinic Foundation, Cleveland, Ohio 44106

There is growing evidence that plasma exchange therapy may be helpful in the treatment of a number of disorders whose pathogenesis is believed to be mediated by circulating immune complexes. Though circulating immune complexes may be identified in a wide variety of conditions, they now appear critical in the pathogenesis of certain forms of necrotizing vasculitis. Our study of the effects of plasma exchange therapy in 17 patients with various forms of vasculitis is described below.

PATIENTS

There was a total of 17 patients who were divided into three groups. The first group (Table 1) included those patients who had vasculitis associated with a connective tissue disease; 8 patients had rheumatoid arthritis and 1 patient had systemic lupus erythematosus. Vasculitis was the predominant clinical feature manifested by either neuropathy, nonhealing ulcers or visceral manifestations.

The second group (Table 2) consisted of 3 patients who had systemic polyarteritis-like disease with multisystem involvement and little cutaneous involvement, high levels of circulating immune complexes, and 2 of the 3 patients had a positive biopsy of either muscle or nerve.

The third group (Table 3) consisted of 5 patients who presented with a picture of hypersensitivity vasculitis. Palpable purpura was the predominant skin lesion and this was associated with multisystem involvement.

METHOD

Each patient was treated with 2–3-liter exchanges, a mean of 7 liters/patient. Replacement fluids consisted of 50% crystalloid and 50% purified protein fraction. Circulating immune complexes were measured by Clq binding and precipitation to polyethylene glycol before and after each exchange. Adjuvant medical therapy is described in the tables and had been initiated prior to and was continued along with plasmapheresis.

TABLE 1. *Group 1: Vasculitis associated with connective tissue disease*[a]

Patient	Connective tissue disease[b]	Target organs	No. plasma exchanges[c]	Adjuvant treatment	Disease clinical course
69-Yr F	RA and Felty's	Nonhealing ulcer	3	5 mg Prednisone	Ulcers healed within 1 mo
50-Yr F	RA	Sensory and motor neuropathy	3	NSAID Plaquenil	No effect on neuropathy
79-Yr F	RA	Neuropathy	3	3 gr IVMP 15 mg IVNM 4 mg Prednisone	Muscle strength improved
59-Yr F	RA	Sensory and motor neuropathy	3	3 gr IVMP 7.5 mg/wk MTX Plaquenil	Paresthesia improved in 3 mos Strength improved in 8 mos
53-Yr M	RA	Finger ulcer, sensory and motor neuropathy	3	100 mg Cytotoxan 20 mg Prednisone 200 mg Plaquenil	Foot drop resolved in 1 mo
39-Yr F	RA	Leg ulcers	2	15 mg Prednisone	Gradual healing over 1 mo
59-Yr F	RA and Felty's	Leg ulcers	5	20 mg Prednisone NSAID	Gradual healing over 2 mos
60-Yr F	RA	Ischemic ulcer obtundation	3	80 mg Prednisone 7.5 mg/wk MTX 3 gr IVMP	Ischemic progression halted within 5 days
30-Yr M	SLE	Ischemic sores and ulcers, CNS obtundation	10	80 mg Prednisone 6 mg IVNM	Obtundation improved over 5 days

[a] *Summary:* Skin (ulceration) improved in 7/7 patients. Neuropathy improved in 3/4 patients.
[b] RA, rheumatoid arthritis; SLE, systemic lupus erythematosus.
[c] Two-liter exchanges.

TABLE 2. *Group 2: Polyarteritis nodosa group*[a]

Patient	Target organ	No. plasma exchanges[b]	Adjuvant treatment	Effect
61-Yr M	Pulmonary infiltrates and acute renal failure	5	80 mg Prednisone	Patient died secondary to respiratory failure
71-Yr F	Sensory neuropathy	3	20 mg Prednisone	Sensory symptoms persist
56-Yr M	Motor sensory neuropathy and renal failure	7	60 mg Prednisone 100 mg Cytotoxan	Transient improvement; patient died of sepsis and renal failure

[a]*Summary:* Two patients with established pulmonary involvement and renal disease, who eventually died. One patient with permanent sensory involvement. There was no immediate benefit.
[b]Two-liter exchanges.

RESULTS

There was a significant decrease of circulating immune complexes prior to and after plasmapheresis. Levels of Clq binding fell from a mean of 133 to 11.8 μg.

Postpheresis rebound defined as a return of the level of immune complexes to 75% of baseline within 4 weeks is listed in the tables for each of the groups. As noted, cytotoxic therapy effectively blocked rebound in those patients with vasculitis associated with connective tissue disease.

No rebound occurred in the 1 patient with polyarteritis who had been receiving cyclophosphamide. Rebound was not observed in 2 patients with hypersensitivity vasculitis.

The side effects related to plasmapheresis were limited. However, 1 patient with systemic lupus required the use of femoral catheters for plasma exchange. One of the catheters became lodged in the femoral vein and had to be surgically removed.

The results for each of the treatment groups are the following. In Group 1, all patients with rheumatoid arthritis and vasculitis skin ulcerations had been refractory to conventional treatment prior to apheresis. Skin ulceration showed gradual healing in 7 of 7 patients. Of the 4 patients with an associated peripheral neuropathy, 3 also showed improvement. The patient with systemic lupus showed a temporary but dramatic improvement with plasmapheresis plus high dose prednisone, but relapsed in conjunction with rebound of anti-DNA. His clinical and laboratory course showed that he again responded to apheresis used in conjunction with low dose nitrogen mustard which effectively blocked rebound phenomena and was eventually associated with maintenance of clinical remission.

Two patients with polyarteritis presented with established renal and pulmonary failure at the outset of therapy. They subsequently died. The third patient with

TABLE 3. *Group 3: Hypersensitivity vasculitis*[a]

Patient	Etiology	Target organs	No. plasma exchanges[b]	Adjuvant treatment	Results
50-Yr M	Bactrim	CNS obtundation	1(3)	3 gr IVMP 80 mg Prednisone	Dramatic improvement in obtundation
34-Yr M	Penicillin	Renal purpura	1(3) 3(2)	3 gr IVMP 80 mg Prednisone	Dramatic improvement in kidney function; healing of vasculitic lesion in weeks
52-Yr F	Unknown	Motor and sensory neuropathy	3(2)	80 mg Prednisone	Ulcers healed and improvement in neuropathy
62-Yr F	Unknown	Purpura and pulmonary infiltrates; azotemia	7(2)	100 mg Cytotoxan 60 mg Prednisone	Resolution of skin lesion and pulmonary infiltrates, and improvement in renal function
69-Yr F	Unknown	Purpura	3(2)	80 mg Prednisone	Skin lesion cleared X-ray infiltrate; infiltrate resolved over 2–3 weeks

[a]*Summary:* Two patients with drug-induced hypersensitivity vasculitis had a dramatic response. Three additional patients also had complete resolution of symptoms within 1 month of treatment.
[b]Number of liters per exchange expressed in parentheses.

neuropathy had a poor response also. The clinical outcome in those patients with hypersensitivity vasculitis was favorable.

It is appreciated that most patients with hypersensitivity vasculitis have a generally self-limited course. However, 2 patients in this group with drug-induced hypersensitivity vasculitis had serious visceral involvement. One patient presented with progressive central nervous system involvement with both focal neurologic signs and obtundation (Fig. 1). The second patient presented with rapidly progressive renal failure. Both of these patients showed a dramatic clinical improvement after as little as 2–4 liters of plasma exchange. In the 1 patient with central nervous system disease, total mental clearing occurred within 24 hr. In the second patient with rapidly progressive azotemia, there was continued improvement in renal function and rapid clearing of mentation within 2 days of initiating plasma exchange. The 3 remaining patients also had complete resolution of symptoms within 1 month of treatment.

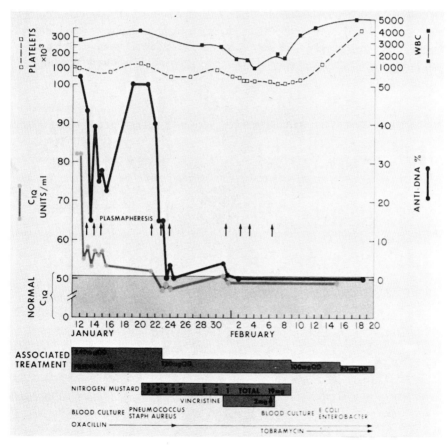

FIG. 1. Thirty-year-old male with systemic lupus erythematosus, small and medium vessel vasculitis with myositis nephritis, myocarditis, GI vasculitis, thrombopenia, and leukopenia.

We recognize some of the limitations of our study; it was retrospective and patients were receiving concurrent medical therapy. However, in those patients with rheumatoid vasculitis, improvement in both skin ulcerations and neuropathic symptoms seem to coincide shortly after the plasma exchange therapy.

We believe the dismal outcome in those patients with polyarteritis was related to their near terminal condition when they presented.

Lastly, those patients with hypersensitivity vasculitis had the best outcome. Although this is generally a self-limited illness, these patients had, in addition to skin involvement, serious internal organ disease. In those 2 patients with acute vasculitis secondary to a known drug, it is possible that apheresis treatment may be performing the dual function of removing both preformed immune reactants and an exogenous antigen, and potentially ending an on-going immune response.

CONCLUSION

Plasmapheresis reduced immune complexes in all patients. Rebound immune complex levels were effectively blocked by cytotoxic medicines but not by prednisone. Plasmapheresis may be helpful in the treatment of immune complex vasculitis, and may be particularly useful in those patients with hypersensitivity vasculitis.

Plasmapheresis, edited by Y. Nosé, P. S.
Malchesky, J. W. Smith, and R. S. Krakauer.
Raven Press, New York © 1983.

Treatment of Steroid Resistant Renal Allograft Rejection with Plasma Lymphapheresis

*§P. R. McCurdy, *§F. W. Darr, †G. B. Helfrich, †T. Philips,
†B. W. Pechan, †M. Alijani, †Z. K. Papadopolou,
and †M. Gelfand

*American Red Cross Blood Services, Washington, D. C. 20006; †Georgetown University
School of Medicine, Washington, D.C. 20007; §George Washington University
School of Medicine, Washington, D.C. 20037

Kidney transplants have been a viable option for at least some patients with end-stage renal disease since the early 1950s. The initial transplants were syngeneic in that they came from identical twins. Later, human leukocyte antigen (HLA)-matched siblings, selectively mismatched parents, and HLA-matched cadaver transplants were done. With standard immunosuppressive therapy using azathioprine and steroids, transplant retention at the end of 1 or 2 years for other than syngeneic organs approximated 50–60% (1,2). Among the maneuvers aimed at improving this graft survival figure are thoracic duct drainage (3) and administration of antithymocyte globulin (1). The former is technically difficult and not always successful, and there are numerous side effects from the latter. Nevertheless each has apparently improved graft survival by 10–20% or to 70–80%. In an attempt to devise an alternative to these techniques, we began to perform a combination of plasma exchange and lymphocytapheresis in patients whose graft rejection was resistant to steroid pulses.

A 1-plasma volume exchange will reduce by approximately 60% all plasma constituents not replaced during the procedure (4). The rate of recovery of intravascular concentration depends upon the synthetic rate and on the total body distribution. For example, IgM is exclusively intravascular whereas IgG is about equal in concentration in both intra- and extravascular spaces. Some graft rejection is due to humoral mechanisms, presumably mediated by immunoglobulins. Plasma exchange is aimed at reducing the intravascular concentration of such immunoglobulins. Preliminary data from other centers suggest that this procedure has some value in protecting against transplant rejection, although the degree of protection is somewhat in doubt (5). Since some transplant rejection involves T cells, we elected not only to do plasma exchange but also to remove as many lymphocytes as possible during the procedure—"plasma exchange with leukocyte removal" or PLEX (6,7).

The procedures were done using the Haemonetics Model 30 Pheresis Machine. The objective was to do five PLEX treatments of approximately 1-plasma volume each, as close together as possible each day after it was determined that the rejection episode was resistant to steroid pulses. Five additional treatments were done on a schedule of approximately three times weekly. At each instance the buffy coat was removed, including a small amount of the upper layer of red cells. Hence, as many lymphocytes were removed as possible. The numbers are of a similar order of magnitude to thoracic duct drainage (3) (Table 1). After several patients were entered into the study, it became apparent that early recrudescence of the rejection phenomenon was possible. Accordingly, most subsequent patients had "maintenance" therapy with weekly, later biweekly, exchanges until it seemed likely that the rejection episode would not recur. It should be noted that the removal of lymphocytes also results in the removal of a large number of platelets; each procedure reduces the platelet count by approximately one-third. Since these were preliminary and pilot studies involving patients with an extremely high risk of completely rejecting the kidney, no concomitant controls were used.

To date, 24 patients were studied; 3 were not evaluable because too few procedures were done. Of the 21 others, 11 have still retained their kidneys whereas transplant nephrectomy was necessary in 10. Follow-up for those who retained their grafts was 6 months or more in 10 patients; thus in this group of very poor risk patients, about half continue to have functioning kidneys (Table 2). If one assumes that the patients studied had an 80–90% chance of completely rejecting the kidney graft, then this level of graft retention is highly significant and approximates the overall 70–80% success rate attained by such measures as antithymocyte globulin and thoracic duct drainage. Following are several illustrative cases.

TABLE 1. *Protocol*

10 Exchanges
5—Daily
5—3/Week
1 plasma volume/exchange (approx. 65% exchange)
Buffy coat including top layer red cells
Lymphocytes: $2.3 \pm 1.5 \times 10^9$/procedure
Platelets: $2.8 \pm 0.6 \times 10^{11}$/procedure

TABLE 2. *Results*

Total patients treated	24
Unevaluable	3
Kidneys retained	11
>6 Mos follow-up	10
<6 Mos follow-up	1
Kidneys lost	10

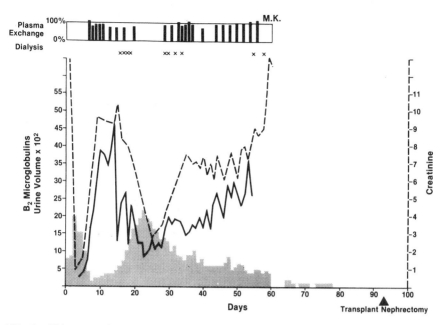

FIG. 1. Thirty-year-old man whose second transplant was placed on day 0. Serum creatinine *(broken line)*, serum β₂-microglobulins *(solid line)*. Plasma exchange expressed as percentage of 1 plasma volume. Steroid pulses *(crosses)* are 1,000 mg methylprednisolone sodium succinate. Transplant nephrectomy indicated by *triangle*.

Case Studies

M. K. is a 30-year-old white man who had recently undergone his second cadaver transplant (Fig. 1). Previously, under the stimulus of pulse steroid therapy, he had a massive gastrointestinal hemorrhage from a peptic ulcer, thus contraindicating such massive steroid therapy at this time. Although his graft began to function well immediately, rejection rapidly supervened as manifested by a sharply reduced urinary output, a rising creatinine, and elevated β₂-microglobulins. A period of intensive plasma exchange accompanied by lymphocyte and platelet removal appears to be followed by rising urinary output, decreasing creatinine, and decreasing β₂-microglobulins. In retrospect, however, the rejection episode continued to smolder, and about 10 days after the last plasma exchange the urinary output began to decrease again and the creatinine and β₂-microglobulins began to rise. Although another series of intensive plasma exchanges may have delayed the final graft rejection, transplant nephrectomy was necessitated on the 93rd day after it was placed.

M. A., a 19-year-old woman, received her first cadaver transplant on day 0 (Fig. 2). Several mild rejection episodes, manifested by decreased urinary output and an increase of both serum creatinine and serum β₂-microglobulins, were treated with large doses of steroids. Despite this, both parameters continued to rise and output to decrease. PLEX therapy was followed by improvement in all parameters which continued over a long period of exchange treatment. Ultimately all parameters normalized and she continues to do well.

This patient, a 32-year-old white man, had his first cadaver transplant at day 0 (Fig. 3). His course was relatively stormy from the beginning, and on day 32 plasma exchanges with

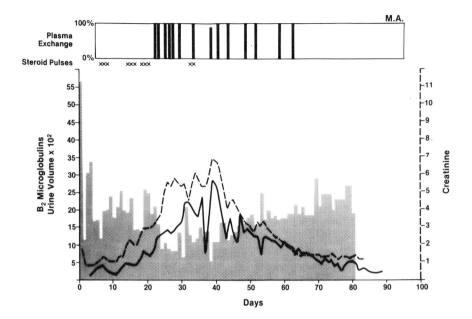

FIG. 2. Nineteen-year-old woman whose first transplant was placed on day 0. Serum creatinine *(broken line)*, serum β₂-microglobulins *(solid line)*. Plasma exchange expressed as percentage of 1 plasma volume. Steroid pulses *(crosses)* are 1,000 mg methylprednisolone sodium succinate.

lymphocyte and platelet removal were begun. Although the response was not immediate or dramatic, it appeared as though the β₂-microglobulins and the serum creatinine gradually began to fall and the urinary output to rise. As of the present writing, 8 months after the transplant, the graft is still in place and functioning well.

Nevertheless, all results were not good. In this patient with his first cadaver transplant (Fig. 4), initial success was followed immediately by diminishing urinary output and later by increasing creatinine and β₂-microglobulins. Despite intensive PLEX therapy, urinary output never recovered, creatinine and β₂-microglobulins remained high, and transplant nephrectomy was necessary.

It is difficult to draw firm conclusions from these studies since there are no concomitant controls. I have learned through bitter experience to be careful in such circumstances (8). Nevertheless, if one assumes an 80–90% graft loss in these patients, there does appear to be a significant improvement in graft survival. About 50% or slightly more kept their graft. Plasma exchange with lymphocyte and platelet removal is expensive therapy in dollars, but few side effects have been noted.

Occasionally a patient will suffer the consequences of too large an extra corporeal volume. One must guard against electrolyte imbalance, although when kidney function is poor, dialysis and hemofiltration techniques are better at controlling these than is plasma exchange. Very little citrate is reinfused to these patients since the majority is removed with the plasma. Nevertheless, an occasional patient will develop symptoms of hypocalcemia, possibly because of imbalance between cal-

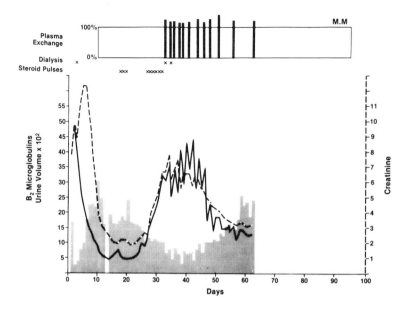

FIG. 3. Thirty-two-year-old man; first cadaver transplant on day 0. Serum creatinine *(broken line)*, serum β₂-microglobulins *(solid line)*. Plasma exchange expressed as percentage of 1 plasma volume. Steroid pulses *(crosses)* are 1,000 mg methylprednisolone sodium succinate.

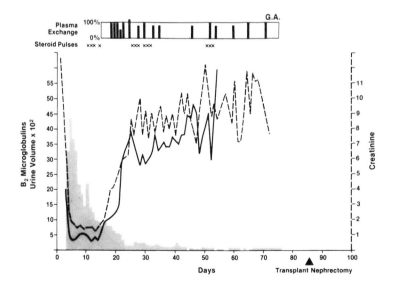

FIG. 4. Thirty-seven-year-old man; first cadaver transplant on day 0. Serum creatinine *(broken line)*, serum β₂-microglobulins *(solid line)*. Plasma exchange expressed as percentage of 1 plasma volume. Steroid pulses *(crosses)* are 1,000 mg methylprednisolone sodium succinate. Transplant nephrectomy indicated by *triangle*.

cium, phosphorus, and sodium. Two insulin-requiring diabetic patients decreased their need for insulin, perhaps due to removal of mildly antagonistic insulin antibodies.

We offer this therapy as a possible less toxic substitute for antithymocyte globulin or a technically less difficult substitute for thoracic duct drainage, and suggest that it may be useful as adjunctive therapy in selected patients rejecting kidney transplants.

REFERENCES

1. Guttmann, R. D. (1979): Renal transplantation. *N. Eng. J. Med.*, 301:975, 1039.
2. Standards Committee, American Society of Transplant Surgeons (1981): Current results and expectations of renal transplantation. *J.A.M.A.*, 246:1330.
3. Sarles, H. E., Smith, G. H., Fish, J. C., and Remmers, A. R., Jr. (1967): Observations concerning human lymphocyte homeostasis during prolonged thoracic duct diversion. *Tex. Rep. Biol. Med.*, 25:573.
4. Orlin, J. B., and Berkman, E. M. (1980): Partial plasma exchange using albumin replacement: Removal and recovery of normal plasma constituents. *Blood*, 56:1055.
5. Cardella, C. J., Sutton, D. M. C., Uldall, P. R., Katz, A., and de Veber, G. A. (1979): Renal allograft rejection and intensive plasma exchange. *Proc. Haemonetics Research Inst. Adv. Component Sem.*, Boston, MA.
6. Wright, D. G., Karsh, J., Fauci, A. S., Klippel, J. H., Decker, J. L., O'Donnell, J.F., and Deisseroth, A.B. (1981): Lymphocyte depletion and immunosuppression with repeated leukapheresis by continuous flow centrifugation. *Blood*, 58:451.
7. Kurland, J., Franklin, S., and Goldfinger, D. (1980): Treatment of renal allograft injection by exchange plasma-lymphocytapheresis. *Transfusion*, 20:337.
8. Cooperative Urea Trials Group (1974): Treatment of sickle cell crisis with urea in invert sugar. *J.A.M.A.*, 228:1125.

Plasmapheresis, edited by Y. Nosé, P. S.
Malchesky, J. W. Smith, and R. S. Krakauer.
Raven Press, New York © 1983.

Therapeutic Plasma Exchange and Lymphocyte Depletion in Aplastic Anemia and Pure Red Cell Aplasia

Neal S. Young, Harvey G. Klein, Patricia Griffith,
and Arthur W. Nienhuis

*Clinical Hematology Branch, National Heart, Lung, and Blood Institute, and
Clinical Center Blood Bank, National Institutes of Health, Bethesda, Maryland 20205*

Several lines of evidence suggest that aplastic anemia may be an autoimmune disorder (1). First, occasional patients receiving immunosuppressive therapy as conditioning for bone marrow transplantation have recovered autologous bone marrow function. Second, simple infusion of bone marrow from a syngeneic twin has occasionally failed to cure aplastic anemia, and immunosuppressive therapy has been required for successful engraftment. Third, *in vitro* studies with cultured bone marrow cells have indicated that a large proportion of aplastic anemia patients may have either serum or cellular inhibitors of normal hematopoietic colony formation. The effectiveness of antithymocyte globulin in European studies (2) has been credited to its toxic effect on suppressor cells (3).

If aplastic anemia is an autoimmune disorder, it might be anticipated that medical therapy directed toward the immune system would be beneficial. Cyclophosphamide and prednisone in combination with either plasma exchange or lymphocyte depletion appear to be beneficial in a variety of disorders with immune etiologies, including myasthenia gravis (4), Goodpasture's syndrome (5), immune thrombocytopenia (6), cold agglutinin disease (7), and antibody formation directed against Factor VIII (8). In contrast to antithymocyte globulin, this form of immunotherapy is reproducible among patients and treatment centers, and therefore potentially offers significant advantages over antithymocyte globulin. We have treated 6 aplastic anemia patients with cyclophosphamide, prednisone, and either plasma exchange or lymphocyte depletion in order to test the hypothesis that aplastic anemia is autoimmune in origin. Three patients with pure red cell aplasia were also treated to test the effectiveness of this regimen in patients with a better documented autoimmune disorder (9). The presence of cellular or humoral suppressors of hematopoiesis was determined in an attempt to correlate the effects of treatment with laboratory measurements.

MATERIALS AND METHODS

The protocol was approved for use in patients by the Clinical Research Subpanel of the National Heart, Lung, and Blood Institute. Patients with aplastic anemia fulfilled the criteria for severe disease (10) and were not candidates for bone marrow transplantation. Patients with pure red cell aplasia were dependent on transfusions; these patients either had failed to respond to or had relapsed on conventional immunosuppressive therapy.

Treatment Protocol

All patients received cyclophosphamide, 2 mg/kg/day orally, and prednisone, 1 mg/kg/day orally, for the 1-month period of treatment. All patients with pure red cell aplasia received plasma exchange in combination with cyclophosphamide and prednisone. Patients with aplastic anemia were randomized to receive either a 3-liter plasma exchange, three times weekly, or depletion of 4×10^9 lymphocytes three times weekly, for a period of 1 month. Fresh frozen plasma was selected as replacement solution in order to maintain near normal levels of plasma coagulation factors in these severely thrombocytopenic patients. The anticoagulant used was ACD–NIH formula A. Plasma exchange was performed with either a continuous-flow or discontinuous-flow cell separator.

Blood counts, including reticulocytes and white cell differentials, clotting studies, and calcium were monitored three times weekly at the time of exchange. Complete serum chemistries, quantitative immunoglobulins, and complement levels were determined weekly. Skin testing using Keyhole limpet hemocyanin, tuberculin protein derivative, dermatophytin, and mumps antigens was performed at the initiation of the study, immediately following the 1-month period of treatment, and 2–3 months later. Peripheral blood was obtained weekly for determination of colony number.

In Vitro Analysis of Hematopoiesis

Serum samples were obtained at intervals before, during, and following treatment for determination of inhibition of normal hematopoietic colony growth; coculture of patients and normal bone marrow samples were performed if adequate bone marrow could be aspirated from the aplastic patients. The erythroid and myeloid hematopoietic colonies were grown in methylcellulose as previously described (11).

Results of both serum and coculture inhibition are presented as percentage inhibition of the normal bone marrow colony formation in the absence of serum inhibitor or added bone marrow cells from patients.

RESULTS

Clinical Effects

The population of patients treated was heterogeneous by clinical criteria (Table 1). The duration of time between the onset of symptoms and diagnosis and the

TABLE 1. *Clinical characteristics of treated patients*

Pt. no./ sex/age	Diagnosis	Etiologic associations	Time: onset symptoms to diagnosis	Time: diagnosis to apheresis	Previous R$_x$ and response
1/M/44	PRCA	Idiopathic	4 mos	98 mos	Pred and Chlor; transient response
2/F/40	PRCA	Evolved from AIHA	104 mos	192 mos	Refractory to pred; Cyclo
3/M/63	PRCA	Thymoma	5 mos	25 mos	Refractory to pred; Cyclo;
4/F/31	AA	Chemical exposure?	3 mos	20 mos	Androgens: failed
5/M/59	AA	Eosinophilic fasciitis	3 mos	5 mos	Pred, Vin: failed
6/F/21	AA	Hepatitis	6 days	4 wks	
7/M/22	AA	Idiopathic	2 wks	5 wks	
8/M/20	AA	Trinitro-toluene	4 mos	14 mos	Androgens, steroids: failed
9/M/23	AA	Idiopathic	2 mos	2 wks	

PRCA, pure red cell aplasia; AA, aplastic anemia; AIHA, autoimmune hemolytic anemia; Pred, prednisone; Chlor, chlorambucil; Cyclo, cyclophosphamide; Vin, vincristine.

interval between diagnosis and treatment by apheresis was highly variable. Some patients were treated immediately after diagnosis. Others had been clinically stable for years following diagnosis and prior to entry into the study, despite severe pancytopenia and dependence on red blood cell and platelet transfusions. Some of the patients with aplastic anemia had been treated with an androgen without improvement. The 3 patients with pure red cell aplasia had all been treated with chlorambucil or cyclophosphamide with either no effect or only a transient response. All patients with aplastic anemia fulfilled the criteria for severe disease by peripheral blood counts and bone marrow cellularity. One patient with pure red cell aplasia had had an unusual hematologic picture, having evolved from autoimmune hemolytic anemia to pure red cell aplasia with mild depression of her platelet count; her bone marrow cellularity was hypoplastic on biopsy, possibly related to a previous course of intensive treatment with cyclophosphamide.

Peripheral blood counts before and immediately after treatment for all the patients are shown in Fig. 1. All 3 patients with pure red cell aplasia responded to therapy. A large increase in reticulocyte number was seen for 2 of the 3 patients with pure red cell aplasia. In patient 1, who showed the most dramatic response, the hematocrit and bone marrow returned to normal and the serum inhibitor disappeared. In patient 2, a response was demonstrated by a prolonged, sustained decrease in red blood cell transfusion requirement by about 25%; her reticulocyte count and bone marrow morphology did not change. In the third patient, who died of cirrhosis shortly after the discontinuation of a 2-week course of plasma exchange, cyclophosphamide,

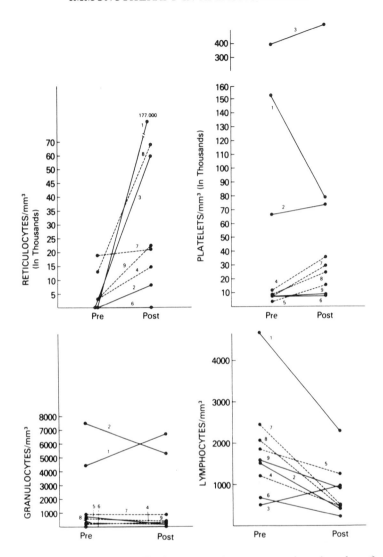

FIG. 1. Blood counts in patients. Pretherapy counts are averaged numbers from the week preceding treatment, posttherapy counts are averaged for the 2-week period after discontinuation of apheresis. Patients 1, 2, and 3 were diagnosed as having pure red cell aplasia; patients 4–9 had aplastic anemia. *Solid lines,* patients treated with plasmapheresis; *broken lines,* patients who underwent lymphocyte depletion. All patients were treated with cyclophosphamide and prednisone.

and prednisone, a reticulocytosis and reappearance of normoblasts in the bone marrow was apparent.

In contrast, most of the patients with aplastic anemia did not respond to immunotherapy. As shown in Fig. 1, granulocyte counts did not change and platelet counts increased only slightly. In 1 patient (no. 5), in whom aplastic anemia was associated with eosinophilic fasciitis, there was no response either to a course of plasma exchange in combination with vincristine performed at another hospital or to treatment with lymphocyte depletion on this protocol (Table 2). A single patient (no. 8) did show a sustained improvement in blood counts following treatment. He had an usual course prior to therapy, which included fluctuating reticulocyte counts, hemoglobin, and white blood counts on intermittent prednisone therapy.

Tolerance of Immunotherapy

The drug and apheresis regimens were remarkably well tolerated by all patients, even those with severe pancytopenia at the onset of treatment. No significant bleeding was associated with the apheresis procedures. Only 1 patient demonstrated an allergic response to plasma, and he was then treated with lymphocyte depletion (no. 8). Arteriovenous fistulae were placed in 2 patients prior to the initiation of therapy to improve venous access; these patients were maintained on low dose salicylate therapy for its anticoagulant effect during the course of treatment without excessive bleeding. Complications of therapy are listed in Table 2.

Immunosuppressive Effects

Three of the six patients with aplastic anemia and two of the three patients with pure red cells aplasia were anergic prior to treatment. In patients in whom skin test reactivity was present prior to treatment, all skin tests were negative at the termination of immunosuppressive therapy. In all patient groups, there was a decline in the absolute number of lymphocytes (Fig. 1, lower right graph), but no change in the relative proportion of T and B lymphocytes as determined by E-cell rosetting. Immunoglobulin levels were either unchanged or mildly decreased in patients following plasma exchange, due to replacement with fresh frozen plasma. IgG and IgM levels were mildy decreased following lymphocyte depletion alone, but these differences were not statistically significant.

TABLE 2. *Clinical course*

Pt. no./R_x	Complications	Outcome
1/PE	None	Return to normal of hemoglobin and bone marrow for 6 wks, then relapse
2/PE	None	↓ Transfusion requirement for 2 mos
3/PE	None	Reticulocytosis, normoblasts in BM. Death due to cirrhosis after 2 wks of plasmapheresis
4/LD	None	Mild decrease in white count
5/LD	None	Death due to aortic aneurysm rupture
6/PE	A-V shunt infection	Death due to sepsis
7/LD	None	Partial recovery >10 mos after R_x
8/LD	Allergy to plasma	Partial recovery 2 wks after R_x
9/PE	Hepatitis	No change

PE, plasma exchange; LD, lymphocyte depletion.

In Vitro Studies

The number of colonies present in bone marrow and peripheral blood in patients with aplastic anemia was small, as has been reported in other studies (1) (Table 3). Erythroid but not myeloid colonies were also decreased in number in the 3 patients with pure red cell aplasia. No patients, even those who improved clinically by peripheral blood counts and bone marrow appearance, showed a significant change in the number of BFU-E or CFU-E in peripheral blood or bone marrow.

The distribution of serum inhibitors and cellular inhibitors of normal hemopoiesis was heterogenous among the patients treated (Table 3). Some patients showed only evidence of serum inhibition, others only evidence of cellular inhibition, and some patients showed evidence of both or neither. Improvement in patients with pure red cell aplasia could be correlated with the decline or disappearance of a serum inhibitor of bone marrow erythroid colony formation. For example, patient 1 showed a decline in an inhibitor of BFU-E derived colony formation from 68% pretreatment to 30% posttreatment inhibition and patient 2 from 69% to 20%. Decrease in serum inhibitors in the patients with aplastic anemia were not related to clinical changes. Moderate decreases in inhibitors were measured in patients 6 and 8 (82–68% and 69–48% inhibition of bone marrow burst formation). Both patients were untransfused at the time of the initial serum sampling. In patient 4, who had received frequent transfusions before treatment, serum inhibition of normal hematopoiesis declined from 53% to 0. None of these patients showed a clinical response to therapy.

Coculture inhibition experiments were not performed in all patients because of difficulty in obtaining adequate bone marrow specimens. Nevertheless, in the single patient with aplasia whose blood counts improved following treatment, coculture inhibition of normal hematopoiesis, present prior to therapy, could not be demon-

TABLE 3. *Colony studies*

Pt. no.	Bone marrow (colonies/10^5 nuc cells)[a]			Serum inhibitor (% normal bone marrow growth)		Coculture inhibition (% nl bone marrow growth only)	
	CFU-E	BFU-E	CFU-C	BFU-E	CFU-C	BFU-E	CFU-C
1	192	26	nd	32	nd	nd	nd
2	nd	19	nd	31	—	64	0
3	0	16	14				
4	0	4	nd	47	nd	DT	DT
5	0	7	nd	95	nd	DT	DT
6	0	0	0	18	nd	19	18
7	192	6	2	31	nd	DT	DT
8	12	0	nd	75	100	63	43
9	4	1.5	11	76	89	39	45

nd, not done; DT, dry tap.
[a]Bone marrow colonies, normal range: CFU-E, 413 ± 293; BFU-E, 62 ± 47; CFU-C, 65 ± 24

strated during remission on testing against the same normal target bone marrow cells.

DISCUSSION

An empirical trial of immunotherapy was undertaken to test the hypothesis that aplastic anemia has an immune basis. Previous studies have shown that this form of treatment is effective in patients with autoimmune disorders. Apheresis and immunosuppressive drugs have obvious advantages compared with antithymocyte globulin, various nonstandardized preparations of which have been administered in different doses and schedule regimens. Interpretation of studies performed with antithymocyte globulin has also been confused by concurrent treatment with androgens and infusion of heterologous mismatched bone marrow in some patients.

Due to randomization between the two arms of the protocol, lymphocyte depletion and plasma exchange, only a small number of patients were treated with each therapy, and extrapolation to large groups must be undertaken with caution. However, other studies have suggested that the effects of these two therapies on immunological function and pathologic processes are similar. Both lymphocyte depletion and plasma exchange have been reported to produce equivalent effects on plasma proteins (12,13), and clinical improvement has been reported in some series following either plasma exchange or lymphocyte depletion (14).

In the current study, all 3 patients with pure red cell aplasia demonstrated a hematologic response. However, none showed the sustained, dramatic improvement reported in a single patient following a few courses of plasma exchange by Messner et al. (15). The complete recovery of their patient after a more limited number of plasma exchanges is especially notable as their therapy did not include cylophosphamide and prednisone. In contrast, in our study improvement was complete but transient in only 1 patient and incomplete in the others. These results suggest that plasma exchange may not be curative in most patients with pure red cell aplasia refractory to conventional treatment.

Our results also are in contrast to those of Abdou et al. (16). Their studies compared the results of a variety of treatments in a heterogenous population of patients with aplastic anemia. Of 21 patients, 3 exhibited serum activity, which inhibited myeloid colony formation. Each was treated with plasmapheresis consisting of six exchanges on alternative days followed by cytotoxic drug therapy. Partial or complete remissions were reported in all 2 of these patients. However, two had associated defined immunological disorders, systemic lupus erythematosus and cryoglobulinemia. In our own study, a desire to initiate treatment as soon as possible and a lack of confidence in the predictive reliability of *in vitro* assays forestalled matching treatment protocol with assay results. However, we treated 2 patients in whom a serum inhibitor was documented. One with eosinophilic fasciitis (17) diagnosed on muscle biopsy failed to respond to either plasmapheresis or lymphocyte depletion. A second patient with hepatitis-associated aplastic anemia had a potent plasma inhibitor of colony formation, but also failed to respond to plasmapheresis.

A single patient with aplastic anemia did show clinical improvement following lymphocyte depletion, cyclophosphamide, and prednisone. As noted above, this patient had several atypical features including prior improvement in hematocrit and reticulocyte count on prednisone alone, although reversal of bone marrow inhibition of colony formation observed during our treatment protocol is consistent with the possibility that his remission was related to the removal of a suppressor population of lymphocytes. Three other patients treated with lymphocyte depletion exhibited no response, although coculture studies *in vitro* were not done in all cases. Both this study and that of Abdou et al. (16) reflect the heterogeneity of aplastic anemia and the unpredictability of various forms of therapy.

Unfortunately, the reasons for failure of a particular therapeutic regimen may be multiple. It is possible that patients with aplastic anemia do have an autoimmune-mediated suppression of their bone marrow, but that this suppression results in either quantitative or qualitative effects on stem cells makes recovery of normal bone marrow function unlikely. The reported success of treatment with antithymocyte globulin would argue against this hypothesis, however (1). Second, the nature of the immune phenomena in aplastic anemia may be different from antibody-mediated diseases such as pure red cell aplasia, myasthenia gravis, and Goodpasture's syndrome. For example, a cell–cell effect that is local to the bone marrow may not be affected at all by administration of drugs or depletion of peripheral blood of T lymphocytes. Third, the basis of the response in other disorders to plasmapheresis or lymphocyte depletion may not be related to the obvious removal of lymphocytes or antibody, but secondary to some other effect, such as unblocking of the reticuloendothelial system.

In conclusion, plasma exchange and lymphocyte depletion in combination with cyclophosphamide and prednisone cannot be recommended for patients with aplastic anemia. It may have a role in the treatment of some patients with refractory pure red cell aplasia, but uniformly dramatic recovery should not be anticipated. Second, patients with aplastic anemia can tolerate a significant degree of immunosuppression. Finally, caution must be exercised in the interpretation of *in vitro* culture studies for both the pathogenesis and therapy of aplastic anemia.

REFERENCES

1. Young, N. : Aplastic anemia: Research themes, clinical issues. In: *Progress in Hematology, Vol. XII*, edited by E. Brown, p. 227. Grune and Stratton, NY.
2. Speck, B. (1979): Treatement of aplastic anemia by antilymphocyte globulin with or without marrow infusion. *Clin. Hematol.*, 7:611.
3. Nissen, C., Cornu, P., Gratwohl, A., and Speck, B. (1980): Peripheral blood cells from patients with aplastic anemia in partial remission suppress growth of their own bone marrow precursors in culture. *Br. J. Haematol.*, 45:233.
4. Dau, P., Lindstrom, J., Cassel, C., Denys, E., Shev, E., and Spitler, L. (1977): Plasmapheresis and immunosuppressive drug therapy in myasthenia gravis. *N. Engl. J. Med.*, 297:1134.
5. Rosenblatt, S. G., Knight, W., Bannayer, G. A., et al. (1979): Treatment of Goodpasture's syndrome with plasmapheresis. *Am. J. Med.*, 66:68.
6. Branda, R. F., McCullough, J. J., Tate, D. Y., and Jacobs, H. S. (1978): Plasma exchange in the treatment of fulminant idiopathic (autoimmune) thrombocytopenic purpura. *Lancet*, i:688.

7. Taft, E. G., Propp, R. P., and Sullivan, S. A. (1977): Plasma exchange in cold agglutinin hemolytic anemia. *Transfusion*, 17:173.

8. Pineda, A. A., Taswell, H. F., and Bowie, E. J. W. (1975): Treatment of life-threatening haemorrhage due to acquired factor VIII inhibitor. *Blood*, 46:535.

9. Krantz, S. B., and Zaentz, S. D. (1977): Pure red cell aplasia. In: *The Year in Hematology—1977*, edited by A. S. Gordon, R. Silber, and J. LoBue, p. 153. Plenum, New York.

10. Camitta, B. M., Thomas, E. D., Nathan, D. G., et al. (1976): Severe aplastic anemia: A prospective study of the effect of early marrow transplantation on acute mortality. *Blood*, 48:63.

11. Ogawa, M., Parmley, R. T., Bank, H. L., and Spicer, S. S. (1976): Human marrow erythropoiesis in culture. I. Characterization of methylcellulose colony assay. *Blood*, 48:407.

12. Karsh, J., Wright, D. G., Klippel, J. H., Decker, J. L., Deisseroth, A. B., and Flye, M. W. (1979): Lymphocyte depletion by continuous flow centrifugation in rheumatoid arthritis: Clinical effects. *Arthritis Rheum.*, 22:1055.

13. Koepke, J. A., Wu, K. K., Hoak, J. C., and Thompson, J. S. (1976): Effects of long-term plasmapheresis on plasma proteins. *Transfusion*, 16:191.

14. Wallace, D. J., Goldfinger, D., Gatti, R., Lowe, C., Fan, P., Bluestone, R., and Klinenberg, J. R. (1979): Plasmapheresis and lymphoplasmapheresis in the management of rheumatoid arthritis. *Arthritis Rheum.*, 22:703.

15. Messner, H. A., Fauser, A. A., Curtis, J. E., and Dotten, D. (1981): Control of antibody-mediated pure red-cell aplasia by plasmapheresis. *N. Engl. J. Med.*, 304:1334.

16. Abdou, N. I., Verdirame, J. D., Amare, M., and Abdou, N. (1981): Heterogeneity of pathogentic mechanisms in aplastic anemia. *Ann. Intern. Med.*, 95:43.

17. Hoffman, R., Dainiak, N., Sibrack, L., Pober, J. S., and Waldron, J. A., Jr. (1979): Antibody-mediated aplastic anemia and diffuse fasciitis. *N. Engl. J. Med.*, 300:718.

Plasmapheresis, edited by Y. Nosé, P. S.
Malchesky, J. W. Smith, and R. S. Krakauer.
Raven Press, New York © 1983.

Plasma Exchange in Myeloma Renal Failure

J. P. Pourrat, J. M. Dueymes, J. J. Conte, *O. Pourrat,
*D. Alcalay, *G. Touchard, and *D. Patte

*Service de Néphrologie et d'Hémodialyse, C.H.U. Toulouse-Purpan, and *Service de
Réanimation Médicale et de Néphrologie, C.H.U. Poitiers, France*

Renal failure is reported to occur in about 50% of patients with multiple myeloma (1–3) and to be associated with poor prognosis. Renal disease often progresses to end-stage renal insufficiency and eventually hemodialysis (4,5); uremia is the cause of death in 14–21% of autopsied myeloma cases (1,3).

Multiple factors have been incriminated in myeloma renal failure, but nephrotoxicity of circulating monoclonal light chains appears to be the prominent mechanism (2,6). Therefore a therapeutic effect might be expected from plasma exchange.

Plasma exchange therapy has already been reported to be efficient in myeloma renal failure (7–12), but the precise role of plasma exchange in the observed beneficial effects remains unclear, since exchanges have been usually associated with other treatments. The purpose of this study was: (a) to report results of plasma exchange therapy in 13 patients with myeloma renal failure: (b) to delineate the role of plasma exchanges from the role of the associated treatments; and (c) to define the conditions of therapeutic effect in order to design an optimal protocol for a further controlled study.

PATIENTS AND METHODS

Patients

Thirteen consecutive patients presenting with severe renal failure (plasma creatinine > 350 μmoles/liter) were included in the study. They included 10 men and 3 women, aged 62 ± 13 years (33–78 years). All patients fulfilled diagnostic criteria for multiple myeloma (South-West Oncology Group) (13).

A monoclonal abnormality was found in serum of all patients, and was identified as IgGκ, IgGλ, IgAλ or κ-light chain in, respectively, 4, 4, 2, and 3 patients. Bone marrow aspirations showed more than 10% abnormal plasma cells in all patients, and more then 30% in 7/13. Lytic bone lesions were found in 11/13 patients by roentgenogram of the skull. Hypercalcemia was present in 7 patients (2.60–3.75 mmoles/liter). All patients were anemic (5.5–12.0 g/dl hemoglobin), and 4 had thrombocytopenia below 150,000 elements/mm^3.

Bence Jones proteinuria was found in all patients but 1, and corresponding light chain could be found in the serum of 7. The only patient without urinary light chain presented with a proteinuria (1.2 g/24 hr) composed mostly of the monoclonal IgG.

Renal function was severely impaired in all patients (350–1,580 μmoles/liter; mean : 705). Two patients presented with oliguria, and one patient was anuric. Three patients needed an urgent hemodialysis for life-threatening disorders, but only one had to be dialyzed a second time.

In 9 patients the diagnosis of renal failure and myeloma were made simultaneously. In the other 4, multiple myeloma had been previously diagnosed but only 2 patients were treated with chemotherapy. One more patient presented in association untreated chronic myeloid leukemia with phi-chromosome.

In all patients renal failure had been discovered shortly before referral (less than 1 week), and no recent precipitating factor (e.g., radiocontrast agent) could be found.

Treatment

Patients were treated with chemotherapy in all cases. Schedules were always of the intermittent type and the most frequent were: corticosteroids–melphalan–vincristin–cyclophosphamide (8 cases) and corticosteroids–melphalan (2 cases). In all cases, doses of melphalan were reduced according to the degree of renal failure. Chemotherapy was started as soon as possible in all cases, and daily doses were given after the completion of every procedure when a course of daily exchanges was proceeding.

In all patients the possibility of functional renal failure was considered, and treatment included volume repletion (monitored by central venous pressure measurement in 9/13), urate oxidase in the 12 patients with hyperuricemia, and symptomatic measures against hypercalcemia, including mithramycin, in 5 cases. At the same time, forced diuresis was started, with the use of furosemide (0.5–1 g/day in 8 patients) and alkali (sodium bicarbonate 100–200 mEq/day in 9 patients). Urinary pH was measured in these patients and kept above 7 when possible.

Plasma Exchanges

Plasma exchanges were only started when creatininemia appeared stable or rising with previous treatment, except in cases of hemodialyzed patients. At every procedure, 60 ml/kg body weight of plasma were exchanged using fresh frozen plasma or albumin solutions of various concentrations (2.6–3.6 g/dl). Cell separators were IBM 2997 (76 cases) and Haemonetics Model 30 (31 cases). In the 13 patients, 107 exchanges were performed in various schedules: 18 courses of 2–12 exchanges in 2–30 days (2 patients had 3 courses each).

RESULTS

All patients tolerated well rehydration and forced diuresis treatment, as well as the first course of chemotherapy. The effect on renal impairment was moderate only, mean creatinine being 629 μmoles/liter before and 616 μmoles/liter after the 2–12 days of this treatment (10 patients).

Plasma exchanges were always well tolerated. Their effect on serum monoclonal component has been measured in 17 occasions: In all cases postexchange values were under 50% of preexchange values. In the absence of exchange on the following days, values returned towards preexchange values in 2–3 days.

The effects of plasma exchanges on creatinine values are summarized in Table 1. Postcourse values were lower than precourse values in all cases but one; this case (patient 5, 3rd course) corresponded to the terminal phase of a κ-light chain myeloma, with chemotherapy resistance and recurrent hypercalcemia resistant to mithramycin.

When restricted to the 13 initial courses of each patient, creatinine values decreased in all cases, from 695 ± 225 to 543 ± 208 μmoles/liter. Hemodialysis could be stopped in all 3 patients who had needed it.

Creatinine values at 3 months after the course of plasma exchange could be evaluated in 10 patients: in 4 patients, a return to or above the starting level was observed. These 4 patients presented other signs of chemotherapy resistance (re-

TABLE 1. *Summary of creatinine values before and after initial treatment, after plasma exchange course, and 3 months later*

Patient			Creatinine values[b]					
No.	Sex/age	MCC[a]	C0	D	C1	N	C2	C3
1	M/70	IgGλ	683	0	683	5	484	191
2	M/50	IgGκ	720	4	700	10	400	293
3	F/74	IgAλ	653	5	806	5	500	
4	M/55	IgGκ	HD	8	HD	6	875	
5	M/32	κ	410	2	375	11	180	670
					980	4	670	
					680	3	920	
6	M/70	IgGλ	1200	2	750	2	410	280
					640	6	599	
7	M/68	κ	450	5	431	12	484	
8	M/62	IgGκ	350	2	365	4	318	980
9	M/56	IgGκ	450	0	450	4	360	170
10	M/50	IgGλ	377	0	377	2	220	150
11	F/62	κ	865	12	784	10	600	650
					950	5	630	
					890	2	755	
12	M/78	IgAλ	761	3	991	10	693	281
13	F/78	IgGλ	877	3	962	6	680	739

[a]MCC, monoclonal component.
[b]Creatinine values (μmoles/liter) before treatment (C0), after initial treatment (C1), after plasma exchange course (C2), and 3 months later (C3). D, duration (days) of preplasmapheresis treatment. N, number of plasma exchanges; HD, hemodialysis.

current hypercalcemia in 3/4 and rising monoclonal peak in 4/4), and died within 9 months after plasma exchange, not having needed hemodialysis.

At the present time, 7 of the patients are dead, and the 1-year survival rate is 45%.

DISCUSSION

Renal biopsy was obtained in only 1 patient who showed typical lesions of "myeloma kidney" (2,3,12). However we believe that all 13 patients of this study probably presented such lesions, as indicated by the presence of Bence Jones proteinuria, by the degree of renal failure, and by the poor results of initial treatment on the level of creatininemia (2,5).

Previous reports on plasma exchange therapy indicate in most cases a good effect on myeloma renal failure (7–12), and the most important question is that of causal relationship. We believe that the decrease in creatinine level observed in all our patients was due neither to chemotherapy nor to initial rehydration and forced diuresis treatment. Chemotherapy is known to be slow in action, and would not be able to produce an effect on renal function within 2–10 days (the duration of most exchange courses). Furthermore, some patients were treated with only plasma exchange while chemotherapy had been stopped for more than 1 month (Fig. 1).

Rehydration and forced diuresis were not responsible for creatinine decreasing after exchanges since creatinine level was stable or rising before the exchanges started. In 1 case, this delay was extended to 12 days (Fig. 2).

A survival rate of 45% at 1 year may appear poor, but is to be compared with data in matched patients: in Medical Research Council myeloma trials, mean survival in patients with blood urea levels >15 mmoles/liter after initial rehydration was 37 days (third trial) and 140 days (fourth trial) with adjunctive forced diuresis. Individual survival tables illustrate the bad prognosis associated with light chain myeloma (Fig. 3).

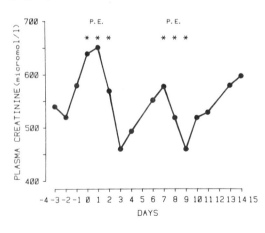

FIG. 1. Variations of creatinine level during a course of plasma exchange in a patient without chemotherapy (because of bone marrow insufficiency) (patient 6; 2nd course).

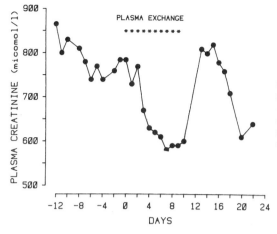

FIG. 2. Variations of creatinine level during a course of plasma exchange (patient 11): the start of plasma exchange was delayed up to 12 days after starting chemotherapy and forced diuresis treatment.

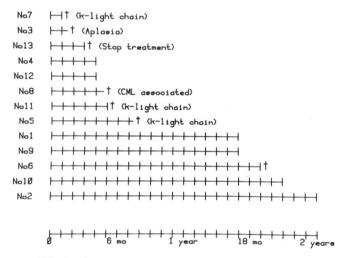

FIG. 3. Summary of individual survivals (+ indicates death).

CONCLUSION

Our results suggest that plasma exchange in itself is an efficient treatment of myeloma renal failure: a decrease in creatinine level is observed within a few days after starting the exchanges, and this decrease is probably not related to chemotherapy or to symptomatic treatment, according to the conditions of the study. The duration of this beneficial effect depends mostly on chemotherapy efficiency.

Plasma exchange therapy appears useful in cases of myeloma with severe renal failure: the need for hemodialysis is avoided, and any improvement in renal function may be important for the patient, in terms of chemotherapy tolerance and the duration of hospital stay. A suitable protocol might include two daily plasma exchanges of 60 ml/kg body weight performed as soon as possible after starting chemotherapy.

ACKNOWLEDGMENTS

The authors thank Prs. M. Alcalay, D. Bontoux, A. Fournie, J. Pris, J. Monnier, and Drs. Letourmy and Yver for referring patients, and Pr. J. Ducos, Dr. S. Bierme, and J. P. Calot for help in plasmapheresis.

REFERENCES

1. Kyle, R. A. (1975): Multiple myeloma: Review of 869 cases. *Mayo Clin. Proc.*, 50:29.
2. Defronzo, R. A., Cooke, C. R., Wright, J. R., and Humphreyy, R. L. (1978): Renal function in patients with multiple myeloma. *Medicine (Balt.)*, 57:151.
3. Kapadia, S. B. (1980): Multiple myeloma: A clinico-pathologic study of 62 consecutively autopsied cases. *Medicine (Balt.)*, 59:380.
4. Johnson, W. J., Kyle, R. A., and Dahlberg, P. J. (1980): Dialysis in the treatment of multiple myeloma. *Mayo Clin. Proc.*, 55:65.
5. Cosio, F. G., Pence, T. V., Sharpiro, F. L., and Kjellstrand, C. M. (1981): Severe renal failure in multiple myeloma. *Clin. Nephrol.*, 15:206.
6. Stone, M. J., and Frenkel, E. P. (1975): The clinical spectrum of light chain myeloma. *Am. J. Med.*, 58:601.
7. Feest, T. G., Burge, P. S., and Cohen, S. L. (1976): Successful treatment of myeloma kidney by diuresis and plasmapheresis. *Br. Med. J.*, 1:503.
8. Isbister, J. P., Biggs, J. C., and Penny, R. (1978): Experience with large volume plasmapheresis in malignant proteinaemia and immune disorders. *Aust. N. Z. J. Med.*, 8:154.
9. Powles, R. L., Smith, C., Kohn, J., and Hamilton-Fairley, G. (1971): Method of removing abnormal protein rapidly from patients with malignant paraproteinaemias. *Br. Med. J.*, 3:664.
10. Russel, J. A., Toy, J. L., and Powles, R. L. (1977): Plasma exchange in malignant paraprotein-aemias. *Exp. Haematol.*, 5(Suppl.):105.
11. Russel, J. A., Fitzharris, B. M., Corringham, R., Darcy, D. A., and Powles, R. L. (1978): Plasma exchange versus peritoneal dialysis for removing Bence Jones protein. *Br. Med. J.*, 4:1397.
12. Misiani, R., Remuzzi, G., Bertani, R., Licini, R., Levoni, P., Crippa, A., and Giuliano, M. (1979): Plasmapheresis in the treatment of acute renal failure in multiple myeloma. *Am. J. Med.*, 66:684.
13. Durie, B. G. M., and Salmon, S. E. (1977): Multiple myeloma, macroglobulinemia and mono-clonal gammapathies. In: *Recent Advances in Haematology*, edited by A. V. Hoffbrend, M. C. Brain, and J. Hirsh, no. 2. Churchill Livingstone, London.

Plasmapheresis, edited by Y. Nosé, P. S. Malchesky, J. W. Smith, and R. S. Krakauer. Raven Press, New York © 1983.

Treatment of Renal Failure with Elevated Levels of Circulating Immune Complexes: Technical and Clinical Considerations

A. Murisasco, *D. Bernard, G. Leblond, E. Montas, and †R. Elsen

*Hôpital Sainte Marguerite, 13274 Marseille, France; *Laboratoire d'Immunologie, Hôpital Nord, Marseille, France; †Cordis Dow, 1160 Brussels, Belgium*

MATERIAL

The plasma filter used during the present investigation is an experimental device manufactured by Cordis Dow Corporation and corresponds to the following device description. The Cordis Dow plasma filter is a 0.7-m^2 hollow fiber membrane device. The jacket and headers are the same as those in the commercial C-DAK 3,500 hemodialyzer. The membrane is of the microporous polyoleofin type; polyurethane resin is used to pot the fibers. The number of fibers in the device is 5,500, and the internal diameter of the fiber is about 270 μ. Total blood volume is about 75 ml. The experimental devices were sterilized using formaldehyde or gamma radiation, saline filled. The manufacturer specifies the following performance characteristics based on whole blood *in vitro* studies:

Sieving coefficients: S albumin = 0.8, S globulin = 0.8, S globulin = 0.9, S total protein = 0.8.

Typical *in vivo* plasma filtration rate is approximately 20–40 ml/min at Q_B = 200 ml/min and TMP = 50 mmHg. Blood volume is 75 ml average.

METHODS

We have made some modifications to conventional dialysis equipment to allow plasma filtration with the same degree of safety as dialysis. With these modifications the machine can still be used for hemodialysis. The disposable extracorporeal blood circuit is identical as for hemodialysis. The eliminated plasma is collected in a sterile plastic bag. The infusion is made through the venous bubble trap (Fig. 1). The infusion fluid is brought to body temperature using a heat exchanger with circulating dialysate fluid.

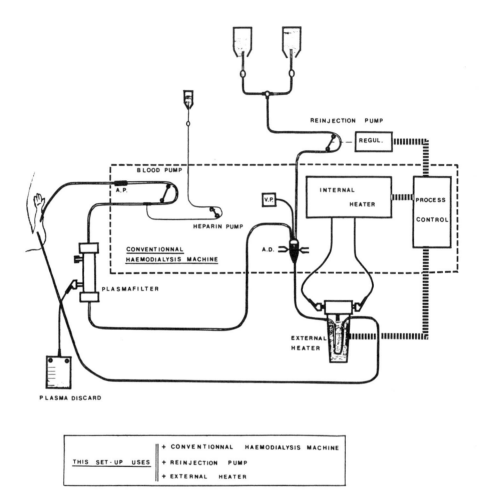

FIG. 1. Schematic of plasma filtration circuit using conventional hemodialysis machine.

A safety control cuts off dialysate circulation in the heat exchanger when the temperature is outside the limits of 35–41°C. Other alarms included are shown in Fig. 2.

Preparation of the session includes the following steps. (a) The plasma filter is primed with saline, avoiding infusion of air into the filter. The last bottle of priming saline is rewarmed to 37°C and contains 4,000 IU heparin. (b) During the session of plasma filtration, we stop the filtration for 2 min while changing the infusing bottle. This procedure improves the filtration rate from the average specified by Cordis Dow (between 20 and 40 ml/min) to 50–60 ml/min.

ALARMS	REACTIONS		
	BUZZER SOUNDS	REINJECTION PUMP BLOOD PUMP STOP	BY PASS DIALYSATE
AIR DETECTOR	✸	✸	
ARTERIAL PRESSURE	✸	✸	
VENOUS PRESSURE	✸	✸	
HIGH TEMPERATURE DIALYSATE	✸		✸
LOW TEMPERATURE DIALYSATE	✸		✸

FIG. 2. Outline of alarm conditions and system response.

The filtration is at a constant rate; this allows isovolumetric elimination of plasma and infusion of plasma substitute. This regular infusion is controlled manually at present. The Y connection reduces bottle manipulation, and changes of bottles can be carried out in good conditions with less risk of contamination. Substitution fluids used are 6% albumin, Ringer's lactate, or dissolved lyophilized plasma. Blood flow rate in the ECC is 200 ml/min. We administer continuous heparinization at the inlet of the plasma filter. The duration of the plasma filtration session is from 30 to 60 min.

RESULTS

We report the clinical course of 2 patients treated by this technique.

Case 1

A 27-year-old man, Mr. R., was admitted to the hospital for acute renal disease with oliguria. He had been unwell for several weeks, with arthralgia, fever, and biological inflammation syndrome. Raised erythrocyte sedimentation rate (100) at the first hour, hyperfibrinemia, and hyper-α_2-globulinemia were found. Also, a marked deterioration of general health (asthenia, anorexia, sweating, loss of weight, normochromic anemia, normal renal function, and microscopic hematuria) was noted before the acute onset of renal failure.

The patient had no history of previous illness apart from repeated sore throats since childhood. Chest X-ray before admission showed a patchy infiltrate in both apices suggesting pulmonary TB, but no tubercule bacilli were found and a Mantoux test was negative at 10 units. Serial blood tests showed a deterioration in renal function and led to the patient's admission to the hospital.

This patient was initially treated symptomatically, particularly by hemodialysis. Several diagnoses were considered including Goodpasture's syndrome and rapidly progressive glomerulonephritis. Blood tests confirmed previous findings but no firm diagnosis could be made.

He subsequently developed a Mickulicz syndrome, with circulating immune complexes, indicating the involvement of autoimmune process. He was therefore treated with prednisone

1 mg/kg/day. Other immunological tests were normal: immunoglobulin levels, complement levels, and lupus erythematosus cells. A KVIEM test ultimately proved negative.

The investigation of the proteinuria when the diuresis reappeared showed an important defect of glomerular permeability (nonselective proteinuria with light chains).

In view of this clinical picture, 22 sessions of plasma filtration were carried out in 4 months in association with hemodialysis and corticotherapy (Fig. 3). Circulating immune complexes disappeared after this time. After 3 months there was complete recovery of renal function with clearing of the chest X-ray appearance. A precise diagnosis was not obtained because the patient refused renal and lung biopsies.

Case 2

The second patient, Mr. B. (29 years old), was admitted to the hospital for severe renal disease. Treatment of this patient included appropriate diet, exchange resins (Kayexalate), and diuretics.

A hemorrhagic pleurisy appeared 15 days later, and the patient was admitted to the nephrology department. He displayed the following clinical symptoms and signs: diffuse arthralgia, abdominal pain, a painful hepatosplenomegaly, axillary and inguinal lymph nodes, blood pressure 120/80 mmHg, normal auscultation of heart and lungs, and diuresis 1,000 ml/24 hr. The biochemical abnormalities found were: urea 0.38 g/100 ml, creatinine 15 mg/

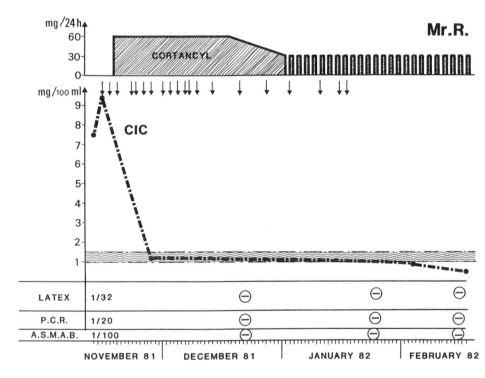

FIG. 3. Course of plasma filtration therapy and resulting changes of circulating immune complexes in patient Mr. R.

100 ml, plasma phosphate 2.2 mg/100 ml, plasma calcemia 7 mg/100 ml, and plasma uric acid 6 mg/100 ml.

This patient was treated by hemodialysis. Further investigation found the following conditions:

Kidneys: Creatinine clearance 6 ml/min. Extraction rate of white blood cells in urine 40,000/ml/min. Normal kidney and urinary tract on ultrasound; quantitative scintigraphy: no renal fixation.

Lung: Restrictive lung insufficiency with reduced alveolocapillary diffusion.

GI system: Gall bladder calculi, hiatal hernia, hypertrophic duodenal folds.

Otorhinolaryngology: Bilateral lack of vestibular response.

Hematology: Mixed normochromic normocytic anemia with renal disease and eterozygotis drepanocytosis.

Marrow biopsy: Rich marrow with granular hyperplasia, delayed maturation and toxic granulation.

Sequestration studies showed intrasplenic uptake with no involvement of the liver.

Immunology: Latex test, antileukocytes and antithrombocyte antibodies, anti-smooth muscle, circulatory immunocomplexes were positive. C3, C4, C3pa, IgA, and IgM were decreased, IgG was increased.

There was some improvement with hemodialysis 18 hr weekly. After 3 months a severe hyperthermic syndrome developed with no evidence of infection. Nevertheless, Bactrim was given.

This patient rapidly developed red and white cell lines and marrow dysplasia. At this point we immediately changed his treatment: Bactrim was stopped, and treatment continued with 18 hr hemodialysis/week, prednisone 1 mg/kg/day, and plasma filtration 4,000 ml/week (Fig. 4). There was rapid improvement. The temperature became normal, hepatomegaly and splenomegaly disappeared; weight, asthenia, anemia, and leukopenia were corrected. In addition, circulating immune complexes became negative, complement became normal, and IgG, IgA, and IgM normalized.

This patient is in good condition. The kidney is not functional although diuresis is 1,500 ml/24 hr. The prednisone was progressively reduced and stopped. Only hemodialysis and plasma filtration are continued.

COMMENTS

Case Histories

In both cases we can accept the *a priori* diagnosis of circulating immune complex disease, since the existence of these complexes was established in each case. Nevertheless this point requires discussion, because the specificity of the polyethylene glycol technique is not absolute; in fact, aggregated immunoglobulins, particularly IgM and complement, can give false positive results.

In the first case there was associated lung disease and acute renal disease. The diagnosis suggested was Goodpasture's syndrome, but even if the absence of hemoptysis does not eliminate Goodpasture's syndrome, the apical presentation of the lung lesion is not convincing; finally, Goodpasture's syndrome is not a circulating immune complex disease. But a similar syndrome associated with different lung pictures and renal disease was described with circulating immune complex disease.

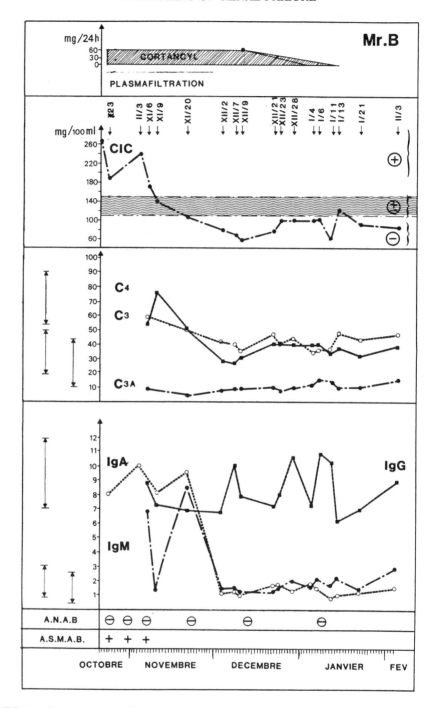

FIG. 4. Course of plasma filtration therapy and resulting changes in circulating immune complexes, complement components, and immunoglobulins in patient Mr. B.

In the second case rapidly progressive glomerulonephritis (proteinuria, progressive renal insufficiency) developed in a few weeks. A generalized disease affecting several organs and tissues suggested general disease with circulating immune complexes. First, the marrow disease should be considered. The discovery of anti-white and anti-platelet antibodies was linked to the marrow disease. It was difficult to ascertain whether the main cause could be attributed to the immunological disorder or to the toxic effect of Bactrim.

Corticotherapy was associated with plasma filtration in 2 cases. The role of each treatment is difficult to ascertain. In the first case, after 22 plasma filtration sessions, an apparently complete recovery of the lung and kidney lesion was obtained. In the second case, with 10 plasma filtration sessions, the biochemical signs disappeared. The patient is in apparently good health with normal-sized kidney, but renal function has not recovered.

CONCLUSION

The association of corticoid therapy, plasma filtration, and hemodialysis allowed removal of circulating immune complexes from the circulation, normalization of complement and immunoglobulin levels, and recovery of diuresis with total recovery of renal function in 1 case. The experimental Cordis Dow plasma filter proved to be a safe and efficient device, and the technique employed, simple and easy to implement.

Plasmapheresis, edited by Y. Nosé, P. S.
Malchesky, J. W. Smith, and R. S. Krakauer.
Raven Press, New York © 1983.

Plasma Exchange in Immune Thrombocytopenic Purpura

*†V. Blanchette, *V. Hogan, and *§G. Rock

*Canadian Red Cross, Blood Transfusion Service, Ottawa Centre,
†Children's Hospital of Eastern Ontario, and §University of Ottawa,
Ottawa, Ontario K1S 3E2, Canada

The role of plasma exchange in the management of patients with immune thrombocytopenic purpura (ITP) remains to be defined. ITP is an immune-mediated disorder in which antibody or immune complex-coated platelets are destroyed prematurely in the reticuloendothelial system, particularly the spleen. It is postulated that plasma exchange by removal of toxic serum factors may unblock the cycle of immunologic injury and result in clinical remission.

To date, however, the reported experience with plasma exchange therapy in ITP is small. In the largest reported series of 14 adult cases, the "exchange protocol" was not intensive and consisted of one to three single volume exchanges with an interval period of 3–10 days between exchanges. The results of that series are encouraging, since approximately 50% of cases with acute ITP entered a prolonged clinical remission and did not require splenectomy. No patients with chronic ITP resistant to splenectomy and steroids responded. Based on reported experience of plasma exchange therapy in other immunological diseases, we initiated a trial of intensive plasma exchange in 8 patients with ITP and found encouraging results in acute cases. Correlation with platelet antibody level was good.

CLINICAL MATERIALS AND METHODS

Patients

Eight patients with ITP (3 chronic, 5 acute) were studied. The diagnosis of ITP was made on the basis of thrombocytopenia, increased megakaryocytes in the bone marrow, and no alternative explanation for the thrombocytopenic state. The patients' clinical courses are detailed in Table 1.

Plasma Exchange Procedures

Patients were exchanged using either a Haemonetics Model 50 or IBM 2997 blood processor. Single plasma volumes were exchanged at each procedure and

TABLE 1. *Plasma exchange in acute ITP*

Patients Case/Age/Sex	Reason for exchange	Platelet count $\times$ 10³/μl		No. of exchanges	Total volume exchanged (liters)[a]
		Pre-exchange	Post-exchange		
1/56/F	Clinical bleeding	1	196	5	13.4 (10)
	Failed steroid R$_x$	3	118	8	24.4 (18)
2/37/F	Failed Steroid R$_x$ Presplenectomy	<10	114	6	18.3 (6)
3/29/F	Failed steroid R$_x$ Presplenectomy	77	156	4	9 (4)
4/63/M	Failed steroid R$_x$ Presplenectomy	50	146	3	9.2 (3)
5/16/M	Steroid dependent	17	18	6	15 (8)
6/17/F	Steroid dependent	16	10	7	20.5
7/67/F	Clinical bleeding	3	318	4	11.7 (5)
8/15/M	Failed steroid R$_x$	26	180	5	12.5 (8)
Mean				5.3	14.9 (8.2)

[a]Numbers in parentheses indicate period over which exchanges were performed (days).

TABLE 2.

Case	Diagnosis	Platelet bound antibody level (PAIgG)[a]		Serum antiplatelet antibody level[b]		Responded to plasma exchange
		Pre	Post	Pre	Post	
1	Acute ITP	89	nd	B/T% 1.1	B/T% 3.8	Yes
2	Acute ITP	90	7.2	2.7	3.3	Yes
3	Acute ITP	32	6.5	1.1	3	Yes
4	Chronic ITP	50	20	3.3	2.5	Yes
5	Chronic ITP	54	43	9	7.1	No
6	Chronic ITP	>100	>100	8.6	6.3	No
7	Acute ITP	nd	nd	nd	nd	Yes
8	Acute ITP	77.5	9	1.5	7.5	Yes

nd, no data.
[a]Pre- and post-exchange values presented. PAIgG measured by complement lysis inhibition assay (N—<15 fg/platelet).
[b]Pre- and post-exchange values presented. Serum antiplatelet antibody measured by ^{125}I-staphylococcal protein A assay (N^{Bound}/total CPM 4–11%).

fresh frozen plasma was used as replacement fluid. Venous access was through peripheral veins in all cases. Details of the plasma exchange procedures together with patient's responses are detailed in Table 2.

Measurement of Antiplatelet Antibody Level

Platelet bound antibody (APIgG): A complement lysis inhibition assay was used to quantitate platelet bound immunoglobulin. Normal range = 8.4 ± 3.4 fg/platelet.

Serum antiplatelet antibody: A ^{125}I-labeled staphylococcal protein A assay was used to quantitate free serum antibody. Normal range (bound/total CPM) = 4–11%. Results are detailed in Table 2.

CONCLUSIONS

Intensive plasma exchange therapy produces a significant response in platelet count in most patients with acute ITP who have not responded to steroid therapy. In certain patients with ITP, the response to plasma exchange therapy is prolonged and the need for splenectomy avoided. Based on our experience, we suggest that an intensive course be used in testing this possibility. Changes in the level of platelet bound antibody, but not free serum antibody, correlate well with the clinical response to plasma exchange.

Plasmapheresis, edited by Y. Nosé, P. S. Malchesky, J. W. Smith, and R. S. Krakauer. Raven Press, New York © 1983.

Plasma Exchange in the Treatment of Rh Disease

*G. Rock, I. Lafreniere, L. Chan, and N. McCombie

*Canadian Red Cross, Blood Transfusion Service, Ottawa Centre, Ottawa, Ontario K1S 3E2 Canada; *Department of Medicine, University of Ottawa, Ottawa, Canada*

Women who are sensitized to the Rh antigen have few therapeutic avenues open to them should they become pregnant. Early delivery with neonatal exchange transfusion is possible only if the fetus survives the pregnancy without significant damage. While intrauterine transfusion can be used to provide the fetus with red cells during the pregnancy, the procedure has a high fetal mortality even in experienced hands. Early attempts to treat Rh-sensitized women with plasmapheresis were unsuccessful in reducing the titer of anti-D; however, the procedure was successful in reducing the titer in nonpregnant donors. This study utilized the Haemonetics Model 50 plasmapheresis machine to perform repeated plasma exchanges on sensitized women, and achieved gradual decreases in both antibody titer and quantity as well as in amniotic fluid spectrophotometric values which resulted from the treatment.

MATERIALS AND METHODS

Plasma exchange was initiated as early as possible, with 1.5–2-liter exchanges performed two to three times per week. Exchanges utilized fresh frozen plasma. Amniocentesis ± intrauterine transfusion was as indicated.

Antibody was quantitated according to the autoanalyzer technique of Moore et al.

IgG subclass was determined according to a modification of the method of Chown and Lewis, using specific subclass antisera obtained from the Central Laboratory of the Netherlands.

RESULTS

Antibody titer and quantity of antibody progressively decreased during treatment (Fig. 1, Table 1).

Serial monitoring of hematological and biochemical parameters indicated no significant change in hemoglobin, platelet count, prothrombin time, or partial throm-

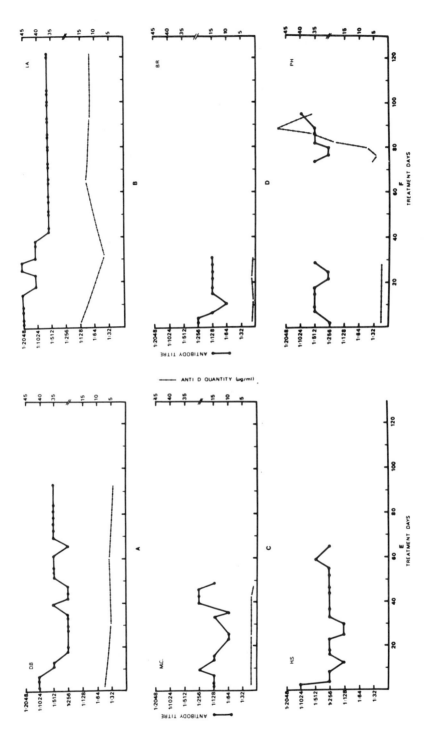

FIG. 1. Changes in antibody titer and quantity during the plasma exchange program.

TABLE 1. *Changes in hematological parameters following a plasma exchange program*

	Patient				
	M.C.	H.S.	I.A.	D.B.	B.R.
Blood group	A neg	A neg	B neg	A neg	A neg
Previous stillbirth(s) due to hemolytic disease of newborn	2	0	1	2	0
Father	A pos CDe/cde	O pos CDe/CDe Kell pos	B pos cDe/dce	A pos CDe/cDE	B pos CDe/cde
Beginning of therapy					
Weeks' gestation	27	26	11	13	34
Antibody	D	K	D,G	D	D
Titer	1:128	1:1024	1:2048	1:1024	1:256
Type	IgG	IgG	IgG	IgG	IgG
Quantity (μg/ml)	1.0	—	15.0	7.0	0.7
IgG subclass	1,2	1,2,3	1,2	1,2,3,4	1
At termination					
Weeks' gestation	33	35	28	26	39
Antibody	D	K	D,G	D	D
Titer	1:128	1:256	1:512	1:512	1:128
Type	IgG	IgG	IgG	IgG	IgG
Quantity (μg/ml)	0.6	—	9.0	4.0	0.4
IgG subclass	1,2	1,2,3	1,2	1,2,3,4	1
Liters exchanged	15.8	25.5	40.5	32.7	14.1
Child	A pos	A pos	B pos	A pos	B pos

boplastin time throughout the exchange program. Total protein and albumin decreased progressively in 2 patients. Little change in immunoglobulin level was noted and there was no change in IgG subclass.

TABLE 2. *Results of amniocentesis*

Pt	Gestation (weeks)	Titer	Quantity (μg/ml)	Liley classification zone	ΔOD	Ovenstone factor
M. C.	20	—	—	2B	0.15	21
	25	—	—	2A	0.19	29
	27	1:128	1.0	2A	0.18	26
	29.5	1:128	1.0	2A	0.13	20
	31	1:64	1.0	2A	0.10	17
I. A.	26.5	1:512	9	IB	0.42	58
D. B.	20	1:256	5	2A	0.34	43
	20.5	1:512	5	2A	0.37	48
H. S.	26	1:256	—	2B	0.14	20
	29.5	1:256	—	2A	0.11	16
	31	1:256	—	2B	0.07	14
B. R.	37	1:128	0.5	3	0.01	19

TABLE 3. *Fetal outcome*

Pt	IUT	Time	Fetal outcome
I. A.	1	26 weeks 6 days	Stillbirth 28 weeks 5 days, minimal but definite ascites
	2	28 weeks 4 days	
D. B.	1	22 weeks	Live birth 26 weeks 4 days, died sepsis in 48 hours, mild–moderate erythroblastosis
	2	23 weeks	
	3	26 weeks	
M. C.	0		Viable fetus, C section 33 weeks, 25 ml transfusion, cord: Coombs 3+
H. S.	0		Viable fetus, induction 35 weeks, 420 ml O neg K neg, cord: Coombs 3+
B .R.	0		Viable fetus, induction 39 weeks, 150 ml transfusion, cord: Coombs 3+

IUT, intrauterine transfusion.

No patients developed additional red cell antibodies or became positive for HB_sAg.

Results of amniocentesis (Table 2) showed improvement of change in optical density (ΔOD) in several patients during the treatment program. Four of the six patients delivered viable fetuses with Coombs positive cord blood specimens. Two of the patients had unsuccessful pregnancies with fetal death within 48 hr of intrauterine transfusion (Table 3).

CONCLUSIONS

Repeated plasma exchange is effective in reducing the antibody titer in sensitized women at risk of developing hemolytic disease of the newborn. There is a concomitant decrease in the quantity of antibody found in the plasma. None of the women developed additional antibodies during the plasma exchange program. None of the patients experienced marked alteration in hematological parameters. All patients remained negative for HB_sAg and anti-HB_sAg at the end of the exchange program. Therefore, plasma exchange is a worthwhile therapeutic consideration for the sensitized gravid woman who has few medical options.

Plasmapheresis, edited by Y. Nosé, P. S. Malchesky, J. W. Smith, and R. S. Krakauer. Raven Press, New York © 1983.

Plasmapheresis and Kidney Transplant Rejection

B. Amir-Ansari and A. M. Joekes

Institute of Urology, London University, London W.C.2, United Kingdom

The loss of transplanted kidneys due to rejection uncontrolled by conventional pulse high-dose methylprednisolone remains a clinical problem. Plasma exchange has been reported to be of benefit in this situation (1).

PATIENTS AND METHODS

Plasma exchange was carried out on 12 occasions in 11 patients who had not responded to at least 1 g of methylprednisolone intravenously on 2 consecutive days. There was a great variation in the time after transplantation that plasmapheresis was carried out (Table 1). The blood processor used was the Haemonetics 30 (Haemonetics Corporation, Braintree, MA) and the replacing fluid was plasma protein fraction (PPF) or Buminade 5% (Travenol Laboratories Ltd., Thetford,

TABLE 1. *Patient data and time intervals*

Patient (no.)	Sex	Original diagnosis	T_x	HLA match	Date of T_x	Pheresis time after T_x(mos)
A. E. (1)	F	GN	Live	3	14.8.79	3
	F	GN	Live	3	14.8.79	8
A. M. (2)	M	GN	Live	2	3.9.79	6
J. M. (3)	M	GN	Cad.	1	12.7.80	[a]
M. G. (4)	F	Polycyst.	Cad.	1	11.9.74	81
A. B. (5)	M	?	Live	3	23.5.81	1
H. E. (6)	M	GN	Live	3	7.7.81	3
A. A. (7)	M	GN	Cad.	2	26.7.80	3
A. N. (8)	M	?	Live	4	20.5.80	1
V. H. (9)	F	GN	Live	2	6.5.80	[b]
G. N. (10)	M	CR	Cad.	3	8.9.77	36
A. W. (11)	F	Congen.	Cad.	2	19.9.79	29[c]

T_x, transplant; CR, childhood reflux; GN, glomerulonephritis.
[a]Plasmapheresis 48 hr post-transplant.
[b]Plasmapheresis 36 hr post-transplant.
[c]Plasmapheresis 2 months post-delivery.

371

UK). Heparin, 20,000 IU, in 1,000 ml of normal saline was used as anticoagulant. The plasma volume replaced in each exchange was 3 liters, and each complete procedure consisted of three exchanges. There were no side effects in any of the patients.

RESULTS

Immunoglobulins and complements were measured before and after each exchange. Apart from a general reduction in immunoglobulins, especially IgM, after exchange, no specific pattern was recognized. Immune complexes (2) were measured in 2 of the patients who responded and there was no difference in the level before and immediately after exchange.

Table 1 presents the patients' age, sex, and primary renal disease (when known), and notes the use of cadaver or live transplant and the interval after transplantation of plasma exchange.

Four patients (nos. 1, 2, 5, 10) showed renal functional improvement following exchange. Individual graphs for each of these four patients are given in Figs. 1–4.

In patient 7 the renal function data were incomplete; 3 months after transplantation the creatinine clearance was 23 ml/min and had been stable for 2 weeks following 2 doses of methylprednisolone on consecutive days. Ten days later the clearance had fallen to 14 ml/min and plasma exchange was carried out on six occasions over the next 13 days. One week after the last exchange the creatinine clearance had risen stepwise to 26 ml/min and has remained unaltered for 3 months.

Patient 4 had a successful cadaveric transplant with good function for 7 years. She then developed leukopenia and renal function rapidly deteriorated following temporary withdrawal of azathioprine; steroids having been withdrawn because of bilateral hip necrosis some months before. Plasmapheresis failed to affect the progressive deterioration in renal function.

Patient 8 had a live kidney transplant. Initial normal function was followed by a severe prolonged rejection, and recovery of function at 1 month was followed by a steady, slow deterioration unaffected by plasmapheresis and transplant nephrectomy 2 months after transplantation.

Patient 11 had received a cadaveric transplant some 20 months before becoming pregnant. At the time of conception, her creatinine clearance was 23 ml/min. After a caesarean delivery at 32 weeks because of deteriorating renal function and hypertension, renal function continued to deteriorate, unaffected by plasmapheresis, and the patient returned to regular hemodialysis.

Patient 6 received a live kidney transplant which never worked satisfactorily. Plasmapheresis at 3 months had no effect on renal function which has continued to deteriorate over the following 5 months.

In patients 3 and 9 a hyperacute rejection was thought to have occurred. No benefit was obtained following plasma exchange starting 48 and 36 hr after transplantation. Transplant nephrectomy was performed in both patients without renal function having been recovered. In patient 3 cytotoxic antibodies were found ret-

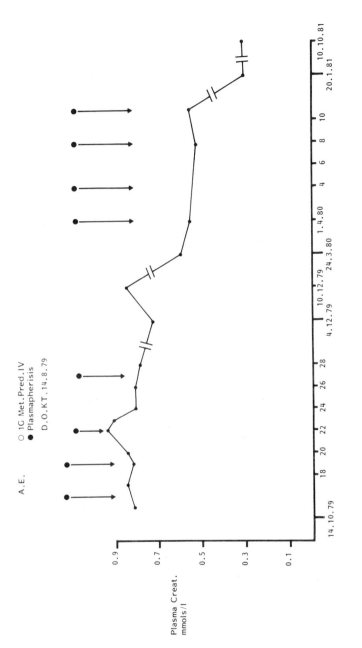

FIG. 1. Renal function following plasma exchange. A. E., female, live transplant.

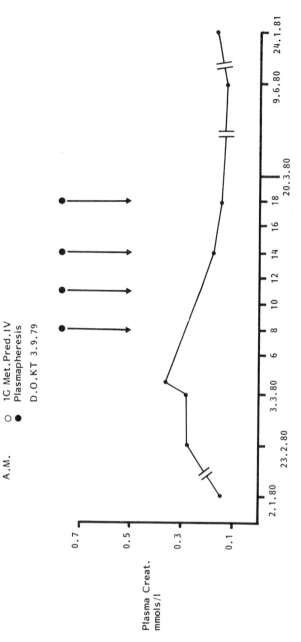

FIG. 2. Renal function following plasma exchange. A. M., male, live transplant.

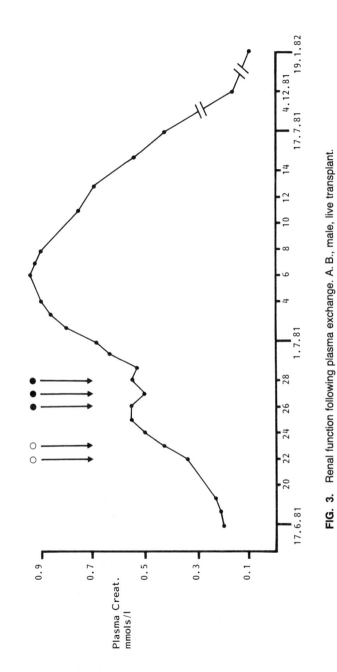

FIG. 3. Renal function following plasma exchange. A. B., male, live transplant.

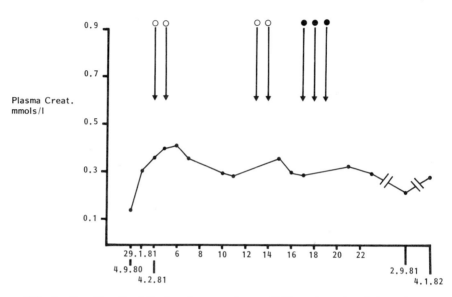

FIG. 4. Renal function following plasma exchange. G. N., male, cadaveric transplant.

rospectively in an immediately pretransplant serum, although a 3-week-old serum had shown a negative crossmatch with donor cells.

DISCUSSION

Conventional antirejection therapy, although effective against the cellular component of the rejection, does not seem to lower antibody levels sufficiently nor modify antibody-mediated injury. Plasma exchange has been shown to be an effective procedure for removal of serum antibodies and, in Goodpasture's syndrome, to be followed by improved renal function (3,4). On that basis it has also been used in conjunction with immunosuppressant drugs to treat uncontrolled transplant rejections (5).

The effectiveness of removal by plasmapheresis of any protein including immunoglobulin, complement, and immune complexes depends on the rate of synthesis and equilibration between intravascular and extravascular compartments. Antigen may also be removed. Immune complexes differ from other proteins in that they have a predominantly intravascular distribution (6). It is also clear that apart from direct removal there may be an indirect effect on their formation (plasma exchange may affect the intrinsic mechanisms so as to enhance their clearance further) (7). In our patients who improved with a time lag, it is possible that a continued elimination without new formation of complexes may have allowed renal functional recovery.

CONCLUSIONS

A minority of patients with transplant rejections may benefit from plasmapheresis. So far there are no indications that can predict the response to treatment. The immunological factors affected by plasmapheresis are not defined but are presumably humoral rather than cellular.

ACKNOWLEDGMENT

This work was supported in part by the St. Peter's Research Trust.

REFERENCES

1. Cardella, C. J., Sutton, D., Uldall, P. R., and deVeber, G. A. (1977): Intensive plasma exchange and renal transplant rejection. *Lancet*, i:264.
2. Devey, M. E., Taylor, J., and Stewart, M. W. (1980): Measurement of antigen antibody complexes in mouse sera by conglutimin Clq and rheumatoid factor solid phase binding assay. *J. Immunol. Methods*, 34:191.
3. Lockwood, C. M., Rees, A. J., Pearson, T. A., Evans, D. J., Peters, D. K., and Wilson, C. B. (1976): Immunosuppression and plasma-exchange in the treatment of Goodpasture's syndrome. *Lancet*, i:711.
4. Walker, R. G., d'Apice, A. J. F., Becker, G. J., Kincaid-Smith, P., and Crasswell, P. W. J. (1977): Plasmapheresis in Goodpasture's syndrome with renal failure. *Med. J. Aust.*, i:875.
5. Cardella, C. J., Sutton, D., Falk, J. A., Katz, A., Uldall, P. R., and deVeber, G. A. (1978): Effect of intensive plasma exchange on renal transplant rejection and serum cytotoxic antibodies. *Transplant Proc.*, 10:617.
6. Pinching, A. J. (1980): Plasma exchange in immunologically mediated disease. *Rec. Adv. Clin. Immunol.*, 12:318.
7. Lockwood, C. M., Worlledge, S., Nicholas, A., Cotton, C., and Peters, D. K. (1979): Reversal of impaired splenic function in patients with nephritis or vasculitis (or both) by plasma exchange. *N. Engl. J. Med.*, 300:524.

Plasmapheresis, edited by Y. Nosé, P. S.
Malchesky, J. W. Smith, and R. S. Krakauer.
Raven Press, New York © 1983.

Hemolytic Uremic Syndrome Successfully Treated with Plasma Exchange

R. Bambauer, G. A. Jutzler,
H. G. Hartmann, D. Stolz, *K. Schmengler,
†M. Koehler, and §M. Wahlen

*Departments of Nephrology, *Cardiology, †Hematology, and §Pediatrics,
University of Saarland, D-6650 Homburg/Saar, Federal Republic of Germany*

The hemolytic uremic syndrome (HUS), the etiology and pathogenesis of which still remain a partial mystery, also presents therapeutic problems. Therapeutic attempts with heparin as well as streptokinase have not improved the often poor prognosis. Although the introduction of acute dialysis has reduced the lethality of HUS it has been unable to bring about complete healing. A turning point in the therapy of HUS appears to have been reached with the use of plasma exchange. First reports on this new therapy are very promising (1–4).

In 1955 Gasser et al. (5) first described a complex of symptoms consisting of acute renal failure, thrombocytopenia, and hemolytic anemia, symptoms now generally known as hemolytic uremic syndrome. HUS usually occurs sporadically in infants and young children (6,7). It has, however, also been described in adolescents and adults (8,9). In women it can mainly be seen post-partum (10) and while taking oral contraceptives (11,12).

We report below on a 14-month-old boy and a 19-year old female patient who were suffering from severe acute HUS and whom we treated with plasma exchange. The therapy concept developed from this treatment is presented.

CASE STUDIES

Case 1

M. M., 14 months old: Clinical treatment 4/30/81–9/9/81.
April 1981: Infection of the upper respiratory tracts, diarrhea.
One week later: Tonic–clonic convulsions for 15–20 mins.
Referral as inpatient: Further convulsions, encephalitis with tonic–clonic cramps, oligoanuria, hemolysis, thrombocytopenia, consumption coagulopathy. Patient unconscious, intubated, pale, edematously swollen.
Clinical diagnosis: HUS (no kidney biopsy).
Laboratory data on referral: Hgb 5.2 g/dl, Hct 18%, leukocytes 11,000/μl, thrombocytes 18,000/μl, potassium 6.1 mmoles/liter, SGOT 115, SGPR 67 mU/ml, creatinine 3.3, urea 199 mg/dl.

Treatment

Insertion of a Shaldon catheter in the right femoralis vein. Plasma exchange (PE) of 1,000 ml. PE on two following days. Total volume exchanged: 2,100 ml. Thereafter, daily hemodialysis (HD), frequent decreases in blood pressure, bradycardia. Ten days after beginning PE, Scribner shunt placed in left upper arm because of infection at the place of entry of the Shaldon catheter in the area of the right groin. Frequent shunt problems (thrombosis, infections, etc.). Further developments: deterioration of cerebral situation, increased tendency to convulsions. From June 1981, slow improvement. By middle of June 1981, slow recovery of renal function. Final HD treatment end of June 1981 (total of 56 HD).

Middle of June 1981: ^{131}I-hippuran clearance 39 ml/min.

Beginning September 1981: Creatinine 1.0 mg/dl, urea 45 mg/dl. Continuance of the cerebral symptoms with slow regressive tendencies. Normal renal function.

Case 2

M. U., 19 years old: Clinical treatment 1/2/81–2/6/81. Apart from chronic bronchitis the patient had never been seriously ill.

12/31/80: Beginning of acute disease with diffused pains in the upper abdominal region and joints, headache and fever up to 39.6°C.

1/2/81: Hospitalization with suspected acute appendicitis.

1/3/81: Transferred to our department with hemolysis and oligoanuria.

Findings on admission: Patient pale and somnolent, blood pressure 160/110 mmHg, sporadic petechia on both calves. Hemolysis, oligoanuria, thrombocytopenia.

Diagnosis: HUS. Laboratory findings are shown in Table 1.

Treatment

Low-dose heparinization (250 E/hr). Shaldon catheter placed in the right internal jugular vein followed by HD.

TABLE 1. *Laboratory data of the 19-year-old patient with HUS*

Parameter		Admission (1/31/81)	1st PE (1/4/81)	After 3 PE (1/7/81)	After 5 PE (1/9/81)	Discharge (2/6/81)
Potassium	(mg/dl)	3.7	4.6	4.8	5.0	4.4
Urea	(mg/dl)	—	296	196	194	36
Creatinine	(mg/dl)	13.3	10.9	11.5	10.2	1.3
Bilirubin	(mg/dl)	—	—	2.4	—	0.3
LDH	(U/liter)	2,840	—	1,905	480	230
HBDH	(U/liter)	1,482	—	1,037	—	125
Hgb	(g/dl)	9.6	8.3	9.6	7.9	8.9
Hct	(%)	28	24.1	27.6	23.4	26.6
Leukocytes	(cells/μ³)	5,200	4,900	8,700	9,100	5,500
Thrombocytes	(cells/μ³)	18,060	25,000	38,000	72,000	232,000
PT	(%)	92	98	65	40	90
PTT	(sec)	30	37	36	47	29
TT	(sec)	27	46	22.5	17	16
Fibrinogen	(mg/dl)	275	146	275	160	350
Coagulase	(sec)	29	29.5	23.6	20.5	—

LDH, lactic acid dehydrogenase; HBDH, hydroxybutyric dehydrogenase; Hgb, hemoglobin; Hct, hematocrit; PT, prothrombin time; PTT, partial prothrombin time; TT, thrombin time.

1/4/81: PE treatment was carried out. Over a period of 5 days, five PE with a volume totaling 9 liters of plasma were performed. The working hypothesis here was that hemoglobin and other decomposition products which were present in the blood due to the severe hemolysis and consumption coagulopathy, and which additionally may damage the kidney, had to be eliminated. PE was performed with a simplified technical process after the "single needle" method with a double pump and a substitution pump (double pump BL 760, substitution pump BL 709, Bellco, D-7800 Freiburg/Br., FRG), and a plasma filter Plasmaflo (13) (Plasmaflo, Plasma separator, Asahi Medical Co., Inc., Tokyo, Japan).

No additional heparin was necessary for the first two PE. To bridge over the acute renal failure a total of 11 HD were required, the first two being immediately attached to the plasmapheresis. Prednisolone was administered over 14 days in decreasing doses, beginning with 120 mg/day. The coagulation conditions normalized visibly. Two days later the polyuria phase started, which lasted for about 3 weeks. At this time the serum concentration of creatinine and urea gradually decreased and all other pathologically increased laboratory parameters (Table 1) normalized.

Thirty-two days after referral we were able to discharge the patient, cured. A slight reduction of the tubular function of both kidneys can still be observed (^{131}I-hippuran clearance 383 ml/min, normal 400 ml/min) with normal total glomerular function (99 m-Tc DTPA clearance 94 ml/min, normal 80 ml/min), and creatinine with the normal value of 1.3 mg/dl (Fig. 1).

1/22/81: Kidney biopsy was performed. According to Professor Dr. Med. A. Bohle, the findings were: "In the light microscope only slight changes are seen in terms of a mesangial proliferative glomerulonephritis with remnants at the renal tubules in terms of hyperplasia of epithelial cells [Fig. 2]. The electronic microscopic section taken from a glomerulus [Fig. 3] shows, apart from changes typical for a mesangial proliferative glomerulonephritis, a detachment of the basement membrane with a transition of endothelial cells or macrophages into the subendothelial space. They indicate an almost complete disappearance of the hemolytic uremic syndrome."

The patient has been regularly examined as an outpatient up to December 1981 and appeared to be in good health with renal function now fully normalized.

DISCUSSION

The pathogenesis of HUS is still as unclear as its etiology. Until fairly recently HUS was considered to be the consequence of a disseminated intravascular coagulation. It was, however, possible to show by corresponding coagulation analysis that with HUS no large-scale generalized consumption coagulopathy takes place, but rather that a more or less isolated thrombocyte consumption occurs with an almost normal fibrinogen rate (14).

Consideration has also been given as to whether HUS may primarily be a renal disturbance along the lines of a microangiopathy triggered off by viral and/or bacterial toxins. On the other hand such viral and/or bacterial toxins could also trigger off intravascular coagulation through direct damage of the erythrocytes and thrombocytes. During the course of hemolysis substances are set free, among others adenosinephosphate, lipide, and thrombokinase, which via a disseminated intravascular platelet aggregation lead to a higher thrombocyte consumption and thus to a microthrombus formation in the arterioles and glomerular capillaries (15).

This hypothesis is supported by the observations made by Poschmann and Fischer (16) that, for example, following a pneumococcus septicemia, immunohemolytic

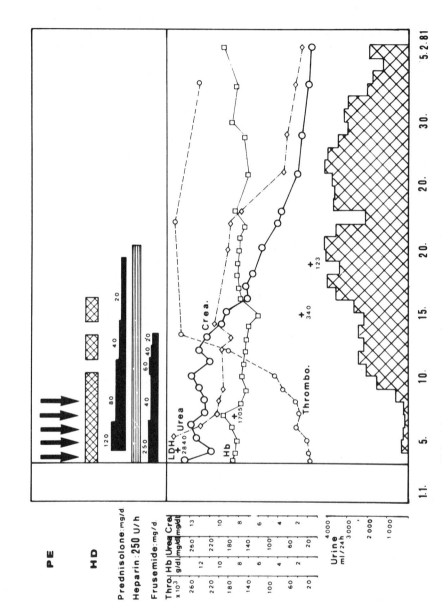

FIG. 1. Development of HUS in a 19-year-old female patient.

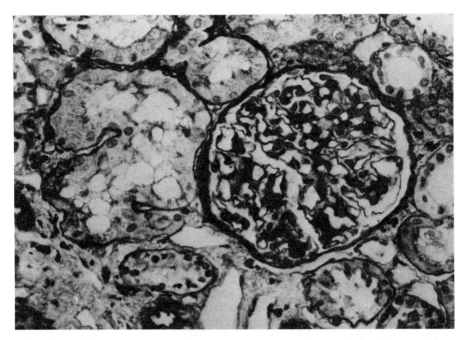

FIG. 2. Histology of a kidney biopsy about 3 weeks after the beginning of the disease.

anemia can be induced by neuraminidase set free from erythrocyte membranes and probably also from endothelial cells of the renal capillaries.

In 1978 Remuzzi et al. (3) discovered that possibly the lack of a not yet defined plasma factor can be held responsible for the triggering of HUS. This factor, which is probably inactivated by toxic substances, stimulates the synthesis of prostacyclin. In turn prostacyclin is able to prevent thrombocyte aggregation and moreover to dilate vessels. If prostacyclin is absent, or not present in sufficient quantities in the blood, disseminated intravascular coagulation can take place more or less unhindered with a high thrombocyte consumption.

It can be concluded from these pathogenetic considerations that HUS may have many causes. Exogenous toxins such as viruses and bacteria (17), following oral contraception (11,12,18), postpartum (10), and perhaps genetic factors probably initiate an immunological process which leads to HUS. Experience in this problem is still, however, very sparse. Immunohistological and electronmicroscopic investigations over the last years were also not able to confirm an immunological basis for HUS (19).

Spontaneous healing of the disease has often been described but this usually only occurs in the less severe cases, although exact statistics are not given in the literature. The prognostically most unfavourable course of the disease is the severe acute form. From the literature available to us we were unable to find any confirmation of spontaneous healing from this group.

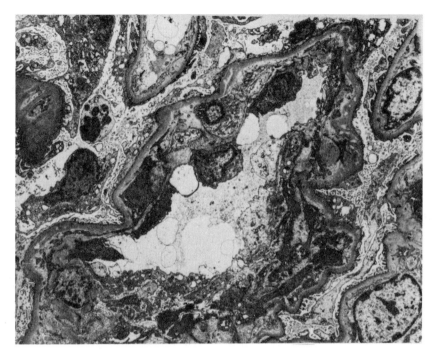

FIG. 3. Electronmicroscopic section taken from a glomerulus (3 weeks after the beginning of the disease).

Over the last few years very different therapy concepts resulted from the different etiological and pathogenetical presentations. Bergstein et al. (8) and Monnens et al. (20) report on very good results with streptokinase with an early lethality of about 30%. Treatment with heparin has been reported as very promising (16,21,22). The overall lethality of HUS could, however, not be reduced by the heparin therapy, and remained at the previous level of 30–40% (15%).

It was the introduction of dialysis for treating HUS which first considerably reduced the lethality to about 20% (7,23). When treated promptly with this process, two-thirds of the cases are healed without consecutive symptoms. The combination treatment of acute dialysis, streptokinase, heparin, and aggregation inhibitors appears to be promising (15).

With the concept that immunological processes are at least involved with HUS, Remuzzi et al. (3) successfully carried out exchange transfusions and plasma infusions.

Vialtel et al. (4), Gillor et al. (2), and Beattie et al. (1) went one step further; they reported on the successful treatment of HUS with PE. Also here an immunopathogenesis is discussed. PE permits the removal of circulating immune complexes and other toxic substances, thereby interrupting pathogenetic chain reactions. Complexes of high molecular weight other than fibrinogen and decomposition products of fibrinogen which may stimulate or inhibit coagulation are also rapidly eliminated.

TABLE 2. *HUS therapy concept*

1. Plasma exchange treatment
   Depending on severity, daily or twice daily exchange of 1–4 liters
   Substitution solution
     a. Electrolytic solution with human albumin (20%) enriched to 3–6%
     b. Conserved serum protein (5%) ⎱ immunoglobulin
     c. Fresh frozen plasma ⎰
   Between treatments possibly substitution of immunoglobulins (2.5–5.0 g/day)
2. Heparinization
   Low dose (250–500 E heparin/hr)
3. Aggregation inhibitor
   E.g., salicylic acid, 1–1.5 g/day, and/or dipyridamole, 300–400 mg/day
4. Prednisone
   80–120 mg/day in decreasing doses

In the case of ARI and/or ARF
5. High dose furosemide: over 4 hr 1 g
     a. As continuous infusion, 4 mg/min
     b. As short infusion, 4 × 250 mg
6. Bicarbonate alcaluria therapy
   Quick infusion of 50–100 ml NaHCO$_3$ (8.4%) portions up to base excess
     (BE) +4–+6 of bicarbonate concentration in blood 26–28 mäq/liter
7. Dialysis procedure
     a. Hemodialysis (2 hr daily)
     b. Hemofiltration
8. Dialysis procedure combined with PE

We were able to show that PE treatment provides the possibility of curing HUS in adults as well as in children. Based on clinical and laboratory findings these patients suffered from severe acute HUS. Apart from the immunological parameters discussed above, the kidney was further damaged by free hemoglobin and other decomposition products which were released by the hemolysis. PE enabled us to quickly remove these substances from the blood without great risk to the patient.

Encouraged by the success of the therapeutic PE in the case of 2 patients, we have developed a therapy concept for HUS (Table 2). Accordingly, PE treatment should begin as soon as the disease is suspected. The other measures stated, such as heparinization, application of aggregation inhibitors, and prednisone are accompanying measures, the use of which, however, are very differently assessed.

In the case of dialysis requiring acute renal insufficiency with or without accompanying acute renal failure, the active kidney replacement therapy should begin at the earliest possible time in the form of HD, which, if required, can be combined at the same time with PE. A Shaldon catheter, placed by the Seldinger technique in the internal jugular vein or subclavian vein (13), offers a particularly effective method of acute vascular entrance.

ACKNOWLEDGMENT

We would like to thank Professor Dr. Med. A. Bohle, Director of the Pathological Institute of the Eberhard-Karls-University, Tübingen, W. Germany, for photomicrographs and histopathologic results.

REFERENCES

1. Beattie, T. J., Murphy, A. V., and Willoughby, M. L. N. (1981): Plasmapheresis in the haemolytic–uraemic syndrome in children. *Br. Med. J.*, 282:1667.
2. Gillor, A., Bulla, M., Bussmann, K., Schrör, K., and Tekook, A. (1981): Plasma-exchange as a therapeutic measure in hemolytic-uremic syndrome in children. *Third International Symposium on Paediatric Dialysis*, May 2–3, Cologne, Germany.
3. Remuzzi, G., Marchesi, D., Mecca, G., Misiani, R., Livio, M., de Gaetano, G., and Donati, M. B. (1978): Haemolytic–uraemic syndrome: Deficiency of plasma factor(s) regulating prostacyclin activity? *Lancet*, ii:871.
4. Vialtel, P., Chenois, F., Dechelette, E., Elsener, M., Bayle, F., and Cordonnier, D. (1980): Adult hemolytic uremic syndrome treated with plasma exchange. *Plasma Therapy*, 1:51.
5. Gasser, C., Gautier, E., Steck, A., Siebenmann, R. E., and Dechslin, R. (1955): Hämolytisch–urämisches Syndrome bilateraler Nierenrindennekrosen bei akuten erworbenen hämolytischen Anämien. *Schweiz. Med. Wochenschr.*, 85:905.
6. Gianantonio, C. A., Vitacco, M., Mendellaharzu, J., Mendellaharzu, F., and Ruttey, A. (1962): Acute renal failure in infancy and childhood clinical course and treatment in 41 patients. *J. Pediatr.*, 61:660.
7. Kaplan, B. S., Thomson, P. O., and de Chaderevian, J. P. (1976): The hemolytic uremic syndrome. *Pediatr. Clin. North Am.*, 23:761.
8. Bergstein, J., Michael, A. F., Kjellstrand, C., Simmons, R., and Najarian, J. (1974): Hemolytic-uremic syndrome in adult sisters. *Transplantation*, 17:487.
9. Karlsberg, R. P., Lacher, J. W., and Bartecchi, C. E. (1977): Adult hemolytic uremic syndrome. *Arch. Int. Med.*, 137:115.
10. Finkelstein, F., Kashagarian, M., and Hayslett, J. P. (1974): Clinical spectrum of postpartum renal failure. *Am. J. Med.*, 57:649.
11. Brown, C. G., Robson, A. P., Robson, J. G., Cameron, J. S., Thomson, D., and Ogg, C. S. (1973): Hemolytic–uremic syndrome in women taking oral contraceptives. *Lancet*, i:1479.
12. Tobon, H. (1972): Malignant hypertension, uremia and hemolytic anemia in a patient on oral contraceptives. *Am. J. Obstet. Gynecol.*, 40:681.
13. Bambauer, R., Jutzler, G. A., Mauch, H., Keller, H. E., and Zaun, H. (1981): Ein vereinfachtes Plasmapherese-Behandlungsverfahren und erste klinische Ergebnisse. *Nieren- Hochdruckkrankheiten*, 10:126.
14. Slichter, S. J., and Harker, L. A. S. (1972): Platelet and fibrinogen consumption in man. *N. Engl. J. Med.*, 287:999.
15. Wehinger, H., Sutor, H. A., Schindera, F., and Kunzer, W. (1974): Zur Therapie des hämolytisch-urämischen Syndroms. *Dtsch. Med. Wochenschr.*, 99:840.
16. Poschmann, A., and Fischer, F. (1974): Hämolytisch-urämisches Syndrom. *Med. Klinik*, 69:1821.
17. Musgrave, J. E., Talwalkar, G. B., Puri, H. C., Campbell, R. A., and Loggan, B. (1978): The hemolytic–uremic syndrome. A clinical review. *Clin. Pediatr.*, 15:218.
18. Schoolwerth, A. C., Schindler, R. S., Klahr, S., and Kissane, J. M. (1976): Nephrosclerosis postpartem in women taking oral contraceptives. *Arch. Intern. Med.*, 136:178.
19. Brandis, M. (1979): Die Klinik des hämolytisch-urämischen Syndroms. *Klin. Wochenschr.*, 57:1081.
20. Monnens, L., Kleynen, F., van Munster, P., Schretlen, E., and Bonnerman, A. (1972): Coagulation studies and streptokinase therapy in the haemolytic–uraemic syndrome. *Helv. Paediatr. Acta*, 27:45.
21. Brain, M. C., Baker, R. J., McBride, J. A., Rubenberg, M. L., and Dacie, J. v. (1968): Treatment of patients with microangiopathie hemolytic anaemia with heparin. *Br. J. Haematol.*, 15:603.
22. Proesmans, W., and Eckels, R. (1974): Has heparin changed the prognosis of the hemolytic–uremic syndrome? *Clin. Nephrol.*, 2:169.
23. Bläker, F., Altrogge, H., Hellwege, H. H., Menke, B., and Thimm, K. (1978): Dialysebehandlung des schweren hämolytisch-urämischen Syndroms. *DMW*, 103:1229.

Plasmapheresis, edited by Y. Nosé, P. S.
Malchesky, J. W. Smith, and R. S. Krakauer.
Raven Press, New York © 1983.

Clinical Evaluation of Different Plasmapheresis Techniques in IgM-Paraproteinemia

Hans-Hartwig Euler, Rosemarie Béress, Klaus Gülzow,
Lutz Kleine, *Claus Laessing, *Hans-Christian Burck,
and Helmut Löffler

*II Medizinische Universitätsklinik Kiel and *Abteilung für Intensivmedizin und Dialyse,
Städtisches Krankenhaus Kiel, D-2300 Kiel, Federal Republic of Germany*

One of the first diseases in which plasmapheresis was employed therapeutically was the hyperviscosity syndrome due to macroglobulinemia in 1956 and 1957 (1,2). Several long-term studies have confirmed that plasmapheresis is an effective therapeutic measure for treating hyperviscosity in IgM-paraproteinemia (3–5). The technique initially employed used discontinuous flow centrifugation. Later, continuous flow centrifugation was increasingly used (6). A new approach towards simplifying the plasmapheresis treatment, provided hemofiltration equipment is available, involves the newly available hollow fiber membrane plasmapheresis filters (7). The effectiveness of filters with medium-sized pores is limited by large quantities of high molecular weight substances (8). Thus a good way to test the clinical value of the different techniques is to compare the results achieved with the various plasmapheresis techniques in patients with high-concentrated high-molecular substances. Patients with IgM-paraproteinemia lend themselves particularly well to such investigations.

PATIENTS

Three patients with hyperviscosity syndromes due to paraproteinemia resulting from IgM secreting lymphoplasmacytoid immunocytomas were treated a total of 20 times with different plasmapheresis techniques.

H. G., male, 55 years old: The hyperviscosity syndrome manifested itself in the form of a high-grade depression of the general condition along with peripheral polyneuropathy and paresthesia. Initially the serum of the patient contained 87.2 g/liter monoclonal IgM (kappa) with a total protein level of 137 g/liter. The IgM was not precipitable in distilled water (SIA test negative), cryoglobulins were present.

O.B., male, 80 years old: The hyperviscosity symptoms consisted of high-grade congestive cardiac failure, visual impairment in connection with fundus paraproteinemicus with bleeding into the retina, and severe fatigue. Laboratory data at the beginning of plasmapheresis treatment: total protein level 138 g/liter, monoclonal IgM 80 g/liter (kappa), SIA test positive, no cryoglobulins.

D.H., female, 81 years old: The hyperviscosity symptoms appeared mainly in the form of fatigue and congestive pneumonia. Total protein 122 g/liter, monoclonal IgM 65 g/liter (kappa), SIA test negative, no cryoglobulins.

METHODS

The plasmapheresis treatment was repeated when renewed signs of hyperviscosity appeared clinically. Between the treatments the patients were able to leave the hospital. Cytostatic therapy was continued.

Centrifugation plasmapheresis was performed via cubital vein-to-vein accesses or via femoral Seldinger catheters, depending on the situation of the blood vessels. Filtration plasmapheresis was performed via femoral venous access, to assure sufficient blood flow.

Replacement was performed with 1.5–4.5% human albumin in physiological saline solution, depending on the degree of hyperproteinemia to be corrected. A dose of 500 ml fresh plasma (FFP) followed. To correct the hypervolemia—associated with hyponatremia and low hematocrit—that often accompanies IgM paraproteinemia, up to 800 ml less fluid was replaced than was eliminated, depending on the central venous pressure.

IgM was measured by laser nephelometry with LN antisera (Behring, Marburg, FRG) every 10 min in the inlet line and in the filtrate. The sieving coefficient (s.c.) for IgM was calculated from the quotient of $IgM_{filtrate}/IgM_{inlet\ line}$. Total protein was determined according to Lowry. The relative viscosity of the citrate plasma was measured according to Leonard, diameter of needle 0.8 mm, with the modification that the temperature was held constant at 37°C. Additional laboratory parameters determined before and after each plasmapheresis treatment and in the filtrate were hematocrit, platelets, electrolytes, and fibrinogen.

Discontinuous Flow Centrifugation

In the single bowl centrifugation technique (4) per plasmapheresis treatment 8–12 × 400 ml blood was drawn into vacuum bottles with 80 ml ACD per bowl and centrifuged at 4°C for 10 min at 750 × g (Cryofuge 6-6, Heraeus-Christ, Osterode, FRG). The supernatant was drawn off by suction; the sediment was resuspended with replacement fluid and reinfused.

Continuous Flow Centrifugation

Continuous flow centrifugation was performed with a Celltrifuge II (Aminco, Fenwal, Deerfield, IL) at 1,600 rpm. For anticoagulation 1 ml ACD and 10 units of heparin per 40 ml blood flow were given. The plasma flow rate was adjusted with the aid of the automatic interface detector to approximately 50% of the blood flow rate, depending on the hematocrit. Replacement occurred isovolumetrically via a second channel of the plasma pump.

Hollow Fiber Membrane Filtration

Four different hollow fiber filters were used in a hemofiltration machine (Haemoprocessor 40005, Sartorius, Göttingen, FRG): Plasmaflo and Plasmaflo Hi-05 (Asahi, Tokyo, Japan), and Plasmaflux and Plasmaflux P2 (Fresenius, Bad Homburg, FRG). The technical data of the filters are summarized in Table 1. The filters were prerinsed with 500 units of heparin in 4 liters of 0.9% NaCl solution. Once the desired blood flow rate was reached, the filtrate side was slowly opened by means of a clamp over a period of 5 min from 0 to the maximum filtrate flow rate. For anticoagulation 500 units of heparin per hour were given.

RESULTS

In all cases the elimination of paraproteins (on the average 130 g IgM per plasmapheresis treatment) definitely reduced the hyperviscosity symptoms. The general condition, fatigue, visual impairment, and cardiac edema all improved. The changes in the laboratory parameters are presented in Figs. 1 and 2. Patient H. G. died 4 months after two plasmapheresis treatments had been performed, of tumor growth that did not respond to therapy. Patient O. B. died 10 days after the last plasmapheresis treatment of a necrotizing pneumonia with agranulocytosis due to cystostatic drugs. Patient D. H. is being treated as an outpatient. The plasmapheresis treatments are performed at 5-week intervals in addition to chemotherapy.

Comparison of the Different Techniques

The technical results are summarized in Table 2. The reason for the described clamp procedure in the filtration techniques was that when we immediately opened

TABLE 1. *Specifications of hollow fiber filters*

Filter	Material	I.D. (μm)	Wall thickness (μm)	Max pore size (μm)	Effective surface (m²)	Priming Vol. (ml)
Plasmaflo (Asahi)	Cellulose diacetate	370	160	0.2	0.65	200
Plasmaflo Hi-05 (Asahi)	Cellulose diacetate	330	75	0.2	0.50	65
Plasmaflux (Fresenius)	Polypropylene	330	140	0.5	0.50	290
Plasmaflux P2 (Fresenius)	Polyproplene	330	150	0.5	0.50	128

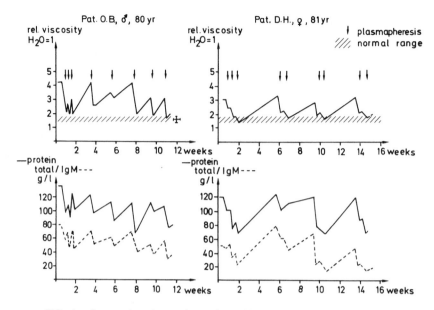

FIG. 1.   Serum viscosity, total protein, and IgM in patients O. B. and D. H.

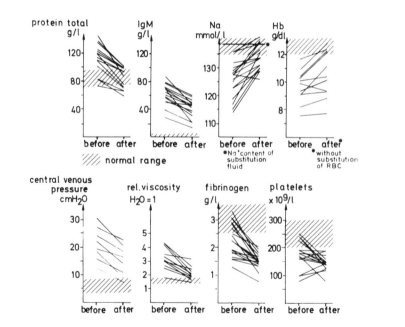

FIG. 2.   Comparison of clinical and laboratory data before and after plasmapheresis.

TABLE 2. Comparison of different plasmapheresis techniques in IgM-paraproteinemia

Methods	N	Vascular access[a]	Max. blood flow (ml/min)	Aver. TMP (mm Hg)	Aver. filtrate flow (ml/min)	s.c. for paraproteinemic IgM	"Clogging"	Aver. length of procedure (4-liter exchange) (min)	Work involved	Cost of disposable material
Continuous flow centrifugation (Celltrifuge II, Aminco)	6	p/c	100[b]	—	50[e]	(1.0)	Ø	80	++	Low
Discontinuous flow centrifugation (single bowl system)	2	p/c	—	—	—	(1.0)	Ø	240	++++	Very low
Plasmaflo (Asahi)	3	c	250[c]	10–30[d]	35→11[f]	0.8→0.4	++	240	+	High
Plasmaflo Hi-05 (Asahi)	4	c	250[c]	10–30[d]	65[f]	0.95	Ø	60	+	High
Plasmaflux (Fresenius)	2	c	250[c]	10–30[d]	50[f]	0.95	Ø	110	+	High
Plasmaflux P2 (Fresenius)	3	c	250[c]	10–30[d]	100[f,g]	0.98	Ø	40	+	High

[a]p, peripheral; c, central.
[b]Limited by collapsing of the tubes, technically 150 ml/min.
[c]Not limited, but further increase did not result in an increase in the filtrate flow rate.
[d]Further increase did not result in increase of the filtrate flow rate (100 mm Hg TMP possible).
[e]With low hematocrit higher.
[f]The maximum filtrate flow rate was reached approximately 5 min after the beginning of the procedure by slowly opening a clamp attached to the filtrate side.
[g]Higher filtrate flow rate possible, but not desired for reasons of therapeutic safety.

the filtrate side completely at the beginning of treatment, hemolysis occurred, followed by a lower filtrate flow rate, probably because of secondary membrane formation due to too high initial polarization concentration. When the filtrate flow was slowly increased, a state of balance was reached within 5 min in which neither an increase in the transmembrane pressure (TMP) nor an increase in the blood flow rate caused an increase in the filtrate flow rate. Only with the filter Plasmaflux P2 would a filtrate flow rate over 110 ml/min have been possible. For reasons of therapeutic safety we did not attempt this. The filtrate flow rates remained constant throughout the treatment with one exception: With the filter Asahi Plasmaflo the filtrate flow rate continually decreased. Since this was accompanied by a decrease in the s.c. for IgM, a pronounced loss of effectivity occurred with this filter. The s.c. of the other filters were close to 1.0. No drop in the s.c. was observed.

With the continuous flow centrifugation techniques the technical upper limit of the blood flow rate is 150 ml/min. The maximum value of 100 ml/min indicated here was determined by the collapse of the inlet line. Since no sieving occurs, s.c. is constantly 1.0 in both centrifugation techniques. No drop in the filtrate flow rate can occur.

Comparing all techniques there are considerable differences in the time, work, and costs involved (Table 2).

DISCUSSION

In the centrifugation techniques there should be no basic differences between plasmapheresis of patients with IgM paraproteinemia and patients with other diseases, because all dissolved serum proteins are removed equally after separation from corpuscular blood components (9). Accordingly, our results coincide with those of other authors (4,10–12). Because single-bowl centrifugation involved a considerable amount of work, we came to prefer continuous flow centrifugation, which produced the same therapeutic results in a much shorter time. The clinical results of the new continuous flow centrifuge used by us, which is technically easy to handle, correspond to the results obtained by other authors with previously available equipment (3,5,13–15). In addition to the low cost of disposable material, the relatively short time involved and a high degree of effectivity, the centrifugation method has the advantage that it is possible to perform cytapheresis or combined lymphoplasmapheresis with the same equipment.

On the filtration plasmapheresis techniques the s.c. plays an important role. For complete plasmapheresis a constant s.c. of 1.0 for all proteins in the solution must be aspired to. The first filters did not yet fulfill this condition. Several authors confirmed that with these filters the s.c. for substances with a high molecular weight (or large steric structure) is lower than that for substances with lower molecular weight (16,17). If high molecular weight substances are present in a high concentration—as in our patients with IgM-paraproteinemia—the s.c. decreases in the course of treatment combined with a decrease in the filtrate flow rate (8,17), until the pores are almost completely clogged.

With the new filters Plasmaflo Hi-05, Plasmaflux, and Plasmaflux P2 no drop in the s.c. or in the filtrate flow rate is observed, due to a higher cutoff (18,19). In our study these filters had s.c. between 0.95 and 0.98, even for highly concentrated IgM. Since in the serum no larger molecular weight proteins than IgM occur (except for β-lipoprotein, IgA polymers in IgA paraproteinemia, and large circulating immune complexes), these filters should be suitable for almost all cases in which plasmapheresis is clinically indicated. The same holds true for continuous flow centrifugation. There were definite differences between these filters in the average filtrate flow rate, and thus in the total length of time of treatment. With the polypropylene filter Plasmaflux P2 the average time necessary for a plasma exchange of 4 liters was only 40 min. Another factor that may influence the choice of the method to be used is the vascular access of the patient.

CONCLUSION

The comparison of the different plasmapheresis techniques studied here, using IgM-paraproteinemia as an example, showed that the most suitable techniques are continuous flow centrifugation and hollow fiber membrane plasmapheresis via filters with a high flow rate and high s.c.

REFERENCES

1. Reynolds, W. A. (1981): Late report of the first case of plasmapheresis for Waldenström's macroglobulinemia. *J.A.M.A.*, 245:606.
2. Skoog, W. A., and Adams, W. S. (1959): Plasmapheresis in a case of Waldenstrom's macroglobulinemia. *Clin. Res.*, 7:96.
3. Russell, J. A., Toy, J. L., and Powles, R. L. (1977): Plasma exchange in malignant paraproteinaemias. *Exp. Hematol.*, 5(Suppl.):105.
4. Solomon, A., and Fahey, J. J. (1963): Plasmapheresis therapy in macroglobulinemia. *Ann. Intern. Med.*, 58:789.
5. Buskard, N. A., Galton, D. A. G., Goldman, J. M., Kohner, E. M., Grindle, C. F. J., Newman, D. L., Twinn, K. W., and Lowenthal, R. M. (1977): Plasma exchange in the long-term management of Waldenström's macroglobulinemia. *Can. Med. Assoc. J.*, 117:135.
6. Oon, C. J., and Hobbs, J. R. (1975): Clinical applications of the continuous flow blood separator machine. *Clin. Exp. Immunol.*, 20:1.
7. Sieberth, H. G., Editor (1980): *Plasma Exchange. Plasmapheresis—Plasma Separation.* Schattauer Verlag, Stuttgart, New York.
8. Euler, H. H., Gutschmidt, H. J., Herrlinger, J. D., Kokenge, F., and Löffler, H. (1981): Elimination-characteristics of high-concentrated IgM by hollow-fibre plasmapheresis filters. *Proc. Eur. Soc. Artif. Organs*, 8:115.
9. Borberg, H. (1980): Comparison of cell-plasma separation with different centrifuge techniques. In: *Plasma Exchange. Plasmapheresis—Plasma Separation*, edited by H. G. Sieberth, p. 59. Schattauer Verlag, Stuttgart.
10. Godal, H. C., and Borchgrevink, C. F. (1965): The effect of plasmapheresis on the hemostatic function in patients with macroglobulinemia Waldenström and multiple myeloma. *Scand. J. Clin. Lab. Invest.*, 17(Suppl. 14):1.
11. Schwab, P. J., and Fahey, J. L. (1960): Treatment of Waldenström's macroglobulinemia by plasmapheresis. *N. Engl. J. Med.*, 263:574.
12. Skoog, W. A., Adams, W. S., and Coburn, J. W. (1962): Metabolic balance study of plasmapheresis in a case of Wandenström's macroglobulinemia. *Blood*, 19:425.
13. Blacklock, H. A., Hill, R. S., Bridle, M., Simpson, I. J., Matthews, J. R. D., and Woodfield, D. G. (1980): Therapeutic plasmapheresis by continuous flow centrifugation. *N. Z. Med. J.*, 92:145.
14. Lawson, N. S., Nosanchuk, J. S., Oberman, H. A., and Meyers, M. C. (1977): Therapeutic

plasmapheresis in treatment of patients with Waldenström's macroglobulinemia. *Transfusion,* 8:174.

15. Pineda, A. A., Brzica, S. M., Jr., and Taswell, H. F. (1977): Continuous- and semicontinuous-flow blood centrifugation systems. *Transfusion,* 17:407.

16. Glöckner, W. M., Sieberth, H. G., Dienst, C., Vaith, P., Mitrenga, D., Kindler, J., and Borberg, H. (1980): Elimination kinetics of antibodies and immune complexes in membrane plasma separation. In: *Plasma Exchange. Plasmapheresis—Plasma Separation,* edited by H. G. Sieberth, p. 121. Schattauer Verlag, Stuttgart.

17. Schindhelm, K., Roberts, C. G., and Farrell, P. C. (1981): Mass transfer characteristics of plasma filtration membranes. *Trans. Am. Soc. Artif. Intern. Organs,* 27:554.

18. Yamazaki, Z., Inoue, N., Fujimori, Y., Takahama, T., Wada, T., Oda, T., Ide, K., Kataoka, K., and Fujisake, Y. (1980): Biocompatibility of plasmaseparator of an improved cellulose acetate hollow fiber. In: *Plasma Exchange. Plasmapheresis—Plasma Separation,* edited by H. G. Sieberth, p. 45. Schattauer Verlag, Stuttgart.

19. Gurland, H. J., Samtleben, W., Blumenstein, M., Randerson, D. H., and Schmidt, B. (1981): Clinical applications of macromolecular separations. *Trans. Am. Soc. Artif. Int. Organs,* 27:356.

Plasmapheresis, edited by Y. Nosé, P. S. Malchesky, J. W. Smith, and R. S. Krakauer. Raven Press, New York © 1983.

Acute Copper Deficiency in Patients Undergoing Plasma Exchange

William H. Roberts, Ronald E. Domen, Gregory P. Wanger, and Melanie S. Kennedy

Department of Pathology, The Ohio State University, Columbus, Ohio 43210

Copper is an essential nutrient, being required for heme synthesis, connective tissue metabolism, nerve function, and bone formation. It is also a required cofactor in several metalloenzymes (e.g., cytochrome oxidase) (1,2).

To date, no direct study of serum copper levels in patients undergoing plasmapheresis (plasma exchange) has been reported. A recent paper indirectly studied the effects of plasmapheresis on copper through the measurement of ceruloplasmin (3). We have recently studied 10 patients undergoing plasmapheresis and observed a marked decrease in the serum copper concentration in 8 of the 10 patients.

MATERIALS AND METHODS

The patients included in this study had glomerulonephritis, acute renal allograft rejection, or acute Guillain–Barré syndrome. None of the patients had nephrotic syndrome or severe urinary protein loss. A patient with thrombotic thrombocytopenic purpura (TTP) who received fresh frozen plasma (FFP) during exchange was used for comparison.

Blood samples were collected in chemically clean serum tubes. Copper was determined by atomic absorption spectrophotometry in serum deproteinized by 5% trichloroacetic acid containing 0.25% lanthanum chloride. Absorption was measured at 324.7 nm on a Perkin-Elmer model 306 atomic absorption spectrophotometer (Perkin-Elmer Corporation, Norwalk, CT) (4). Normal serum copper ranged from 63 to 131 µg/dl.

Plasma exchange was performed using a Haemonetics Model 30 blood processor (Haemonetics Corporation, Boston, MA). Approximately 2.0 liters of plasma was exchanged with 1.5 liters of 5% albumin and 300–400 ml normal (0.9%) saline during each of four procedures performed within a 2-week period. Anticoagulation was achieved with 300–400 ml ACD-B solution. The control patient was exchanged with FFP.

The copper content was also determined on four different lots of 5% human serum albumin, on the ACD-B solution, and on the normal saline. No copper was detected in the normal saline or in the ACD-B solution and only minute amounts in the albumin solution (Table 1). Statistical analysis was performed by Student's *t*-test for paired samples (5).

RESULTS

Table 2 illustrates the serum copper levels in the patients studied before and after four plasma exchanges. Prepheresis, the mean serum copper was 120.1 ± 42.2 µg/dl. The mean serum copper postpheresis was 63.9 ± 30.0 µg/dl. The difference in the means was significant at the $p = 0.05$ level of confidence by the *t*-test for paired samples. Five patients were found to have normal copper levels before the procedure. Four had elevated serum copper levels and one a borderline low copper level. All patients showed a decrease in their copper level after four plasma exchanges with a range of 13–95 µg/dl and a mean of 56 µg/dl. Additional studies (complete blood count, serum iron, and total iron binding capacity) were performed, but no identifiable association of anemia or neutropenia with copper depletion was observed.

A single patient was replaced with FFP during plasmapheresis for TTP and failed to show a decrease in serum copper after four plasma exchanges. His course versus that of patient 9 is plotted in Fig. 1.

TABLE 1. *Concentration of copper in replacement solutions (µg/dl)*

5% Human albumin (different lots)	2
	4
	5
	10
Normal (0.9%) saline	0
ACD–B	0

TABLE 2. *Serum copper levels in 10 patients before and after four plasmaphereses with replacement by serum albumin*

Patients	Prepheresis copper level (µg/dl)	Postpheresis (×4) copper level (µg/dl)
1	85	40
2	140	120
3	115	49
4	140	67
5	62	47
6	110	65
7	205	112
8	100	30
9	160	65
10	84	44

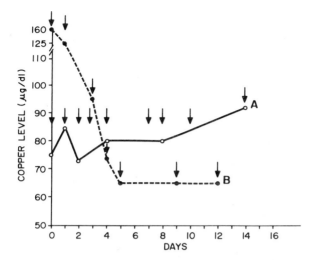

FIG. 1. Copper levels in 2 patients undergoing intensive, multiple plasma exchanges. **Curve A** is the control patient with TTP who was exchanged with FFP. **Curve B** is a representative study patient (patient 9) who was exchanged with 5% albumin solution. The arrows represent individual plasma exchanges. All blood samples were drawn just prior to each exchange.

DISCUSSION

Copper deficiency is a rarely observed phenomenon. Hypocupremia has been observed in the genetically linked Mencke's syndrome, in malnourished infants and in patients receiving total parenteral nutrition (6–10). Some of these patients manifested anemia and neutropenia. Animal studies have implicated copper deficiency in neurologic abnormalities and in depressed immune response (11,12).

Five of our ten patients decreased to hypocupremic levels after four plasma exchanges performed within a period of 14 days. Three other patients dropped to the lower limits of the normal range. Two patients with elevated copper levels decreased to the normal range. Since all the patients had inflammatory conditions, the decrease in copper may represent a decrease in ceruloplasmin, a known acute phase reactant (13,14). Ceruloplasmin would fall as the inflammatory process subsided due to antiinflammatory and immunosuppressive drugs. Also, the ceruloplasmin would be directly removed by the plasma exchange (15,16). The patient with the highest copper level (205 μg/dl) was noted to have grossly green plasma and hyperceruloplasminemia. The green color disappeared following successive plasma exchanges with simultaneous decreases in the ceruloplasmin and copper levels.

The stabilization of the serum copper level observed in patient 9 after five to six plasma exchanges suggests an initial depletion of a readily available serum copper pool and slow equilibration with other copper stores. Intense, protracted plasmapheresis might therefore result in depletion of total body copper stores.

Acute copper depletion in patients undergoing plasma exchange with 5% albumin requires further study, both as a complication of plasmapheresis and for its relationship to the course of immunologic and inflammatory diseases.

REFERENCES

1. Mertz, W. (1981): The essential trace elements. *Science*, 213(4514):1332.
2. Mason, K. E. (1979): A conspectus of research on copper metabolism and requirements of man. *J. Nutr.*, 109(11):1979.
3. Wallace, D. J., Goldfinger, D., Thompson-Breton, R., Martin, V., Louk, C. M., Bluestone, R., and Klinenberg, J. R. (1980): Advances in the use of therapeutic pheresis for the management of rheumatic diseases. *Semin. Arthritis Rheum.* 10(2):81.
4. Ichida, T., and Nobuka, M. (1969): Determination of serum copper by atomic absorption spectrophotometry. *Clin. Chim. Acta*, 24(2):299.
5. Daniel, W. W. (1978): *Biostatistics: A Foundation for Analysis in the Health Sciences*, 2nd edition. John Wiley, New York, p. 135.
6. Dunlap, W. M., James, G. W., and Hune, D. M. (1974): Anemia and neutropenia caused by copper deficiency. *Ann. Intern. Med.*, 80(4):470.
7. Al-Rashid, R. A., and Spangler, J. (1971): Neonatal copper deficiency. *N. Engl. J. Med.*, 285(15):841.
8. Aguilar, M. J., Chadwick, D. L., Okuyama, K., and Kanoshita, S. (1966): Kinkyhair disease: Clinical and pathological features. *J. Neuropathol. Exp. Neurol.*, 25(4):507.
9. Vilter, R. W., Bozian, R. C., Hess, E. V., Zellner, D. C., and Petering, H. G. (1974): Manifestations of copper deficiency with systemic sclerosis on intravenous hyperalimentation. *N. Engl. J. Med.*, 291(4):188.
10. Wheeler, Z. M., and Roberts, P. F. (1976): Menke's steely hair syndrome. *Arch. Dis. Child.*, 51(4):269.
11. Dipaolo, D. V., Kanter, J. N., and Newberne, P. M. (1974): Copper deficiency and the central nervous system myelination in the rat: Morphologic and biochemical studies. *J. Neuropathol. Exp. Neurol.*, 33(2):226.
12. Prohaska, J. R., and Lukasewycz, D. A. (1981): Copper deficiency suppresses the immune system in mice. *Science*, 213(4507):559.
13. Prasad, A. S. (1978): *Trace Elements and Iron in Human Metabolism*. Plenum, New York, p. 17.
14. Brown, D. H., Buchanan, W. W., El Ghobarcy, F., Smith, W. E., and Teape, J. (1979): Serum copper and its relationship to clinical symptoms in rheumatoid arthritis. *Ann. Rheum. Dis.*, 38(2):174.
15. Orlin, J. B., and Berkman, E. M. (1980): Partial plasma exchange using albumin replacement: Removal and recovery of normal plasma constituents. *Blood*, 56(6):1055.
16. Friedman, B. A., Schork, M. A., Aln, S. K., Jones, A. S., and Oberman, H. A. (1976): Plasmapheresis induced hemodilution and its effects on serum constituents. *Transfusion*, 16(2):155.

Plasmapheresis, edited by Y. Nosé, P. S.
Malchesky, J. W. Smith, and R. S. Krakauer.
Raven Press, New York © 1983.

Plasmapheresis in Acute Liver Failure

Makoto Yoshiba, †Noboru Inoue, *Takemasa Sanjo,
*Zenya Yamazaki, Yoshihiro Okada, Toshitsugu Oda, and
*Tatasuo Wada

*1st and *2nd Departments of Medicine, Tokyo University Hospital, Tokyo 113;
†Oji National Hospital, Tokyo, Japan*

The liver plays a major role in the metabolism of numerous substances including proteins, lipids, carbohydrates, hormones, amino acids, bile acids, and bilirubin. Massive liver cell necrosis in fulminant hepatitis brings about acute and severe failure in the metabolism of these substances. This gives rise to the complicated clinical manifestations of acute liver failure. Among its various clinical symptoms, hepatic coma resulting from the accumulation of toxic intermediate metabolites and bleeding tendency resulting from the deficiency of coagulation factors create the most serious therapeutic problems. Future liver support systems for acute liver failure should be directed toward support of these various forms of metabolic failure.

We have treated patients with acute liver failure by charcoal plasma perfusion since 1975 (1) and plasma exchange since 1978 (2). After 7 years of experience, we find that our support systems are still incomplete and that many problems remain to be solved. We present here some of the problems hoping that it will serve in the further development of artificial liver support.

MATERIALS AND METHODS

Charcoal Plasma Perfusion

Charcoal plasma perfusion was performed with a system composed of a cellulose acetate hollow fiber plasma separator (Asahi Plasmaflo), a column of uncoated activated charcoal, and an artificial kidney. Detailed techniques using this system are described elsewhere (1). Five liters of plasma was separated and perfused through activated charcoal, and infused back to patients.

Plasma Exchange

Plasma exchange was done with a system composed of the separator and the artificial kidney. Detailed techniques using this system have been described (2). Five liters of plasma was separated and discarded, and an equal volume of fresh plasma or fresh frozen plasma was substituted. The reconstituted blood was infused back to the patients.

Modified Plasma Exchange

The system was composed of the separator and a polyacrylonitrile membrane hollow fiber filter. A diagram of the apparatus and the circuit is given in Fig. 1. Plasma was separated by ultrafiltration through cellulose acetate hollow fiber filter (Asahi Plasmaflo-Hi). Transmembrane pressure across the cellulose acetate hollow fiber filter was maintained between 50 and 100 mmHg. Five liters of plasma separated in 3 hr was discarded. Ringer's solution in a volume equal to the discarded plasma was combined with the separated blood cell fraction, and the diluted blood was filtered through the polyacrylonitrile membrane filter. About 5 liters of filtrate was discarded, and then fresh plasma or fresh frozen plasma in a volume equal to the discarded filtrate was supplemented to the "washed" blood cell fraction. The reconstituted blood was infused back to the patients.

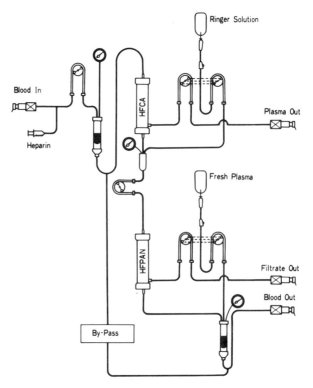

FIG. 1. Circuit diagram for modified plasma exchange.

Experimental Study of the Effect of Charcoal Plasma Perfusion on Blood Coagulation and Fibrinolysis

The study was conducted on normal dogs and on those with acute liver failure with body weight of about 15 kg. Acute liver failure was induced with the intraportal injection of dimethylnitrosamine, 15 mg/kg. Plasma perfusion with both uncoated charcoal and that coated by biocompatible poly-HEMA was done 20 hr after the injection as previously described (1).

Assay Methods

Human and dog prothrombin times were measured on a Fibrometer using Simplastin (General Diagnostics). Concentrations of human plasma proteins such as prealbumin, α_2-HS-glycoprotein, fibrinogen, plasminogen, antithrombin III, α_1-antitrypsin, and α_2-macroglobulin were measured by single radial immunodiffusion methods. Concentrations of dog plasma fibrinogen, plasminogen, and antithrombin III were measured by protein determination (3), caseinolysis (4), and clotting time method (5), respectively. Human and dog serum fibrin degradation products (FDP) were both measured by latex fixation test for human FDP because of the presence of cross-reactivity of dog FDP with human FDP. Plasma total bile acid level was determined by enzymatic method (6), and that of amino acids was measured by LKB 4400 amino acid analyzer.

RESULTS

Clinical Study of Charcoal Plasma Perfusion

Of 26 patients treated by charcoal plasma perfusion in 4 years since 1975, 10 recovered consciousness and 5 survived. Complications due to bleeding were frequent in those patients who ultimately died; the rate was as high as 80%. Their platelet count, which was $197 \pm 76 \times 10^3$ before the treatment, decreased significantly to $71 \pm 46 \times 10^3$ after the treatment. Platelet counts fell to the critically low level of 30×10^3 or less in 3 patients. Most of the patients with thrombocytopenia showed positive tests for serum FDP.

Effect of Charcoal Plasma Perfusion on Blood Coagulation and Fibrinolysis

In normal dogs, changes of prothrombin time, fibrinogen, plasminogen, and antithrombin III levels were transient or insignificant and the serum FDP level was low during plasma perfusion with uncoated charcoal. However, the changes were irreversible and remarkable in dogs with acute liver failure. After the start of plasma perfusion with uncoated charcoal, prothrombin time was too prolonged to be determined. Plasma fibrinogen, plasminogen, and antithrombin III levels were more rapidly decreased than the rate expected from their half-life (Fig. 2). Serum FDP

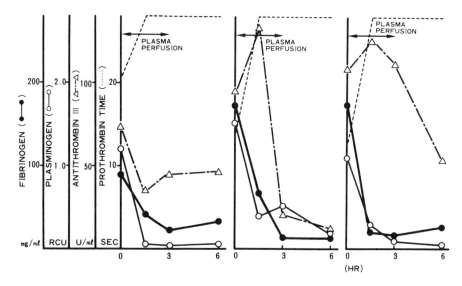

FIG. 2. Changes of prothrombin time, plasma fibrinogen, plasminogen, and antithrombin III levels in dogs with acute liver failure after the start of plasma perfusion with uncoated charcoal. Results in representative 3 dogs out of 10 examined are shown.

levels exceeded 1,000 μg/ml in all 10 dogs. They all died due to sudden hypotension within 20 hr after the experiments. Plasma perfusion with charcoal coated by poly-HEMA was found to cause less effect on blood coagulation and fibrinolysis systems in general. All 8 dogs with acute liver failure treated by this system survived, and their serum FDP level was low. However, changes of the above four parameters were remarkable in 4 dogs with relatively more severe liver failure.

Clinical Study of Plasma Exchange

Table 1 summarizes some clinical characteristics of 12 patients treated by plasma exchange since 1978. Seven recovered consciousness, and four survived. Complications due to bleeding were less frequent and less severe. Thrombocytopenia in case 6 might be ascribed to underlying disseminated intravascular coagulopathy. Most patients died of brain death judged by continuous flat EEG record and the loss of vestibuloocular reflex. Mean survival time of the patients who died was about 14.6 days by plasma exchange, which was significantly longer than 4.6 days by charcoal plasma perfusion.

In order to know the extent to which liver functions were compensated by plasma exchange, the levels of some plasma components were determined serially five times a day in the course of plasma exchange. The study was conducted on case 9, whose liver function was considered completely ruined by severe fulminant viral hepatitis. The patient's coma deepened progressively in spite of daily performance of plasma exchange. She suffered brain death after the fifth plasma exchange, and died after the eighth. The prothrombin time was found to be almost normalized

TABLE 1. *Clinical characteristics of patients treated by plasma exchange*

Patients No./Age/Sex	Coma grade	No. of PE	PE vol. (ml)	Outcome	Bleeding	Thrombo.
1/25/M	IV	6	29,800	Recovered		
2/62/F	IV	1	6,300	Recovered		
3/69/M	IV	1	5,010	Recovered		
4/25/F	III	3	14,000	Recovered		
5/43/M	IV	29	139,200	Died[a]	(+)	
6/60/F	IV	16	78,600	Died[b]	(+)	(+)
7/47/F	IV	5	23,800	Died[b]	(+)	
8/43/F	IV	3	14,400	Died[c]	(+)	
9/15/F	IV	8	38,400	Died[b]		
10/27/F	IV	8	38,800	Died[b]		
11/45/M	III	2	96,000	Died[b]	(+)	
12/37/M	III	3	12,400	Died[b]		

PE, plasma exchange; Thrombo., thrombocytopenia.
[a]Cause of death: renal failure.
[b]Cause of death: brain death.
[c]Cause of death: bleeding.

immediately after each plasma exchange. Plasma levels of prealbumin, α_2-HS-glycoprotein, fibrinogen, and α_2-macroglobulin were maintained in normal ranges, those of α_1-antitrypsin and antithrombin III at half normal values, and that of plasminogen at one-third of normal value after the start of plasma exchange therapy.

Plasma total bile acid levels, which were 20-fold normal levels before the treatment, were continuously lowered to 3-fold after eight plasma exchanges. By contrast, plasma levels of tyrosine, phenylalanine, and methionine were decreased only 30% transiently after plasma exchange (Fig. 3).

Plasma Exchange by the Modified System

Removal of tyrosine, phenylalanine, and methionine was increased by 40–50% and that of bile acids by 15% (Table 2).

DISCUSSION

The results of the experimental study may be of limited value because circulating plasma volume of the dogs is about one-fourth that of patients; however, the findings explain well the reduction of platelet count and the production of serum FDP observed in the clinical study. It was found that plasma levels of plasma fibrinogen, plasminogen, and antithrombin III were decreased far more rapidly than the rate expected from their half-life (7) after the start of experimental charcoal plasma perfusion. A large amount of serum FDP was produced at the same time. These findings indicate that a mechanism consuming both coagulation and fibrinolysis factors works in charcoal plasma perfusion.

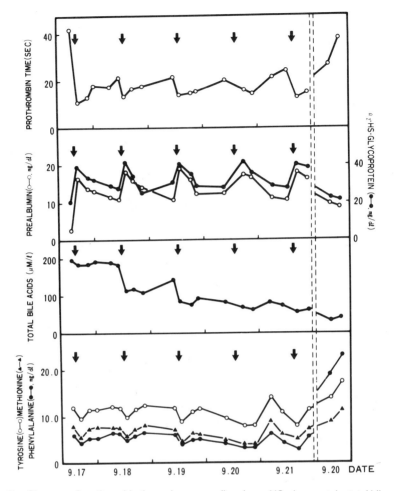

FIG. 3. Changes of prothrombin time, plasma prealbumin, α_2-HS-glycoprotein, total bile acids, tyrosine, phenylalanine, and methionine levels in the course of plasma exchange. *Arrows* signify plasma exchange.

Charcoal, even if coated by biocompatible materials, may act as a foreign body and activate labile coagulation Factor XII, and subsequently activate the entire coagulation and fibrinolysis systems. In the normal state, activated coagulation and fibrinolysis factors are bound to plasma anticoagulants such as antithrombin III, α_2-macroglobulin, and α_2-plasmin inhibitor, and are eliminated from the bloodstream mainly by the reticuloendothelial system (8). In acute liver failure, however, coagulation factors remain activated in blood because of deficient plasma anticoagulants, most of which are synthesized by the liver, and defective reticuloendothelial system. This necessarily results in the continuous activation of the entire coagulation and fibrinolysis systems, and in the consumption of the factors together with platelets.

TABLE 2. *Removal of various components through cellulose acetate hollow fiber (CAHF) and polyacrylonitrile fiber (PANHF)*

Components	CAHF	PANHF
BUN (mg)	1,027	666
Creatinine (mg)	35	16
Tyrosine (nmoles)	874	358
Phenylalanine (nmoles)	579	298
Methionine (nmoles)	229	100
Total bile acids (μmoles)	80	10

It thus becomes clear that biocompatibility of artificial liver support systems should be assessed not only for blood cells but also for the coagulation and fibrinolysis systems.

Plasma exchange demonstrates no bioincompatibility. We have observed no hemolysis, significant thrombocytopenia, increased serum FDP level, or circulatory problems. Most patients died of brain death as a natural outcome of hepatic coma rather than of complications (Table 1). Consequently, patients treated by plasma exchange lived longer than those treated by our plasma perfusion system or by blood exchange as reported by Redeker (9). Taking into account that the aim of artificial liver support for acute liver failure at present is to keep patients alive until their livers regenerate and recover function, this effect of plasma exchange is considered quite meaningful.

On detailed analysis it was found that a daily exchange of up to 5 liters of plasma replaced most plasma proteins synthesized by the liver to satisfactory levels. In addition, this was effective for the removal of accumulated substances with a small body pool, that is, bile acids, even in severe liver failure. Plasma exchange was, however, of limited value for the removal of substances with a large body pool such as aromatic amino acids (Fig. 3). Unidentified toxic substances which affect the central nervous system (CNS) in acute liver failure may have body pools as large as aromatic amino acids, which would account for the progressive deepening of coma in the patient with severe liver failure, in spite of the daily performance of plasma exchange therapy. Therefore, efforts should be concentrated on improving the capability of plasma exchange to eliminate CNS toxins accumulating in hepatic coma. We have shown one such example (Fig. 1). Though the separator is efficient, the amount of separated and discarded plasma is at most 30% of the blood volume flowing through it. The aim of the modified system used is to remove more CNS toxins from the undiscarded plasma and blood cells. By this system 40–50% of aromatic amino acids and 15% of bile acids were additionally removed (Table 2). Because polyacrylonitrile membrane hemodialysis was reported to be effective for recovery from hepatic coma (10), more CNS toxins may be removed by this system.

In conclusion, plasma exchange utilizing hollow fiber plasma separators seems a safe and convenient method for artificial liver support for acute liver failure.

Despite limited removal of CNS toxins accumulating in hepatic coma, plasma exchange allows satisfactory replacement of most of the plasma components synthesized by the liver, and prolongs patients' lives, though mortality rate is unchanged. Future tasks must overcome these limitations and guarantee sufficient time for liver regeneration and recovery of function.

REFERENCES

1. Yamasaki, Z., Fujimori, Y., Sanjo, T., et al. (1977): New artificial liver support systems for hepatic coma. *ASAIO Abstracts*, 6:99.
2. Inoue, N., Yoshiba, M., Yamazaki, Z., et al. (1981): Continuous flow membrane plasmapheresis utilizing cellulose acetate hollow fiber in hepatic failure. In: *Artificial Liver Support*, edited by G. Brunner and F. W. Schmidt, p. 175. Springer Verlag, Berlin.
3. Quick, A. J. (1957): *Hemorrhagic Diseases*, 1st edition. Lea and Febiger, Philadelphia, p. 379.
4. Johnson, A. J., Kline, D. L., and Alkjaesig, N. (1969): Assay methods and standard preparations for plasmin, urokinase in purified systems 1967–1968. *Thromb. Diath. Haemorr.*, 21:259.
5. Dames, P. S., and Rosenberg, R. D. (1976): Antithrombin-heparin cofactor. In: *Methods in Enzymology, Vol. XLV*, edited by L. Lorand, p. 653. Academic Press, New York.
6. Mashige, F., Imai, K., and Osuga, T. (1976): A simple and sensitive assay of total serum bile acids. *Clin. Chim. Acta*, 70:79.
7. Williams, W. J. (1977): Life-span of plasma coagulation factor. In: *Hematology*, 2nd edition, p. 1258. McGraw-Hill, New York.
8. Barnhart, M. I., and Nooman, S. M. (1973): Cellular control mechanisms for blood clotting proteins. In: *Thrombosis: Mechanisms and Control*, p. 59. Schattauer Verlag, Stuttgart.
9. Redeker, A. G., and Yamashiro, H. S. (1973): Controlled trial of exchange transfusion therapy in fulminant hepatitis. *Lancet*, i:3.
10. Opolon, P., Rapin, J. R., Huguet, G., et al. (1976): Hepatic coma treated by polyacrylenitrile membrane hemodialysis. *Trans. Am. Soc. Artif. Intern. Organs*, 22:701.

Plasmapheresis, edited by Y. Nosé, P.S.
Malchesky, J.W. Smith, and R.S. Krakauer.
Raven Press, New York © 1983.

Plasma Exchange in Severe Leptospirosis

S. Landini, U. Coli, S. Lucatello, A. Fracasso, P. Morachiello,
F. Righetto, F. Scanferla, and G. Bazzato

*Nephrology and Dialysis Department, Umberto I Hospital, 50-30174 Venice Mestre,
Venice, Italy*

Leptospiral infections (LI) are caused by a large group of antigenically distinct microorganisms comprising the genus Leptospira. Human infection can occur directly by contact (abraded skin, mucous membrane, etc.) with urine of animals or indirectly through contaminated water or vegetables (1). LI may vary from subclinical to severe and rapidly fatal forms. The most frequent type in our series was due to *L. icterohemorrhagiae*, characterized by severe jaundice, renal failure, hemorrhage, anemia, and disturbances in consciousness.

In anicteric patients mortality is essentially unknown; when jaundice occurs the mortality in various series reaches 40% (2). The case fatality rate in humans rises from 10% in those less than 50 years of age to 56% in those over 51 years (3). The main causes of death are hemorrhagic and neurologic manifestations, supervening infections, and hepatorenal failure.

Conventional treatment includes antibiotics in large doses, correction of fluid and electrolyte disorders, and peritoneal or hemodialysis if acute renal failure develops (1). Hepatic insufficiency and its complications, often lethal, are not well controlled by a merely purifying treatment (dialysis or hemoperfusion).

In our present study we postulated that severe LI requires temporary artificial liver and kidney support. For this reason we present the results of plasma exchange (PE) treatment in 6 patients affected by acute hepatic and renal failure due to severe LI.

PATIENTS AND METHODS

Six patients, aged from 25 to 59 years (average 39 years), affected by LI were admitted to our unit and treated by PE. Serologic tests confirmed in every case icterohemorrhagiae serotype. Laboratory data in all patients showed renal and hepatic failure (bilirubin 49 ± 10 mg/dl, creatinine 8.9 ± 1.4 mg/dl) with oliguria in 5 patients. Four patients were stuporous (EEG coma grade III) and two were comatose (EEG coma grade IV). Thrombocytopenia (platelet count $52,000 \pm 30,000/$ mm^3) and hemorrhages (subconjunctival, petechiae, epistaxis, and hematemesis in one patient) were present at admission. Details of these cases are summarized in Tables 1 and 2.

TABLE 1. *Data from patients affected by severe
leptospirosis*

| Patient | | Plasmapheresis | | |
(age/sex)	Treatment	No.	Vol. (ml)	Outcome
G. V.(59/M)	PE + PD	4	9,000	Survival
F. A.(38/M)	PE + PD	4	10,000	Survival
A. G.(26/M)	PE	5	11,200	Survival
G. B.(25/M)	PE	4	8,800	Survival
R. P.(39/M)	PE	4	8,500	Survival
G. B.(48/M)	PE	4	9,000	Survival

PE, plasma exchange; PD, peritoneal dialysis.

TABLE 2. *Hepatic and renal function in patients
affected by severe leptospirosis treated by PE*

Patient	Creatinine (mg/dl)	Bilirubin (mg/dl)	Platelets (mm³)	EEG Coma grade
1	10.2	52	52,000	IV[a]
2	9.2	58	44,000	III
3	9.5	59	25,000	IV[a]
4	7.5	42	85,000	III
5	8.9	39	62,000	III
6	8.5	44	48,000	III

An intermittent flow cell separator (Progress, Dideco, Mirandola, Italy) was employed. With this machine we separated the plasma from successive batches of patients' blood and returned the red cells to the patient mixed with plasma replaced in adequate quantity (4). Blood access was obtained by venous catheterization between antecubital vein, and in two cases from femoral vein. An average of 40–50 ml/min blood flow rate was achieved.

In order to avoid hypotension and hypovolemia we administered 300 ml of fresh frozen plasma (FFP) at the beginning of the procedure. At each session we exchanged FFP in quantities not less than the plasma removed (about 2.5–3 liters).

All 6 patients underwent PE treatment when bilirubin reached high levels (>30 mg/dl) and the patients were stuporous or comatose.

RESULTS

Blood pressure, serum protein, fibrinogen, and hemoglobin did not change significantly during the treatment. Bilirubin and creatinine decreased about 35% after each session (Fig. 1) in all patients. The removal of about 2.5 liters of plasma led to a reduction of 30–40% of substances present in the bloodstream. Diuresis was observed after the second treatment. Platelet count fell an average of 12% after

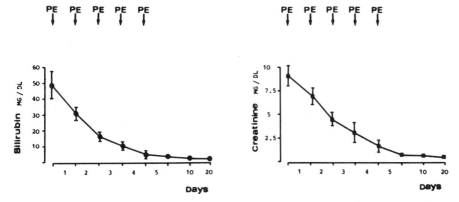

FIG. 1. Effect of PE treatment on bilirubin and creatinine in 6 patients suffering from severe leptospirosis.

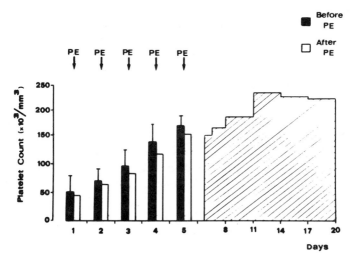

FIG. 2. Platelet count in 6 patients affected by severe leptospirosis and treated by PE.

each treatment (Fig. 2). Nevertheless, we observed an improvement in hemorrhagic state after PE treatment. Total recovery of consciousness was achieved in all patients after the third treatment.

DISCUSSION

In the past 6 years we have treated 14 patients with acute renal and hepatic failure due to LI. The standard therapy in these cases was penicillin and peritoneal dialysis, but in 6 of these patients high serum bilirubin values and hemorrhagic manifestations induced us to try PE with FFP.

In a previous study we described the effectiveness of combined PE and dialysis treatment in severe leptospirosis (4,5). We reported that the progressive increase of serum bilirubin and the worsening of the comatose state were well controlled by intensive PE after unsuccessful intensive dialysis treatment. It has been also suggested by some authors that humoral substances such as bilirubin, bile acids, false neurotransmitters, ammonia, endotoxins, and other unknown agents seem to play an important pathogenic role in renal failure (6).

On the basis of these hypotheses and considering that PE treatment is able to remove all toxic substances not eliminated by the impaired kidney and liver, we have subsequently been treating patients affected by LI with severe hepatorenal failure by PE alone. The 4 patients treated with this methodology showed a quick restoration of diuresis and a return toward normal hepatic and renal function without requiring dialysis treatment. Our results suggest that PE treatment can be considered not only for artificial liver support but also for artificial kidney support (7).

Conventional therapy appeared to us inadequate in severe leptospirosis. Dialysis removes only water soluble substances (8). Hemoperfusion is able to clear many toxins, but in this pathology the loss of platelets and the hypotensive crises provoked by this technique appear to be the limiting factors for its employment in Weil's disease (leptospiral jaundice) (9). Moreover, the development of new specific adsorbents is hindered by the lack of knowledge of the substances to be removed. In contrast, PE not only purifies but also provides the patients with the essential factors not being synthesized by the impaired liver, that is, coagulation factors and immunoglobulins (10).

Thrombocytopenia, often present in these patients, was not significantly worsened by PE treatment in our study. This minimal decrease and the administration of clotting factors during PE prevented the appearance of hemorrhagic episodes often responsible for death in Weil's disease. PE should be viewed as crucial in this pathology if we consider the supposed role of glomerular basement membrane (GBM) antibody in the pathogenesis of renal failure in leptospirosis (11).

CONCLUSIONS

The present study demonstrates that PE with FFP is effective in the management of patients with acute hepatic and renal failure. PE removes all toxic substances, restores volemia, prevents tubulonephrosis, improves the comatose state but, above all, compensates hepatic synthetic defects.

We did not observe in our series any difference between patients treated by PE alone and those treated by PE combined with peritoneal dialysis. In fact, renal function sharply improved because PE is more effective in removing toxic substances than any other purifying treatment.

PE should be considered an artificial liver and renal support because it is able to: (a) remove all toxic substances (bilirubin, false neurotransmitters, creatinine, etc.); (b) normalize the imbalance of humoral agents (bradykinins, prostaglandins, etc.) and correct the impaired ratio between aromatic and branched amino acids (9); and (c) support the liver synthesizing function. PE promotes a shortened healing period; furthermore, it can avoid the often lethal complications, namely hyperbilirubinemic encephalopathy, cholemic tubulonephrosis, hemorrhagic diathesis, and infections.

In our experience the lack of hemorrhage and supervening infections leads us to consider PE the most suitable and safe treatment in severe leptospirosis.

REFERENCES

1. Turner, L. H. (1973): Leptospirosis. *Br. Med. J.*, 537.
2. Sanford, J. P. (1979): Leptospirosis. In: *Textbook of Medicine*, edited by P. B. Beeson, W. McDermott, and J. B. Wyngaarden, p. 532. Saunders, Philadelphia.
3. Heath, C. W., Jr., Alexander, A. D., and Galton, M. M. (1965): Leptospirosis in the United States. *N. Engl. J. Med.*, 273:857.
4. Bazzato, G., Coli, U., Landini, S., and Lucatello, S. (1980): Plasma-exchange and peritoneal dialysis combined treatment in the management of severe leptospirosis. *Plasma-Exchange Int. Symp.*, Cologne. p. 347.
5. Landini, S., Coli, U., Lucatello, S., and Bazzato, G. (1981): Plasma-exchange in severe leptospirosis. *Lancet*, 14:1119.
6. Papper, J. (1975): The hepato-renal syndrome. *Clin. Nephrol.*, 4:41.
7. Landini, S., Coli, U., Lucatello, S., Fracasso, A., Morachiello, P., Michieli, R., Righetto, F., and Bazzato, G. (1981): Acute renal failure associated with liver impairment treated by plasma-exchange. In: *Acute Renal Failure*, edited by H. E. Eliahou, pp. 230–235. John Libbey, London.
8. Frollman, A. P., and Odell, G. B. (1962): Removal of bilirubin by albumin binding intermittent peritoneal dialysis. *N. Engl. J. Med.*, p. 276.
9. Krumlowsky, F. A., Del Greco, F., and Niederman, M. (1978): Prolonged haemoperfusion and haemodialysis in management of hepatic failure and hepato-renal syndrome. *Trans. ASAIO*, 24:235.
10. Lepore, M. J., and Martel, A. J. (1979): Plasmapheresis with plasma-exchange in hepatic coma. *Ann. Intern. Med.*, 72:2.
11. Doudal, P., Mahieu, P., Bloch, B., and Barale, F. (1978): Leptospirose avec immunisation antimembrane basale glomerulare. *Nouv. Presse Med.*, 39:3535.

Plasmapheresis, edited by Y. Nosé, P. S. Malchesky, J. W. Smith, and R. S. Krakauer. Raven Press, New York © 1983.

Intensive Plasma Exchange: A New Treatment for Cholestasis of Pregnancy

Catherine Le Pogamp, *Patrick Le Pogamp, †Pierre Brissot, and §Claudine Le Berre

*Departments of Obstetrics A, *Nephrology, and †Internal Medicine A, University of Rennes School of Medicine; §Regional Blood Bank, 35000 Rennes, France*

Cholestatic jaundice of pregnancy, also known as benign cholestasis of pregnancy, cholestasis hepatosis, and icterus gravidarum, is characterized by pruritus, icterus, or both, during pregnancy. This condition is recurrent, sometimes becoming more severe in subsequent pregnancies. The symptoms of this disease may start any time after the sixth week of pregnancy, and tend to become more severe as the pregnancy progresses; they disappear after termination of the pregnancy.

The percentage of pregnant women presenting with icterus ranges from 0.1 to 6% (1,2). It seems that it is more frequent in the recent literature, perhaps related to diagnostic improvement. Among patients icteric during pregnancy, about 15% have a diagnosis of recurrent cholestasis of pregnancy (3), that is to say 1 or 2 out of 10 icteric pregnancies.

Cholestatic jaundice of pregnancy is regarded as a benign maternal condition, but it is now recognized that this is not the case for the fetus. An important perinatal morbidity is due to prematurity (1/3), hypotrophy, or intrauterine death (4–7).

Because of the risk of fetal complications during pregnancy, it is suggested that those patients who are diagnosed as having cholestatic jaundice should be followed in high risk clinics where continuous obstetrical monitoring is possible. Care should be taken to monitor these patients until the fetus is mature for delivery, and throughout labor and delivery.

With the exception of cholestyramine (8), which is a bile acid exchange resin agent, there is no treatment for the disease. Unfortunately, cholestyramine does not always relieve symptoms in patients with cholestasis of pregnancy; the precocity and severity of fetal distress do not always permit induction of premature labor, or delivery of the fetus by cesarean section. Therefore, for 2 patients with previous severe perinatal morbidity, the precocity of recurrent cholestasis with fetal distress has spurred us to manage them by intensive plasma exchange; this technique has already been used during pregnancy in the treatment of severe rhesus hemolytic disease and in the treatment of cholestasis (9,10), but has never been used in the present condition.

CASE REPORTS

Case 1

The patient was a 30-year-old woman, gravida 4, para 3. Her obstetrical history was remarkable and showed the following:

1971: Premature delivery of a 1,450-g female infant who died at the age of 15 days. During this pregnancy the mother developed pruritus and icterus from the fourth month onwards.

1972: Premature delivery of a 1,700-g male infant who survived but is severely handicapped.

1978: Intrauterine death at the 38th week. She complained of pruritus from the 35th week onwards, and liver function tests revealed cytolysis (i.e., increased transaminases) and cholestasis. Several months after the last pregnancy, liver function tests were performed and showed normal results.

1980: The patient was first seen in the obstetric clinic at the 28th week from her last menstrual period during her fourth pregnancy. She complained of pruritus for the last few days. Liver function tests, which were normal until the 25th week, showed a cholestasis (alkaline phosphatase 2,074 IU/ml; Nl < 210) and a cytolysis (ASAT 210 IU/liter; ALAT 174 IU/liter; Nl < 20). In spite of complete rest and cholestyramine (12 g/day) she experienced severe pruritus and poor general condition (anorexia, asthenia); liver function tests showed aggravation of cholestasis and cytolysis. Uterine contractions and premature labor were hard to control by β-mimetics. Fetal distress was evidenced by reduced active movements, growth retardation, and lower plasma unconjugated estriol levels. Then, at the 30th week of pregnancy, we proposed to the patient to manage her by intensive plasma exchange in order to relieve unknown toxic substances. Ten plasma exchanges, 3 liters each, were performed until the 35th week (Table 1). Cholestasis improved both clinically (pruritus) and biologically (Fig. 1). Fetal distress was relieved as evidenced by diminished uterine contractions and improved estriol levels (Fig. 2). At the 35th week, β-mimetics and plasma exchanges were stopped and, a few days later, natural labor permitted delivery of a 2,370-g healthy female. Amniotic fluid was yellow but did not contain any meconium.

Case 2

The patient was a 32-year-old woman, gravida 6, para 1, abortus 3. Her obstetrical history showed in 1972, 1973, and 1976 three early abortions.

TABLE 1. *Plasma exchange characteristics for case 1*

Day	Plasma exchange (liters FFP)	Side effects	Adjuvant therapy
4/23/80	2.950	Paresthesia	Calcium
4/24/80	3.300	Paresthesia, vomiting	Calcium
4/28/80	2	Paresthesia, cutaneous rash	Polaramine
4/30/80	3	0	Polaramine
5/2/80	2	0	Polaramine
5/5/80	3	0	Polaramine
5/7/80	3	0	Polaramine
5/9/80	3.2	0	Polaramine
5/12/80	3	0	Polaramine
5/14/80	3	0	Polaramine

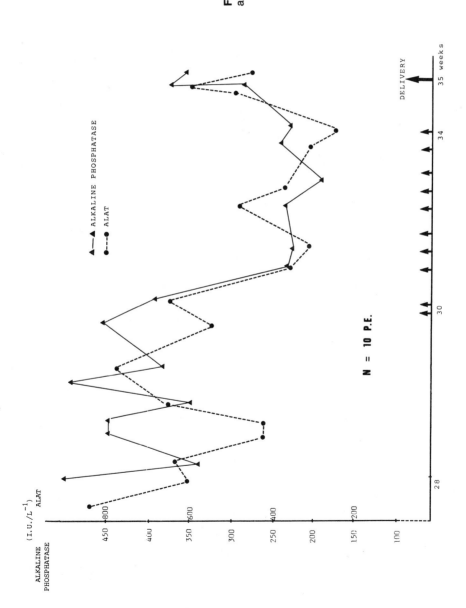

FIG. 1. Evolution of A.L.A.T. and A.P. levels in case 1.

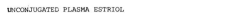

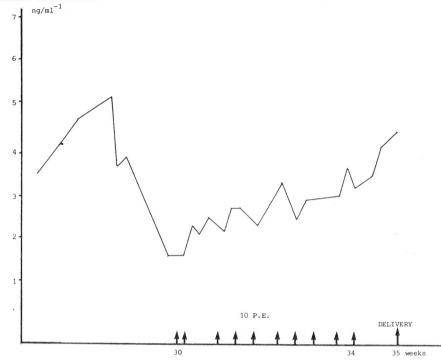

FIG. 2. Evolution of unconjugated plasma estriol in case 1.

1978: A fourth pregnancy was complicated from the seventh month onwards by progressive pruritus; liver function tests showed increased alkaline phosphatase and transaminase. In the eighth month she presented a premature labor despite rest and β-mimetics. At 34 weeks she delivered a meconium stained 1,900-g infant, who died immediately; it presented no obvious abnormalities. After parturition, the mother's pruritus resolved and liver function tests returned to normal within 10 days.

1980: Two years later, after negative exhaustive hepatic investigations, she was authorized to start another pregnancy. Repeated liver function tests and obstetrical survey were normal until the 20th week. Then, a progressive severe pruritus appeared with increased alkaline phosphatase; cholestyramine was ineffective. History, recurrence of the symptoms, and successful treatment of patient 1 led us to propose treatment with plasma exchange. From the 29th week to the 35th week, 15 plasma exchanges were performed (Table 2). Cholestasis improved both clinically (pruritus, more favorable condition) and biologically (Fig. 3). No fetal distress appeared. At the 36th week, after amniocentesis for maturity index, induced labor permitted natural delivery of a 2,285-g healthy infant. The mother was able to breast-feed the infant.

METHODS

Plasma exchanges were carried out on an IBM model 2997 cell separator by continuous flow blood centrifugation. Vascular access was through percutaneous needles in forearm veins. ACD-B was used as anticoagulant. About 3 liters of plasma were exchanged for an equal volume of fresh frozen plasma (FFP) in patient

TABLE 2. *Plasma exchange characteristics for case 2*

Day	Plasma exchange (liters)	Side effects	Adjuvant therapy
6/12/81	2.5 FFP	Paresthesia, vomiting	Calcium
6/16/81	2.5 FFP	Cutaneous rash	Polaramine, soludecadron
6/19/81	2.5 FFP	Rash	Polaramine, soludecadron, calcium
6/23/81	2.2 Albumin diluted 4.6%	0	0
6/25/81	2.6 Albumin diluted 4.6%	0	0
6/29/81	2.6 Albumin diluted 4.6%	0	0
7/1/81	2.5 Albumin + 0.27 FFP	0	Polaramine
7/3/81	2 Albumin + 0.6 FFP	Urticary	Polaramine
7/6/81	2.3 Albumin + 0.31 FFP	0	Polaramine
7/8/81	2.3 Albumin + 0.31 FFP	0	Polaramine
7/10/81	2.3 Albumin + 0.31 FFP	0	Polaramine
7/13/81	2.3 Albumin + 0.31 FFP	0	Polaramine
7/16/81	2.3 Albumin + 0.31 FFP	0	Polaramine
7/20/81	2.3 Albumin + 0.31 FFP	0	Polaramine
7/24/81	2.3 Albumin + 0.31 FFP	0	Polaramine

1 and of human albumin solution for patient 2; FFP was added at the end of plasma exchange, after albumin, in order to supply the patient with coagulation factors. Two or three plasma exchanges were performed weekly.

Patients were followed in a high risk obstetrical clinic. Monitoring of fetal heart rate was performed twice daily and fetal echography once a week. Before each plasma exchange, transaminase, alkaline phosphatase, 5'-nucleotidase, blood cell count, clotting factors and plasma unconjugated estriol were routinely evaluated.

DISCUSSION

In our limited experience, recurrent cholestasis of pregnancy appears to be a new indication for intensive plasma exchange. When there is a severe obstetrical past and precocity of recurrent cholestasis, with or without fetal distress, plasma exchange will permit fetal maturity for delivery (natural, induced, or cesarian section) that is, in the 35th or 36th week. Our observations also show that maternal condition is improved during the course of therapy.

This is an empirical method, since in cholestatic jaundice of pregnancy, potential toxic substances are unknown. Perhaps serum bile acids are involved; they fluctuate during menstrual cycle (11) and increase at the time of intrahepatic cholestatic symptoms (12).

Since toxic substance(s) is unknown, plasma exchange frequency depends on the symptoms. However, SGOT, SGPT, alkaline phosphatase, and 5'-nucleotidase appear to be good biological parameters.

Only mild side effects for the mother are observed. But pregnancy requires careful monitoring of volemia during plasma exchange course. The use of a continuous

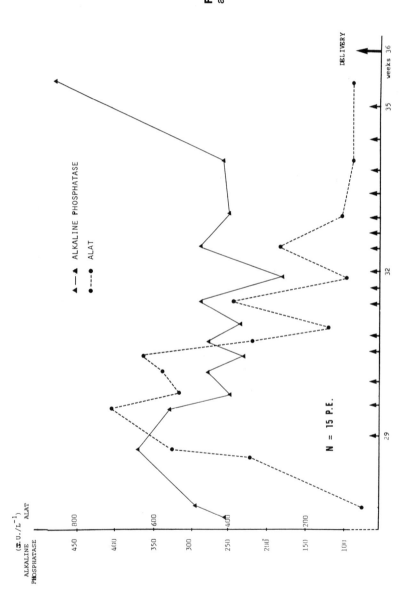

FIG. 3. Evolution of A.L.A.T. and A.P. levels in case 2.

flow cell separator allows performance of plasma exchanges without significant changes in the volemia; maximal extracorporeal blood volume is 300 ml, and this is of interest as far as a pregnant woman is concerned. Moreover peripheral veins are easy to reach.

Prior intrahepatic cholestasis and cytolysis may lead to some difficulties in diagnosing non-A, non-B hepatitis.

The fetus needs continuous obstetrical, clinical, and hematological monitoring while undergoing plasma exchange. It is exposed to volemia and to platelet and coagulation factor impairments. Unconjugated estriol is a good survey index of fetal distress, since it is not modified by cholestasis; but corticoids should not be used since they diminish estriol levels dramatically. Fetal and maternal risks forbid use of plasma exchange after the 36th week.

CONCLUSION

There were two successful pregnancies from the 2 patients with striking obstetrical pasts. This type of treatment has yielded interesting results in the potential therapeutic role of such treatment for selected patients with this disease.

ACKNOWLEDGMENTS

To Robert Reveillard for his thesis and to the "Collège des Gynécologues et Obstétriciens Français" for its material support.

REFERENCES

1. Haemmerli, V. P. (1966): Jaundice during pregnancy with special emphasis on recurrent jaundice during pregnancy and its differential diagnosis. *Acta Med. Scand.*, 179(S 444):111.
2. Querleu, D. (1972): Ictère et grossesse. Intérêt d'une nouvelle classification à propos de 100 observations. *Rev. Fr. Gynecol. Obstet.*, 72:511.
3. Levy, V. G., Chevrel, B., and Caroli, J. (1977): Les ictères au cours de la grossesse; à propos de 93 cas. *Med. Chir. Dig.*, 6:111.
4. Friedlandler, P., and Osler, M. (1967): Icterus and pregnancy. *Am. J. Obstet. Gynecol.*, 97:894.
5. Johnston, W. G., and Baskett, T. F. (1979): Obstetric cholestasis. A 14 year review. *Am. J. Obstet. Gynecol.*, 133:299.
6. Merger, C., Chadeyron, P. A., and Levy, J. (1977): Cholestase gravidique. *J. Gynecol. Obstet. Biol. Reprod.*, 6:357.
7. Wilson, B. R. I., and Haverkamp, A. D. (1979): Cholestatic jaundice of pregnancy: New perspectives. *Obstet. Gynecol.*, 54:650.
8. Laatikainen, T. J. (1978): Effect of cholestyramine and phenobarbital on pruritis and serum bile acid levels in cholestasis of pregnancy. *Am. J. Obstet. Gynecol.*, 132:501.
9. Lauterburg, H., Pineda, A. A., Dickson, E. R., Baldus, W. P., and Taswell, H. F. (1978): Plasma perfusion for the treatment of intractable pruritus of cholestasis. *Mayo Clin. Proc.*, 53:403.
10. Levy, V. G., Julien, P. E., Oppenheimer, M., Denis, J., and Opolon, P. (1981): Traitement de la cholestase par la plasmaphérèse. *Nouv. Presse Med.*, 10:2588.
11. Pennington, C. R., Ross, P. E., Murison, J., and Bouchier, I. A. D. (1981): Fluctuations of serum bile acid concentrations during the menstrual cycle. *J. Clin. Pathol.*, 34:185.
12. Heikkinen, J., Maen Tausta, O., Ylostalo, P., and Janne, O. (1981): Changes in serum bile acid concentrations during normal pregnancy, in patients with intrahepatic cholestasis of pregnancy and in pregnant women with itching. *Br. J. Obst. Gynecol.*, 88:240.

Plasmapheresis, edited by Y. Nosé, P. S. Malchesky, J. W. Smith, and R. S. Krakauer. Raven Press, New York © 1983.

Simultaneous Plasma Collection and Exchange Between Donor Dogs and Dogs with Galactosamine-Induced Hepatic Failure

Z. Yamazaki, Y. Fujimori, I. Iizuka, T. Takahama, F. Kanai, K. Yabe, *N. Inoue, †T. Sonoda, and T. Wada

*Faculty of Medicine, University of Tokyo, Tokyo 113; *Oji National Hospital, Tokyo; †Toray Industries Inc., Tokyo 103, Japan*

Plasma exchange has become a therapeutic tool in an increasing number of intractable diseases (1–4). We have designed a method to collect plasma from the donor and simultaneously exchange it with that of a patient, utilizing two membrane plasma separators, and a triple-channel roller pump in the extracorpoeal circulatory system. This method has been evaluated for its safety and efficiency.

MATERIALS AND METHOD

Simultaneous Plasma Collection and Exchange

Partial extracorporeal circulation was carried out simultaneously in a healthy beagle dog and in another dog with acute hepatic failure induced by galactosamine (5). As shown in Fig. 1, the whole blood of the healthy animal was introduced into the plasma separator where the plasma was separated from the blood and infused into the venous side drip chamber in the recipient's circuit, while the same amount of substitution fluid as that of the separated plasma was fed into the venous side of the donor's circuit by means of the triple-channel roller pump. Meanwhile, the blood was pumped from the animal with hepatic failure into another plasma separator, where the plasma was separated and subsequently discarded by the same triple-channel roller pump. These three channels represent the two plasma and the substitution fluid lines, each with the same diameter. Thus the plasma of the dog with hepatic failure was simultaneously exchanged with the collected plasma from the donor, maintaining a constant balance of circulating plasma volume in the animals.

In this experiment, 2 healthy beagle dogs (8–10 kg) were used for each beagle dog (8–10 kg) with hepatic failure induced by intravenous injection of galactosamine (0.5–0.7 g/kg) 20–24 hr before perfusion. A total of 600 ml from the diseased dog

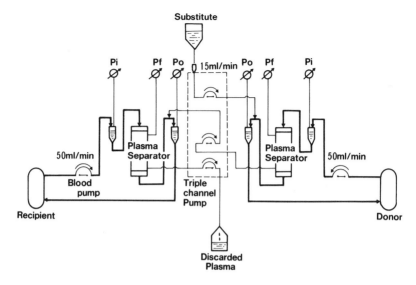

FIG. 1. Circuit for simultaneous plasma collection and exchange.

TABLE 1. *Simultaneous plasma collection and exchange*

Parameter	Healthy dog	Dog with hepatic failure
Blood flow rate	50 ml/min	50 ml/min
Plasma flow rate	10–15 ml/min	10–15 ml/min
Collected volume	300 ml × 2 (animals)	600 ml discarded
Exchanged volume	300 ml × 2 (supplemented)	600 ml
Time required	25–30 min/animal	50–60 min/liter
Plasma separator	Plasmax (0.15 m²)[a]	Plasmax (0.15 m²)[a]

[a]Manufactured by Toray Industries, Tokyo, Japan (6,7).

was exchanged by taking 300 ml of plasma from each donor dog. The experimental conditions are shown in Table 1.

The blood samples for hematological and biochemical analysis were taken immediately before perfusion, when the exchanged plasma was 300 and 600 ml, and at the end of the experiment.

RESULTS

Hemodynamics During Extracorporeal Circulation

Hemodynamics in both the normal dogs and the diseased dogs were maintained stable during extracorporeal circulation, so that the 600-ml plasma exchange was safely and easily performed. A slight decrease in the blood pressure was sometimes observed, but remained stable during the perfusion. Hemodynamic monitoring showed that tachycardia and hypotension, which were often seen in the dog with hepatic failure, approached normal levels after the plasma exchange.

Blood Corpuscular Components

Changes in hematocrit (Hct), platelets, and white blood cells (WBC) are shown in Fig. 2. Hct and platelets were maintained within normal ranges, while WBC lowered temporarily at the outset of the plasma exchange in both the normal and the diseased dogs.

Plasma Biochemical Components

Alterations of plasma sodium, potassium, chloride, urea-nitrogen, creatinine, and alkaline phosphatase remained within normal limits in both the normal and the diseased dogs.

As shown in Fig. 3, decreases in total protein occurred at the outset of the plasma exchange due to dilution effects of physiological saline solution, with which the circuit was primed, for both normal and diseased dogs. However, the plasma exchange subsequently caused an increase in total protein in the dog with hepatic failure. On the other hand, hypoproteinemia was necessarily brought about in the donor dogs because of dilution effect of the substitution fluid, given in the replacement of collected plasma.

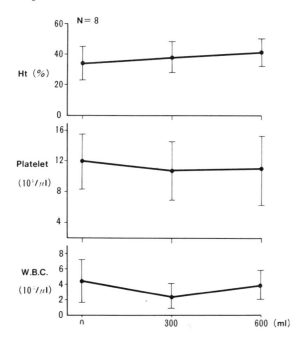

FIG. 2. Alterations of blood cells in the dogs with hepatic failure during simultaneous plasma collection and exchange.

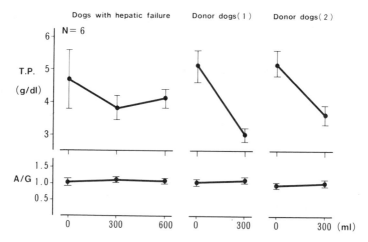

FIG. 3. Alterations of plasma total protein and albumin/globulin ratio (A/G) in the dogs during simultaneous plasma collection and exchange.

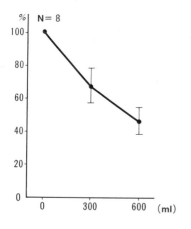

FIG. 4. Rate of decrease in GOT, expressed as percentage, in the dogs with hepatic failure during simultaneous plasma collection and exchange.

The tendency toward lowered plasma GOT was observed in the normal dogs as the amount of collected plasma increased, due to the effect of the substitution solution infused into these animals in the replacement of the collected plasma (300 ml). Plasma glutamic oxaloacetic transaminase (GOT) levels ranged widely from 289 U to 4380 U in the dogs with hepatic failure. In order to compare decreases of the plasma GOT over this wide range during the plasma exchange, the preperfusion levels were expressed as 100% and alteration of GOT levels were expressed in percentages (see Fig. 4). The results of the comparison clearly indicate the effectiveness of the plasma exchange.

DISCUSSION AND CONCLUSION

Our results confirmed that simultaneous plasma collection and exchange was safely and easily performed. Both the normal dogs and the diseased dogs maintained their hemodynamic stability during the procedure so that the exchange of 600 ml of plasma was possible within a period of less than an hour. The analytical studies on hematological and biochemical parameters in the dogs with hepatic failure proved that this plasma exchange therapy was clearly effective in the improvement of these parameters, and improvement in various vital reactions was correspondingly observed.

The present method does not require the cumbersome operations of freezing and thawing the plasma, which are required for its preservation, and completely eliminates the change with time in the plasma components which are inevitable during the preservation of the plasma.

Finally this plasma exchange therapy is undoubtedly the most effective one because the fresh, warm plasma from the donor is given instantly to the recipient without any delay or loss, which would otherwise have been the case if the preservation of plasma had been necessitated.

ACKNOWLEDGMENT

This study was supported by a grant for the hepatic assist system from the Industrial Technical Agency, Ministry of International Trade and Industry, Japan.

REFERENCES

1. Yamagata, J., and Shiokawa, Y. (1980): Plasma exchange for rheumatic disease. In: *Plasma Exchange*, edited by H. G. Sieberth, pp. 265–273. Shattauer Verlag, Stuttgart, New York.
2. Brunner, G., Loesungen, H., and Schmit, F. W. (1980): Plasmapheresis treatment for support of failing and other forms of liver disease. In: *Plasma Exchange*, edited by H. G. Sieberth, pp. 329–333. Shattauer Verlag, Stuttgart, New York.
3. Rees, A. J., Lockwood, C. M., and Peters, D. K. (1980): Plasma exchange in the management of rapidly progressing nephritis. In: *Plasma Exchange*, edited by H. G. Sieberth, pp. 161–167. Shattauer Verlag, Stuttgart, New York.
4. Inoue, N., Yamazaki, Z., Yoshiba, M., Okada, Y., Sanjo, K., Oda, T., and Wada, T. (1981): *Therapeutic Plasmapheresis, Vol. 1*, edited by T. Oda, pp. 57–63. Shattauer Verlag, Stuttgart, New York.
5. Blizer, B. L., Waggonner, J. G., Jones, E. A., Graknick, H. R., Kopin, J. I., Town, D., Butler, J., Weise, V., Walter, I., Teychenne, P. F., Goodman, D. J., and Berk, P. D. (1978): A model of fulminant hepatic failure in the rabbit. *Gastroenterology*, 74:664.
6. Idezuki, Y., Hamaguchi, M., Hamabe, S., Moriya, H., Nagashima, H., Watanabe, H., Sonoda, T., Teramoto, K., Kikuchi, T., and Tanzawa, H. (1981): Removal of bilirubin and bile acid with a new anion exchange resin: Experimental background and clinical experiences. *Trans. Am. Soc. Artif. Intern. Organs*, 27:428.
7. Wernski, A., Malchesky, P. S., Sueoka, A., Asanuma, Y., Smith, H., Kayashima, K., Herpy, E., Sato, H., and Nosé, Y. (1981): Membrane plasma separation: Toward improved clinical operation. *Trans. Am. Soc. Artif. Intern. Organs*, 27:539.

Subject Index

427